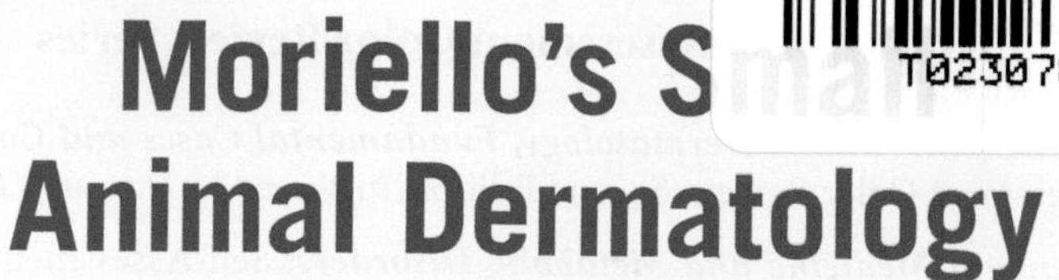

T0230781

Moriello's Small Animal Dermatology

Fundamental Cases and Concepts

Self-Assessment Color Review

Second Edition

Veterinary Self-Assessment Color Review Series

Moriello's Small Animal Dermatology, Fundamental Cases and Concepts: Self-Assessment Color Review, Second Edition, *authored by Darren J. Berger*

Small Animal Medicine and Metabolic Disorders: Self-Assessment Color Review, *authored by Craig Ruaux*

Canine Infectious Diseases: Self-Assessment Color Review, *authored by Katrin Hartmann, Jane Sykes*

Small Animal Imaging: Self-Assessment Review, *authored by John S. Mattoon, Dana Neelis*

Avian Medicine and Surgery: Self-Assessment Color Review, Second Edition, *authored by Neil A. Forbes, David Sanchez-Migallon Guzman*

Veterinary Cytology: Dog, Cat, Horse and Cow: Self-Assessment Color Review, Second Edition, *authored by Francesco Cian, Kathleen Freeman*

Small Animal Clinical Oncology: Self-Assessment Color Review, *authored by Joyce E. Obradovich, DVM, DACVIM*

Ornamental Fishes and Aquatic Invertebrates: Self-Assessment Color Review, Second Edition, *authored by Gregory A. Lewbart*

Rabbit Medicine and Surgery: Self-Assessment Color Review, Second Edition, *authored by Emma Keeble, Anna Meredith, Jenna Richardson*

Cattle and Sheep Medicine: Self-Assessment Color Review, *authored by Philip R. Scott*

Veterinary Dentistry: Self-Assessment Color Review, Second Edition, *authored by Frank Verstraete, Anson J. Tsugawa*

Reptiles and Amphibians: Self-Assessment Color Review, Second Edition, *authored by Fredric L. Frye*

Equine Internal Medicine: Self-Assessment Color Review Second Edition, *authored by Tim S. Mair, Thomas J. Divers*

Small Animal Emergency and Critical Care Medicine: Self-Assessment Color Review, Second Edition, *authored by Rebecca Kirby, Rebecca Kirby, Elke Rudloff, Drew Linklater*

For more information about this series, please visit: https://www.crcpress.com/Veterinary-Self-Assessment-Color-Review-Series/book-series/CRCVETSELASS

Moriello's Small Animal Dermatology Volume 1

Fundamental Cases and Concepts

Self-Assessment Color Review

Second Edition

Darren J. Berger

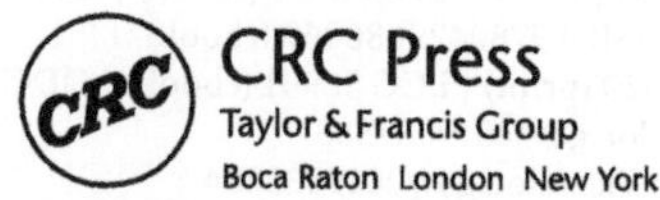

CRC Press is an imprint of the
Taylor & Francis Group, an **Informa** business

CRC Press
Taylor & Francis Group
6000 Broken Sound Parkway NW, Suite 300
Boca Raton, FL 33487-2742

© 2020 by Taylor & Francis Group, LLC
CRC Press is an imprint of Taylor & Francis Group, an Informa business

No claim to original U.S. Government works

Printed on acid-free paper

International Standard Book Number-13: 978-0-8153-7154-0 (Paperback)
978-0-8153-7163-2 (Hardback)

This book contains information obtained from authentic and highly regarded sources. While all reasonable efforts have been made to publish reliable data and information, neither the author[s] nor the publisher can accept any legal responsibility or liability for any errors or omissions that may be made. The publishers wish to make clear that any views or opinions expressed in this book by individual editors, authors or contributors are personal to them and do not necessarily reflect the views/opinions of the publishers. The information or guidance contained in this book is intended for use by medical, scientific or health-care professionals and is provided strictly as a supplement to the medical or other professional's own judgement, their knowledge of the patient's medical history, relevant manufacturer's instructions and the appropriate best practice guidelines. Because of the rapid advances in medical science, any information or advice on dosages, procedures or diagnoses should be independently verified. The reader is strongly urged to consult the relevant national drug formulary and the drug companies' and device or material manufacturers' printed instructions, and their websites, before administering or utilizing any of the drugs, devices or materials mentioned in this book. This book does not indicate whether a particular treatment is appropriate or suitable for a particular individual. Ultimately it is the sole responsibility of the medical professional to make his or her own professional judgements, so as to advise and treat patients appropriately. The authors and publishers have also attempted to trace the copyright holders of all material reproduced in this publication and apologize to copyright holders if permission to publish in this form has not been obtained. If any copyright material has not been acknowledged please write and let us know so we may rectify in any future reprint.

Except as permitted under U.S. Copyright Law, no part of this book may be reprinted, reproduced, transmitted, or utilized in any form by any electronic, mechanical, or other means, now known or hereafter invented, including photocopying, microfilming, and recording, or in any information storage or retrieval system, without written permission from the publishers.

For permission to photocopy or use material electronically from this work, please access www.copyright.com (http://www.copyright.com/) or contact the Copyright Clearance Center, Inc. (CCC), 222 Rosewood Drive, Danvers, MA 01923, 978-750-8400. CCC is a not-for-profit organization that provides licenses and registration for a variety of users. For organizations that have been granted a photocopy license by the CCC, a separate system of payment has been arranged.

Trademark Notice: Product or corporate names may be trademarks or registered trademarks, and are used only for identification and explanation without intent to infringe.

Library of Congress Cataloging-in-Publication Data

Names: Berger, Darren J., author. | Moriello, Karen A. Small animal dermatology.
Title: Moriello's small animal dermatology, fundamental cases and concepts : self-assessment color review / by Darren J. Berger.
Other titles: Small animal dermatology | small animal dermatology, fundamental cases and concepts
Description: Second edition. | Boca Raton, FL : Taylor & Francis, [2020] | Includes bibliographical references and index. | Summary: "This revised fundamental edition includes all new cases and nearly 300 new images. The guide uses a case-based format to deliver a general overview of dermatology of the dog and cat, providing a reference that mirrors the way veterinarians will encounter different scenarios at random in real-life practice. It uses self-assessment problems to review the most common skin diseases encountered every day, plus some more obscure diseases that a veterinarian will face"-- Provided by publisher.
Identifiers: LCCN 2019032383 (print) | LCCN 2019032384 (ebook) | ISBN 9780815371540 (paperback) | ISBN 9780815371632 (hardback) | ISBN 9780429086069 (ebook)
Classification: LCC SF901 .M67 2020 (print) | LCC SF901 (ebook) | DDC 636.089/65--dc23
LC record available at https://lccn.loc.gov/2019032383
LC ebook record available at https://lccn.loc.gov/2019032384

Visit the Taylor & Francis Web site at
http://www.taylorandfrancis.com

and the CRC Press Web site at
http://www.crcpress.com

To Krissy, Gaby, and Quinn, everything is because of you and for you!

Broad classification of cases

Allergic cases
11, 20, 32, 39, 42, 45, 51, 53, 54, 62, 65, 68, 69, 78, 85, 94, 100, 103, 105, 115, 117, 125, 134, 146, 148, 157, 175, 176, 179, 187, 195, 201, 207

Alopecia
4, 17, 29, 35, 47, 67, 80, 83, 111, 151, 177, 188, 199, 205

Autoimmune
26, 56, 60, 63, 102, 118, 130, 153, 171, 186, 198

Bacterial
5, 18, 28, 33, 38, 64, 65, 76, 77, 91, 107, 113, 122, 126, 132, 137, 146, 152, 158, 174, 182, 203

Congenital or breed-related issues
7, 17, 22, 29, 44, 67, 80, 106, 118, 130, 135, 141, 142, 183, 185

Cytology
3, 5, 12, 43, 59, 72, 86, 87, 93, 102, 104, 109, 114, 119, 128, 133, 148, 158, 165, 166, 176, 186, 191, 196, 203, 204, 205

Diagnostic techniques
1, 6, 14, 22, 25, 34, 48, 52, 77, 81, 88, 98, 107, 121, 143, 150, 155, 162, 167, 173, 174, 180, 183, 192

Endocrine
21, 67, 70, 111, 161, 193, 199

Fungal
2, 3, 13, 34, 51, 56, 66, 92, 93, 109, 121, 146, 159, 166, 190, 191

Keratinization cases
15, 39, 101, 115, 141, 142, 169, 170

Miscellaneous
36, 44, 50, 53, 61, 68, 74, 83, 84, 110, 127, 135, 145, 153, 162, 163, 168, 169, 170, 184, 185, 193, 194, 202

Neoplasia
16, 43, 46, 73, 97, 149, 160, 181, 204

Nutrition cases
7, 23

Otitis
22, 46, 50, 61, 87, 95, 112, 129, 155, 168, 197

Parasite cases
1, 6, 8, 9, 19, 24, 30, 32, 33, 37, 39, 40, 42, 45, 47, 54, 57, 62, 71, 72, 79, 88, 89, 96, 105, 106, 114, 123, 124, 131, 138, 139, 156, 172, 179, 183, 189, 201, 206

Pharmacology and therapeutics
10, 23, 27, 28, 41, 55, 58, 63, 75, 76, 82, 90, 95, 99, 100, 108, 113, 116, 120, 136, 140, 144, 147, 148, 153, 154, 161, 164, 174, 178, 187, 200

Structure and function cases
31, 49, 129

Preface

This book has been kept in a similar format established by the original author Dr. Karen Moriello, but the cases and images have been completely revised in an effort to establish a two-volume set. This first book covers cases and concepts that are routinely encountered in everyday general practice.

Acknowledgments

I would like to thank the following people as they have either influenced the way I think about veterinary medicine, contributed images and case material, or provided critical review of the content in this book.

Dr. Matthew T. Brewer, DVM, PhD, DACVM
Iowa State University College of Veterinary Medicine

Dr. Christine L. Cain, VMD, DACVD
University of Pennsylvania School of Veterinary Medicine

Dr. Stephen D. Cole, VMD, MS, DACVM
University of Pennsylvania School of Veterinary Medicine

Dr. Kimberly S. Coyner, DVM, DACVD
Dermatology Clinic for Animals

Dr. Alison B. Diesel, DVM, DACVD
Texas A&M College of Veterinary Medicine

Dr. Michael J. Forret, DVM
Highland Park Animal Hospital

Dr. Shannon Hostetter, DVM, PhD, DACVP
University of Georgia College of Veterinary Medicine

Dr. Thomas P. Lewis II, DVM, DACVD
Dermatology for Animals

Dr. Shelley C. Rankin, PhD
University of Pennsylvania School of Veterinary Medicine

Dr. Karen A. Moriello, DVM, DACVD
University of Wisconsin–Madison School of Veterinary Medicine

Dr. James O. Noxon, DVM, DACVIM
Iowa State University College of Veterinary Medicine

Dr. Anthea E. Schick, DVM, DACVD
Dermatology for Animals

Dr. Austin K. Viall, DVM, MS, DACVP
Iowa State University College of Veterinary Medicine

Author

Darren J. Berger, DVM, DAVCD, is an Assistant Professor of dermatology at Iowa State University's College of Veterinary Medicine. Prior to completing a residency in dermatology, he worked as a small animal general practitioner. His research interests include clinical pharmacology, *Malassezia* dermatitis, and equine hypersensitivity disorders.

1. A 16-week-old female mixed breed puppy presented with a complaint of severe hair loss and "scabs." On physical exam, diffuse alopecia and erythema with the presence of papules, pustules, and crusts were appreciated (**Figure 1a**, **b**) along with a generalized lymphadenopathy. Given the clinical presentation, you are suspicious this puppy has generalized demodicosis.

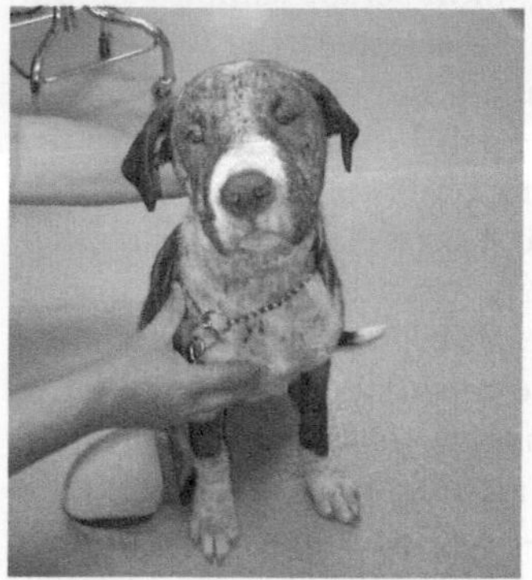

Figure 1a

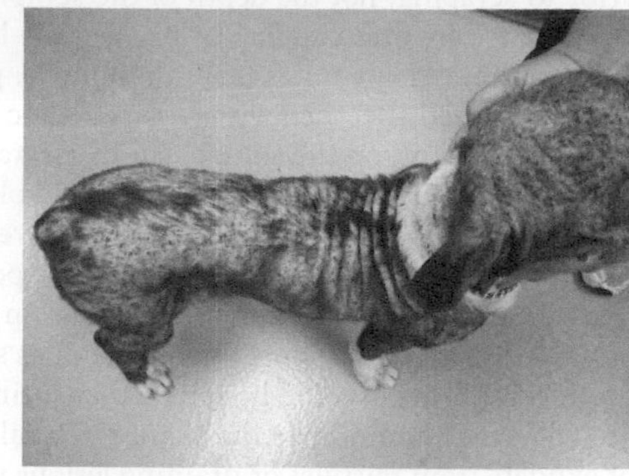

Figure 1b

What are the various diagnostic techniques that can be used to demonstrate the presence of mites in this patient?

2. A 6-year-old castrated male cocker spaniel from the Midwest region of the United States presented for examination of progressive nonhealing wounds on the skin (**Figure 2a**). The lesions were first observed 2 months ago and have failed to respond to prior antimicrobial therapy with cephalexin. The patient is also reported to be anorexic with noticeable weight loss. On physical examination, there were multiple 1–2 cm diameter-crusted nodules, which were moderately painful on palpation. Removal of the crust revealed ulcerated draining tracts with a thick purulent exudate that was easily expressed. In addition, there was generalized lymphadenopathy and increased respiratory noise on auscultation. The patient had a normal rectal temperature but was noted to be quiet and depressed during examination.

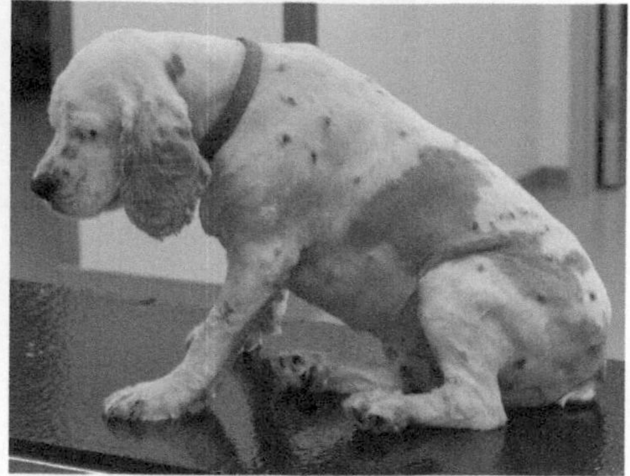

Figure 2a

i. What are the differential diagnoses for this patient?

ii. What are the most logical first diagnostic steps in this patient?

iii. Assuming the cause of the lesions and lymphadenopathy has not been identified, what other diagnostic tests should be performed?

1. Skin scraping is considered the gold standard for demonstrating the presence of *Demodex* mites. Historically, authors have discussed the need for "deep scrapings" (creating capillary bleeding), but this may not be needed and can result in unneeded cutaneous trauma. The author believes the actual important component of the technique is to massage or squeeze the area to be sampled prior to scraping, not the depth of the scraping. Skin scrape samples should be obtained by first clipping or parting the hair coat, squeezing the skin in an effort to extrude mites from the follicle, placing mineral oil on the skin at the squeezed site, then with a scapel blade or spatula at roughly 90° to the skin gently scraping the skin. Next, in a scraping and scooping motion collect the mixture of oil and skin debris and place it on a clean glass slide that should then have a glass coverslip placed over the mixture. Finally, examine the slide microscopically under 4× or 10× power. Trichography may also be used, especially for collection of samples from the paws or periocular region. A downside of this technique is that it is not as sensitive as skin scraping. When used, several sites should be sampled ensuring an adequate number of hairs are collected to minimize the chance of a false-negative result. Examination of exudate from pustules or draining lesions may reveal the presence of mites (**Figure 1c**). The use of a clear acetate tape impression can also be effective in demonstrating the presence of *Demodex* mites (Pereira et al., 2012). This technique specifically highlights the importance of properly squeezing the skin prior to sampling. Finally, mites may also be demonstrated via biopsy, but this is usually not required, and detection by this method is usually accidental when the clinician did not initially suspect demodicosis.

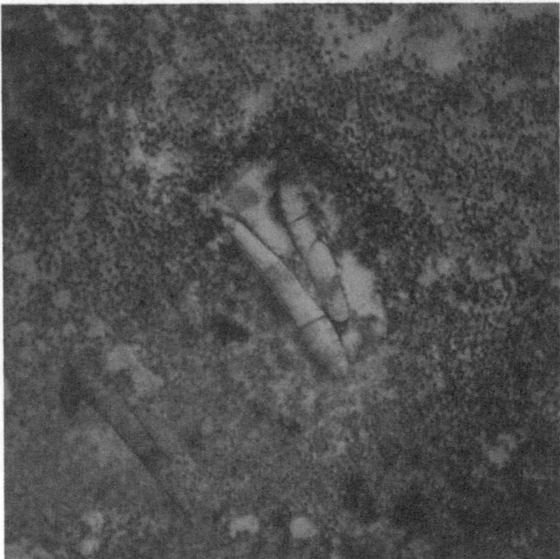

Figure 1c

2. i. The dog's dermatologic problem is multiple draining nodules. Differential diagnoses for nonhealing draining nodules in a dog are somewhat age dependent but would include undiagnosed demodicosis resulting in furunculosis, infectious granulomas (bacterial, mycobacterial, fungal), juvenile cellulitis, adverse drug eruption, sterile nodular dermatoses (i.e., sterile nodular panniculitis), foreign-body reaction, and neoplasia. The concurrent signs of systemic illness (anorexia, depression, weight loss, and lymphadenopathy) suggest that the skin lesions are secondary to an underlying systemic infection, autoimmune disease, or neoplasia.

ii. The first diagnostic steps in a patient such as this should include skin scrapings to rule out demodicosis; impression smears to look for infectious agents; and lymph node aspirates to determine if the lymphadenopathy is reactive, neoplastic, or infectious. These initial diagnostic tests are simple to perform and with practice can be easily interpreted by the veterinarian. In many cases, these simple first-line diagnostics can provide a definitive diagnosis and avoid unneeded patient costs.

iii. If cytologies and aspirates fail to reveal a causative agent, next-level diagnostics involve skin biopsies for dermatohistopathology and tissue culture (bacterial and fungal), serum or urine tests for fungal organisms, and a medical database (complete blood count, serum chemistries, urinalysis, and survey radiographs) to assess the dog's overall health.

3. An impression smear of the exudate from the dog in **Question 2** is shown in **Figure 3a**.

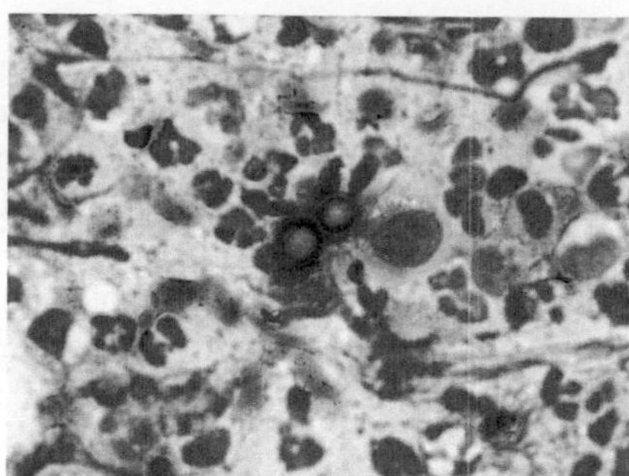

Figure 3a

i. What is the diagnosis, and what are the treatment options?

ii. How did the dog most likely contract this organism? Is this a zoonosis?

iii. What other organ systems are commonly involved, and what is the prognosis for this disease?

4. In January, a 1.5-year-old Chihuahua presented for treatment of "ringworm." The owner reports that the dog has developed a "ringworm" lesion on its leg. There are two other dogs in the house, and none of these animals show signs of skin disease. The dog in question sleeps with the owner, and she does not have skin lesions either. Dermatologic examination reveals a focal area of non-inflammatory hair loss (**Figure 4a**) along the right lateral rear leg. A Wood's lamp examination is negative. The medical record indicates the dog received vaccinations 3 months ago.

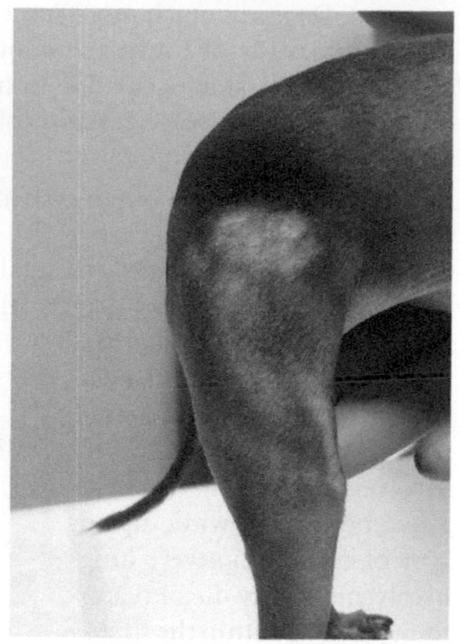

Figure 4a

i. What are the most common differential diagnoses for acquired noninflammatory focal alopecia, and what diagnostic tests should be performed?

ii. The skin biopsy findings revealed atrophic hair follicles, dermal pallor, and nodular lymphohistiocytic panniculitis with areas of necrosis and the presence of a blue-gray amorphous material. What is the most likely diagnosis, and what management recommendations should be made?

3. **i.** Blastomycosis. Note the pyogranulomatous inflammation and the broad-based, thick-walled, budding yeast. Historically, therapy with amphotericin B or ketoconazole as monotherapy or use of sequentially administered therapeutics have been employed. However, the triazoles (itraconazole and fluconazole) have become the drugs of choice. Both are more effective than ketoconazole and far less toxic than amphotericin B. A recent retrospective investigation showed treatment efficacy and relapse rates to be similar in dogs treated with fluconazole or intraconazole (Mazepa et al., 2011). This same study also demonstrated that treatment length was longer for dogs treated with fluconazole (183 days compared to 138 for intraconazole), but overall treatment costs were significantly less. Starting doses for these medications in the dog are 5 mg/kg (by mouth [PO] q12–24h for fluconazole and 5–10 mg/kg PO q24h for itraconazole).

ii. Blastomycosis is a dimorphic fungus, which is a soil saprophyte, and transforms into its yeast form in tissues at body temperature. The organism favors a special environmental niche. Where outbreaks of the disease have been investigated, four common environmental factors seem to be at play, which include moisture, soil type (sandy and acidic), presence of wildlife, and soil disruption. Decaying wood and animal excrement appear to support fungal growth, making sites such as beaver dams ideal. The mode of infection is via inhalation of spores produced by mycelial growth of *Blastomycosis dermatitidis* in the environment. Dogs are much more susceptible to the disease than people.

The disease is of limited zoonotic concern as most cases of animal-to-human transmission occur due to traumatic inoculation. When owners and dogs contract the disease, it is almost always because both were exposed to the same environmental source.

iii. The most common organ system reported to be affected in dogs has been the respiratory system (**Figure 3b**), followed by integumentary, ocular (retinal granuloma, **Figure 3c**), skeletal, nervous, and reproductive systems. In general, the prognosis for dogs is fair to good. The two most important prognostic indicators are whether there is central nervous system (CNS) involvement and severity of lung disease. CNS involvement usually carries a grave prognosis, while up to 50% of dogs with severe lung involvement may die of respiratory failure within the first 7 days of treatment. Treatment should be continued for a minimum of 30 days after clinical resolution of disease, with urine antigen tests used to monitor response to treatment. Roughly 20% of dogs

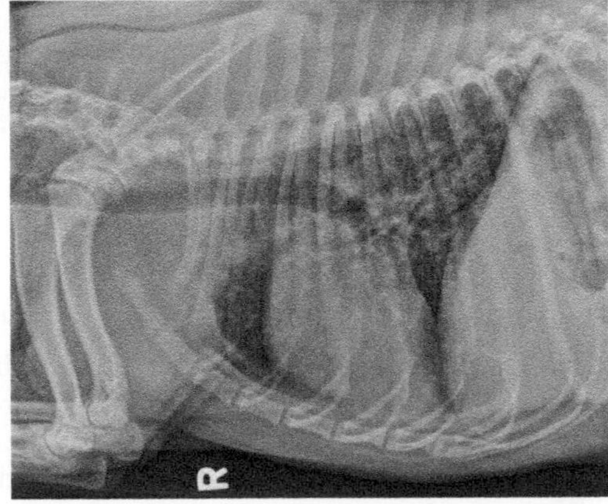

Figure 3b

have been reported to relapse with disease following discontinuation of therapy. Occasionally, enucleation of affected eyes may be required to eliminate a possible nidus of reinfection.

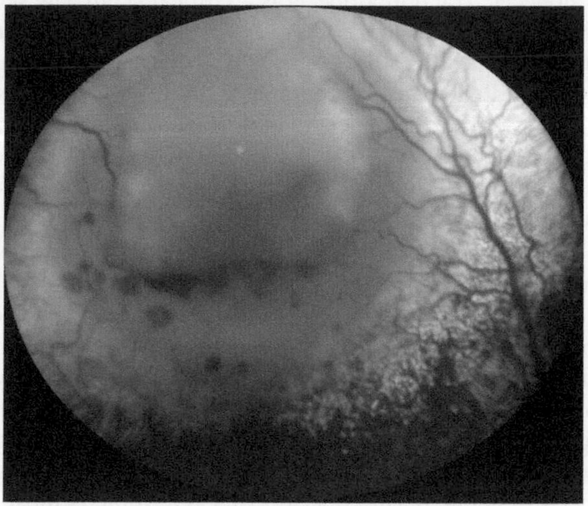

Figure 3c

4. i. Differential diagnoses include alopecia areata, traction alopecia, post-rabies vaccination alopecia, cyclic flank alopecia, and post-glucocorticoid injection site alopecia. Alopecia areata is an uncommon autoimmune skin disease that is characterized by focal or multifocal areas of well-circumscribed nonscarring alopecia. Traction alopecia is a clinical syndrome seen in small breed dogs that have ribbons, barrettes, or bows tied too tightly into their hair coat. The tension on the hair follicles results in damage to the vasculature and permanent loss of hair follicles. Subcutaneous rabies vaccinations can cause vasculitis and a focal area of alopecia at the site of injection. Topical and subcutaneous glucocorticoids are also associated with focal areas of alopecia. The most useful diagnostic tests include skin scrapings, impression smears, dermatophyte cultures, and a skin biopsy.

ii. The skin biopsy findings were consistent with vaccine-induced ischemic dermatopathy. Post-rabies vaccination panniculitis is relatively common and characterized by the focal alopecia shown in this patient. The condition is thought to be due to an idiosyncratic immunologic reaction to rabies antigen. Classically, an area of alopecia develops at the site of rabies vaccination roughly 3 months after administration. Inflammation is commonly absent, and hyperpigmentation may develop with subsequent scarring alopecia. Some dogs can develop a more severe widespread reaction referred to as generalized vaccine-induced ischemic dermatopathy. This syndrome is most commonly encountered with small and toy breed dogs (Gross et al., 2005). The localized form of this condition does not usually require therapy. If inflammation, pain, or the generalized form is present, topical treatment with tacrolimus or systemic medications such as pentoxifylline, glucocorticoids, or cyclosporine can be used, similar to the treatment of dermatomyositis. Revaccination with rabies vaccine is not recommended as subsequent vaccinations may exacerbate the syndrome and lead to the development of the generalized form.

5. Pyoderma is a common condition in small animal medicine that is normally associated with *Staphylococcus* spp. The clinical diagnosis of pyoderma is reliant on cytological demonstration of bacteria from lesional skin.

What is the main cytological characteristic of staphylococci when found on skin cytology?

6. A 10-week-old kitten presented due to head shaking and generalized itching. During examination, you notice blackish-brown debris within the fur along the ventral abdomen (**Figure 6a**). You decide to collect some of this debris, place it on a paper towel that was lightly moistened with water, and gently spread the material out with one of your fingers. The result is shown in **Figure 6b**.

Figure 6a

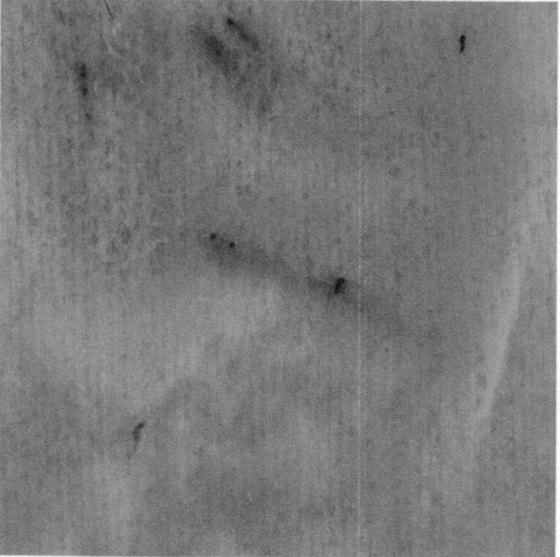

Figure 6b

What is the debris that is present in the fur of the patient?

5. The main cytological feature besides the simple presence of coccoid-shaped bacteria that indicates the causative agent is likely a *Staphylococcus* spp. is that the coccoid-shaped bacteria are found in pairs or tetrads (**Figure 5a**). They may, however, also be observed as singlets and larger groups. Chains of cocci are not seen with this species.

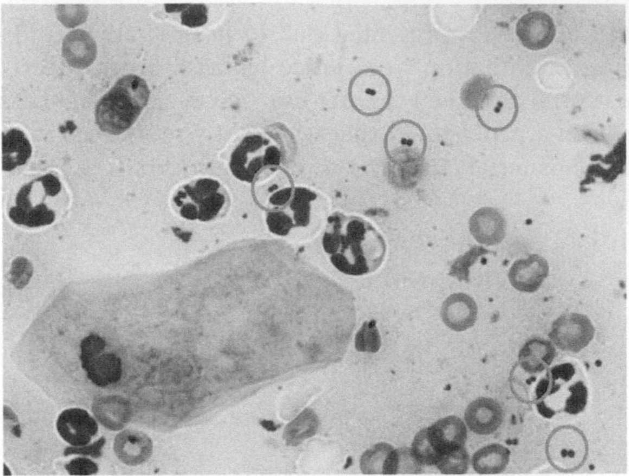

Figure 5a

6. The debris is flea feces or "flea dirt." The reddish discoloration when the material comes in contact with water is characteristic for flea feces due to the presence of blood in the excrement of these biting nuisances. This is different from simple organic material that will leave a brown or black discoloration. The material is best viewed against a white background to help discern the subtle coloration in some cases. A surgical gauze pad or a basic paper towel can be used for this purpose.

7. A 2-year-old castrated male Siberian husky dog presented with a complaint of hair loss and crusting. The owner reports that the lesions were first noted 2–3 months ago and have slowly worsened. On dermatologic examination, symmetrical patches of alopecia with thickened, hyperpigmented skin and crust formation are appreciated around the eyes, the muzzle, and along the perioral margins (**Figure 7a, b**). No other lesions are present, and the dog is healthy otherwise. He is fed a complete and balanced diet.

i. What is the most likely diagnosis, and how should this be confirmed?

ii. How should the dog be treated, and how soon will resolution of clinical signs be expected?

iii. What should be considered or done with this patient if he fails to respond to initial therapy?

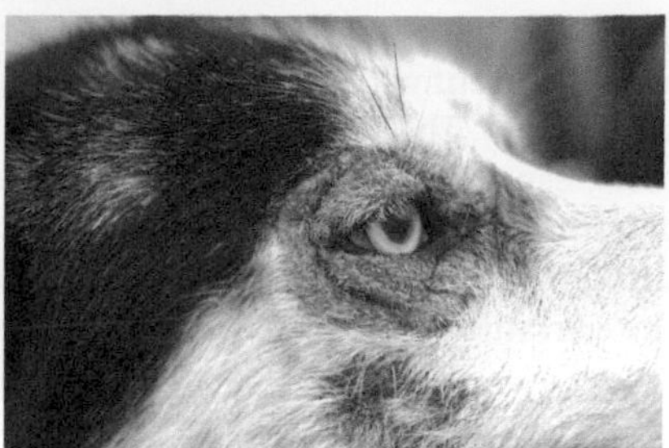
Figure 7a

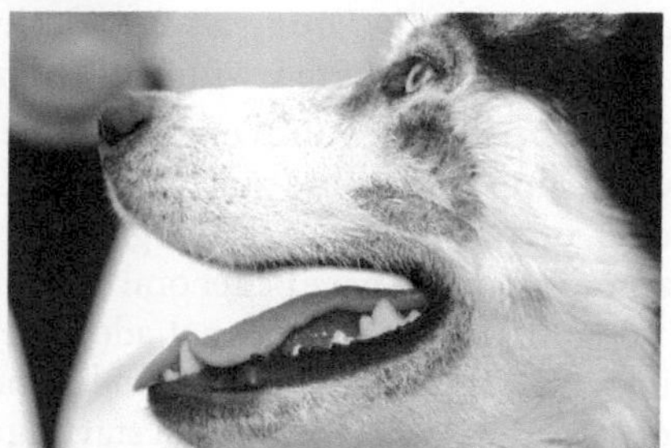
Figure 7b

8. Cats and dogs are atypical hosts for the larva (**Figure 8a**) being removed from a large swelling along the lateral cervical region of a cat.

i. How is this parasite acquired, what is the life cycle in dogs and cats, and where are the lesions commonly located?

ii. What time of year are infestations most commonly seen?

iii. What other body locations has this parasite been reported to affect in dogs and cats?

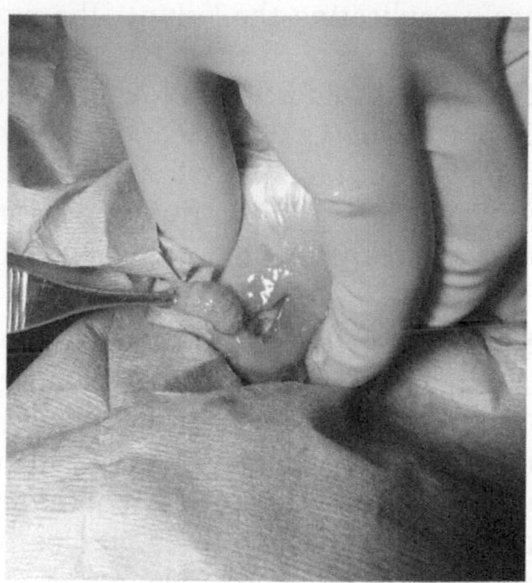
Figure 8a

7. i. This is zinc-responsive dermatosis. The signalment and clinical signs are consistent with this syndrome in dogs. The diagnosis can be confirmed by skin biopsy. The key histopathologic finding is diffuse parakeratotic hyperkeratosis, especially of the follicular epithelium. Although it may seem intuitive to sample blood or hair to determine zinc concentrations in affected patients, this is not routinely performed because of technical issues with sampling and the variable results reported. The Siberian husky and Alaskan malamute are overrepresented as the condition is considered hereditary, arising in part due to a diminished capability to absorb zinc from the gastrointestinal (GI) tract (Hensel, 2010). This form of the disease is commonly referred to as syndrome I. Syndrome II occurs in rapidly growing dogs (usually large breeds) that are fed zinc-deficient diets, diets high in phytates, or food that excessively supplemented with other minerals specifically calcium. Phytates and other minerals are thought to interfere with zinc absorption.

ii. This patient requires oral supplementation with zinc. The most commonly used supplements are zinc sulfate (10 mg/kg/day), zinc gluconate (5 mg/kg/day), or zinc methionine (2 mg/kg/day). The latter two forms of supplemental zinc are noted to have better oral bioavailability and cause less GI upset. Feeding a dog food with "zinc" is not adequate nor are vitamin supplements containing zinc. Therapy is lifelong, and significant clinical improvement should be observed within 4–6 weeks of starting appropriate oral supplementation.

iii. When dogs fail to respond as expected to oral supplementation, the first step is to ensure no secondary infections (*Malassezia* spp. or bacterial) are complicating the lesions. The next option is to try an alternative oral zinc supplement. If these two options do not provide further clinical benefit, then the addition of low-dose glucocorticoid therapy (i.e., prednisone 0.25–0.50 mg/kg PO q48h, potentially long term) to enhance zinc absorption from the GI tract or the use of sterile zinc sulfate solution (10–15 mg/kg IV [intravenous] or IM [intramuscular]) may be required. Injections are administered weekly for a month then given every 1–6 months as needed.

8. i. *Cuterebra* spp. flies do not bite or feed directly on a host but instead lay their eggs on stones, vegetation, or near the openings of animal burrows. Cats and dogs become infested when they come into contact with a contaminated area. The larvae enter the body through ingestion during grooming or via natural openings (eyes, mouth, or nares). The larvae undergo roughly a monthlong aberrant migration prior to localizing in the skin of the head, neck, and trunk. At these locations, the presence of the larvae results in the formation of cyst-like structures with a fistulous opening (breathing hole). It is through the breathing hole that clinicians may visualize the second (cream to gray colored) or third (dark with multiple spines) instar larvae.

ii. *Cuterebra* larvae are typically encountered during late summer or early fall but may be seen year-round in warmer climates.

iii. Erratic larval migration has also been reported to affect the nostrils, pharynx, eyes, and brain of nonnatural hosts.

9. This German shepherd presented for examination with a 6-month history of progress pruritus despite prior therapy with glucocorticoids and oclacitinib maleate (**Figure 9a**). It was one of eight dogs in a kennel and was the only one affected. In addition to skin lesions, the dog was losing weight and was irritable with the owners and other dogs. Close examination of the skin revealed scaling and a generalized papular eruption without evidence of pustules and/or epidermal collarettes. Any manipulation of the skin triggered an episode of intense pruritus. The dog was current with vaccinations, received monthly heartworm prevention, and received a monthly spot-on flea control product that contained fipronil and (S)-methoprene. The owners reported no lesions or discomfort after any handling of the dog. Flea combings were negative. Skin scrapings revealed the results shown in **Figure 9b**.

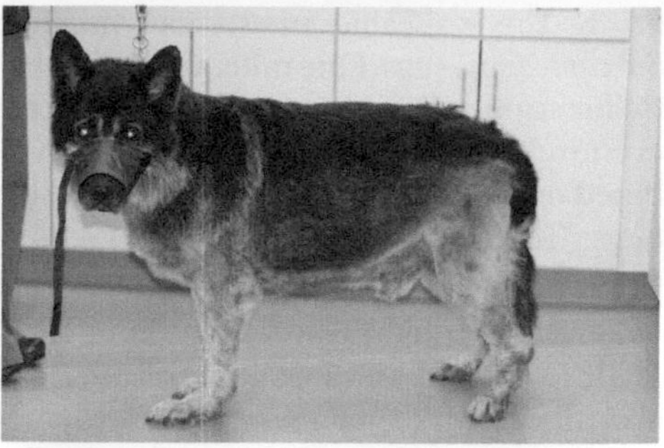

Figure 9a

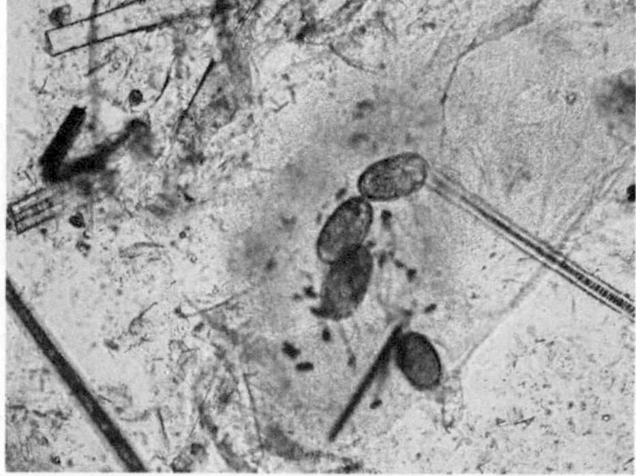

Figure 9b

i. What is the diagnosis?

ii. What are the treatment options for this kennel of dogs?

10. What are the most common side effects of systemically administered glucocorticoids in dogs? What unique adverse events are encountered with cats?

9. **i.** This is a scabies infestation. The structures present on skin scraping are *Sarcoptes* spp. eggs. One mite, an egg, or the presence of fecal pellets is diagnostic for scabies. Definitive evidence of a scabies infestation is not always found, even in "classic cases." The vast majority of dogs with scabies are diagnosed based on response to treatment, hence the old saying with regard to scabies in dogs: "If you suspect it, treat for it."

ii. Scabies mites can live for a short period of time off the host (2–21 days depending on temperature and humidity) (Miller et al., 2013a). The kennel facilities should be thoroughly cleaned and bedding materials washed. Any and all dogs in contact with this German shepherd dog should be treated for scabies. Potential treatment options for this kennel of dogs may include lime sulfur dips once weekly for 6 weeks; amitraz dips applied biweekly for three treatments; ivermectin 0.2–0.4 mg/kg PO q7 days or subcutaneously (SC) q14 days for a total of 6 weeks; doramectin 0.2–0.6 mg/kg SC q7 days for 4–6 weeks; milbemycin oxime 2 mg/kg PO q7 days for 4–6 weeks; Selamectin 6–12 mg/kg applied topically every 2 weeks for three doses; a topical moxidectin/imidacloprid combination product (AdvantageMulti or Advocate) applied at 2-week intervals for three doses; fipronil spray 3 mL/kg applied as a pump spray to the body at 2-week intervals for three doses; or one of the newer isoxazoline antiparasitics (afoxolaner, fluralaner, lotilaner, and sarolaner) at standard flea preventative dosages. It is important to remember that systemic macrocyclic lactones should be used with caution in dog breeds at risk for P-glycoprotein mutations (multidrug resistant [MDR] mutants).

10. Common side effects include polyphagia, polydipsia, polyuria, lethargy, panting, weight gain, behaviorial changes, muscle atrophy, poor dull hair coat with hypotrichosis to alopecia, comedone formation, poor wound healing, exercise intolerance, pot-bellied appearance, secondary skin infections, urinary tract infections, calcinosis cutis, and GI ulceration. Unique adverse events observed in cats are curling of the pinnae, skin fragility syndrome, and the precipitation of congestive heart failure. However, at this time, the association between cardiac dysfunction and glucocorticoid administration in cats remains weak.

11. **Figure 11a** shows some common diets utilized in patients suspected to have a cutaneous adverse food reaction.

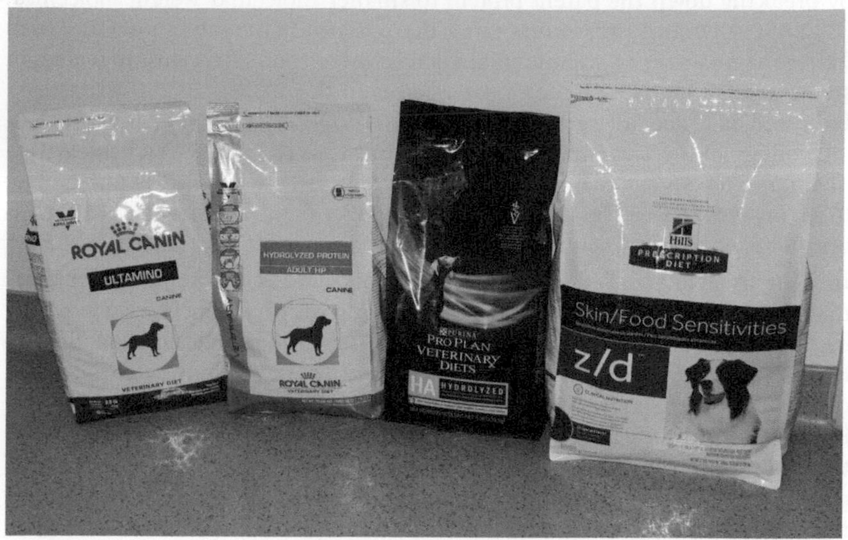

Figure 11a

i. What type of diet do all these examples represent?
ii. What is the theory behind their development, and what advantage do they offer compared to other dietary concepts used in diet elimination trials?
iii. What adverse events and issues have been associated with these diets?
iv. What is the most common reason for diet elimination trial failure in a patient?

12. An impression smear (**Figure 12a**) from the lateral thorax of a dog with circular alopecia and crusting is shown.

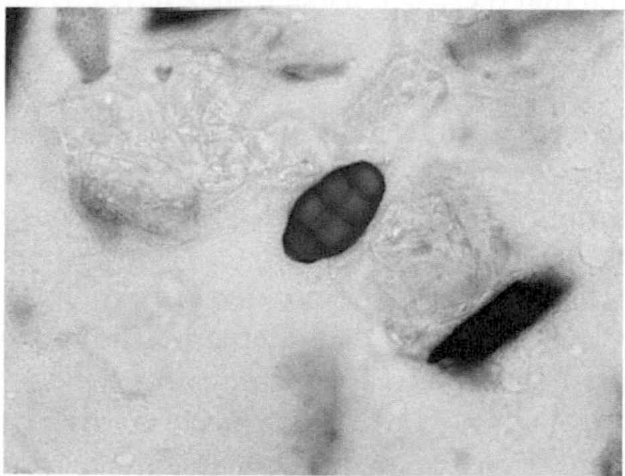

Figure 12a

What is present on cytology?

11. **i.** Hydrolyzed protein diets

ii. The idea behind these diets is to make the protein source "hypoallergenic" by breaking down the parent protein to smaller molecular weight molecules (<12,000 KD) and thus minimizing the potential allergenicity of the diet. This concept arises from human medicine where food allergens are typically stable glycoproteins with molecular weights in the 10,000–70,000 KD range. However, the exact allergens and their corresponding molecular weights that affect dogs and cats are not known at this time (Gaschen and Merchant, 2011). The major advantage that hydrolyzed diets offer is that it is nearly impossible to get an accurate diet history from most owners, so they eliminate the need of finding a "novel" food source that the patient may not yet have been exposed to.

iii. The main adverse event seen with hydrolyzed diets is that some patients may develop osmotic diarrhea while consuming the diet, which resolves when feeding of the diet is discontinued. Another issue has been the palatability of hydrolyzed diets, which leads to some patients being unwilling to eat their chosen diet. There is also the issue of cost. The process of hydrolysis and obtaining purified carbohydrate sources has led to many of these diets costing more than premium maintenance foods, which can be a mental hurdle for some pet owners when these diets are recommended. The final and most significant issue with hydrolyzed diets is persistent immunogenicity. Several studies have revealed subsets of veterinary patients who are known to be allergic to a particular protein and still react when fed the hydrolyzed variant. This last issue contributes to some of the difficulties and controversies surrounding diagnosis of cutaneous adverse food reactions (Bizikova and Olivry, 2016).

iv. The most common reason for a diet elimination trial to fail (besides the fact that the patient may not have a cutaneous adverse food reaction) is owner compliance. The biggest issue with owner compliance is usually insufficient owner education. It is important that when a diet elimination trial is recommended, that the owner and all family members understand why this diagnostic test is being performed, how long the diet trial is going to last, what is included in the "no other food or flavored items," what observations they are supposed to be making at home, and that they should call if they have any questions (and that it is expected they will call).

12. This is an *Alternaria* spp. conidium, which is commonly misidentified as a dermatophyte species macroconidia by inexperienced veterinarians. It is important to remember that dermatophytes only produce macroconidia in culture. Within hair and tissue, dermatophytes produce arthroconidia, which appear as beadlike chains or groups of rounded cells. *Alternaria* spp. is a group of ubiquitous environmental fungi that often grow indoors on carpets or textiles, while outdoors it is associated with moisture, soil, and plant material. *Alternaria* is a documented mold allergen, which can incite human and animal allergic manifestations. However, in this case, it is an environmental contaminant and is considered insignificant.

13. A 1-year-old neutered male Japanese Bobtail cat presented for hair loss, crusting, and pruritus of the head/neck (**Figure 13a**) first noted 3 weeks ago. Physical exam revealed patchy alopecia, erythema, scaling, and crusting along the dorsal head and mild hypotrichosis of the convex portions of the pinnae. Skin scrapings, flea combings, and ear swabs did not reveal the presence of any parasites. A Wood's lamp examination revealed bright green fluorescence of multiple hairs from the periphery of the alopecic regions and along with multiple hairs over the convex pinnae. A microscopic image from the patient's trichogram is shown (**Figure 13b**). Further questioning reveals that the patient lives in a single cat household and was adopted from a local shelter 2 months prior.

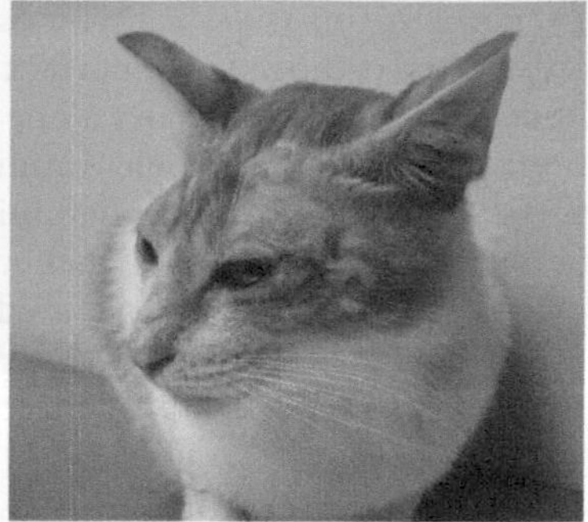

Figure 13a

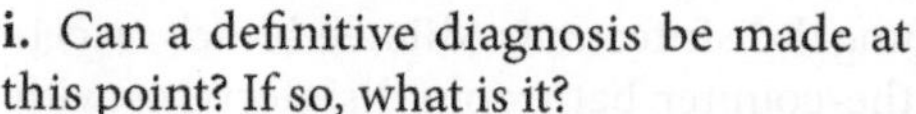

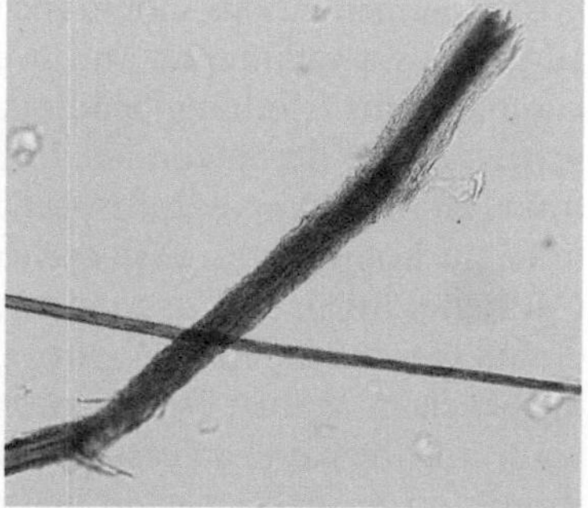

Figure 13b

i. Can a definitive diagnosis be made at this point? If so, what is it?

ii. What environmental cleaning recommendations should be made to the owner as the cat has been present in the home for 2 months prior to diagnosis?

14. A commonly utilized point-of-care diagnostic tool in small animal dermatology is shown in **Figure 14a, b**.

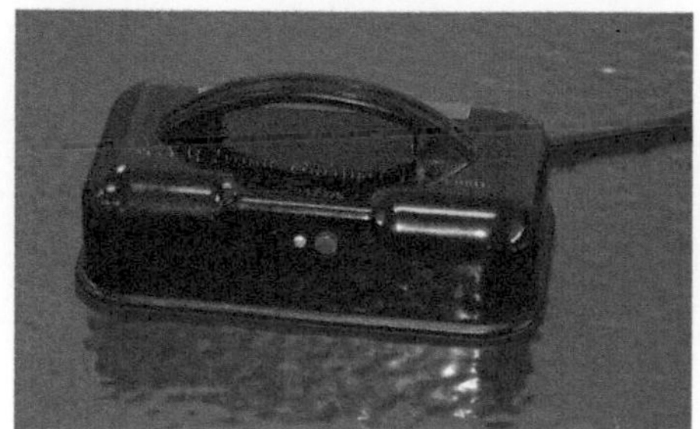

Figure 14a

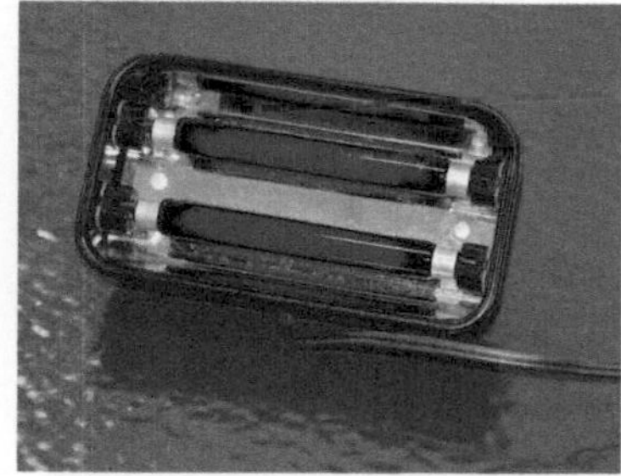

Figure 14b

i. What is the name of this instrument and when was it invented?

ii. What is this instrument principally used for, and how is the test performed?

iii. What substances may lead to falsely interpreted positive reactions?

iv. What causes the positive reaction, and how often are clinical cases positive for this reaction?

13. i. Yes, this is dermatophytosis caused by *Microsporum canis*. This is the only fungal pathogen of importance in veterinary medicine that fluoresces. The finding of fluorescing hairs alone is not diagnostic of a dermatophyte infection; however, microscopic examination of hairs and identification of ectothrix spores and hyphae is definitive. Observe the difference in hair diameter between the affected and nonaffected hair, the linear running fungal hyphae within the shaft, and the fractured end. This is what creates the classic "rotten log" appearance observed with dermatophyte-infected hairs. In addition, note the prominent cuffs of spores near the broken end.

ii. The purpose of environmental cleaning is to eliminate shed keratin material containing spores from around the house minimizing the risk of disease transmission to the people in the household. Second, it eliminates fomite carriage that can complicate treatment monitoring. Good environmental cleaning recommendations should include the following: (1) Mechanically remove all debris via vacuuming and sweeping. (2) Wash all exposed contaminated laundry items (clothing, bedding, etc.). A recent study showed that washable textiles can be decontaminated without the use of bleach or extreme temperatures. The most important aspect to washing contaminated textiles was shown to be the length of the wash cycle and ensuring the machine is not overloaded (Moriello, 2016). (3) Use good antifungal disinfectants (diluted bleach, accelerated hydrogen peroxide, or over-the-counter bathroom disinfectants with a label claim against *Trichophyton* spp.) on compatible surfaces. (4) Consider confining the cat to an easily cleaned room during the early phase of therapy to minimize further contamination of the house. (5) Perform cleaning twice weekly (Moriello et al., 2017).

14. **i.** This is a Wood's lamp, which is different than a "black light." A Wood's lamp emits long-wave ultraviolet (UV) radiation through a special glass filter (barium silicate with nickel oxide) that emits light rays between 320 and 400 nm with a peak around 354 nm. A black light is a clear glass bulb that filters different wavelengths and produces a large amount of blue visible light along with some long-wave UV light, which makes detecting fluorescence difficult. The lamp was invented in 1903 by Robert W. Wood as a light filter used in communications during World War I.

ii. A Wood's lamp is used as a screening tool for dermatophytosis in small animal medicine, which when present, produces a characteristic apple-green fluorescence in the hair (negative fluorescence does not rule out dermatophytosis as a possible cause of disease). Only a limited number of dermatophyte species produce fluorescence, which include *Microsporum canis*, *M. distortum*, *M. audouinii*, and *Trichophyton schoeleinni*. The only one of these species that is of clinical relevance to veterinary medicine is *M. canis*. To perform the screening, the lamp should be turned on and allowed to warm up. The test should take place in a dark room, and the lamp should be held within several centimeters of suspect lesions. Hairs may need to be exposed to the light for several minutes, as some strains are slow to produce the characteristic fluorescence. If fluorescence is observed, the patient should be cultured or hairs plucked for trichogram to confirm the infection. Common mistakes are not using an actual Wood's lamp, not performing the test in a dark enough room, and not taking enough time to perform the test.

iii. False fluorescence has been recognized with lint, topical medications, seborrheic material (keratin), soap residue, and carpet fibers.

iv. Fluorescence in the hair is due to the presence of the water-soluble metabolite pteridine located within the cortex or medulla of the hair that occurs as a result of an infection. The key point is that this reaction only takes place in the hair. Historically, it has been suggested that roughly 50% of *M. canis* strains will fluoresce. Recent published guidelines on the diagnosis and treatment of dermatophytosis suggest, however, that this may be a gross underestimate and that in fact Wood's lamp examination is likely to be positive in most cases of *M. canis*–associated disease if the diagnostic is performed correctly as described earlier (particularly with regard to the time involved in lamp preparation and observation) (Moriello et al., 2017).

15. A 5-year-old male cat presented for the lesion shown in **Figure 15a**. The owner reports that the lesion developed rapidly, and it is unclear if the cat is pruritic. No other cats are present in the household, and he is otherwise reported to be healthy and current with recommended vaccinations.

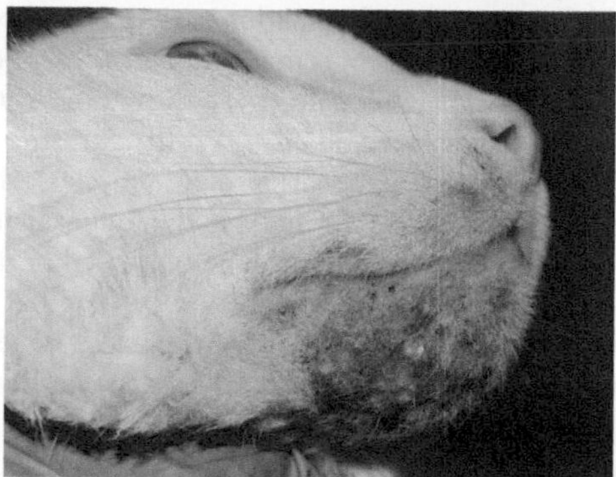

Figure 15a

i. What is the common name for the condition depicted?

ii. What is the etiology? What diagnostics are indicated? How should the lesion be treated?

iii. What are the histological features of this condition?

16. The convex portion of the left pinna of a 6-year-old Jack Russell terrier is shown. The owners present the dog for evaluation of a solitary, alopecic, erythematous well-circumscribed, nodule (**Figure 16a**). The lesion was firm on palpation and was observed to swell and become edematous after manipulation.

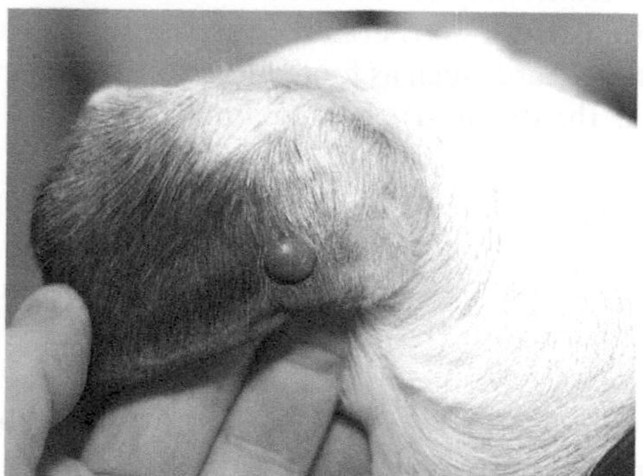

Figure 16a

What skin tumor is most likely to exhibit this behavior?

15. i. Feline acne.

ii. Feline acne is not a "diagnosis" but rather a clinical finding. The classic presentation is a primary disorder of follicular keratinization. In these cats, there is marked comedone production on the chin and lower lip. Feline chin acne may also develop in some cats without a history of lesions as they age. These cats tend to develop scattered comedones that do not become problematic. Dermatophytosis, bacterial pyoderma, *Malassezia*, and demodicosis can trigger feline acne lesions very similar to those shown in **Figure 15a**. In addition, atopic cats may rub their face and chin resulting in similar lesions.

If the lesions are mild (just a few scattered comedones), the best approach may be to practice "watchful neglect" and have the owner bring the cat back if the lesions spread. In cases like the one shown, expressed or draining material should be sampled and smeared on a slide for cytological examination. A dermatophyte culture should be performed if the cat is newly acquired, goes outside, or is from a multicat household. Finally, skin scrapings or trichograms for *Demodex* mites should be performed.

If the lesions are mild and there is no discomfort to the cat, no treatment is required. If the lesions are severe, the previous diagnostics should help determine appropriate treatment. Bacterial infections should be treated for 21–30 days with antibiotics or longer if there is severe furunculosis. Yeast infections respond well to fluconazole or itraconazole (5 mg/kg PO q24h for both drugs) for 30 days. These antimicrobials may need to be given concurrently and should be based on cytologic findings. Topical therapy can vary from daily to every other day wiping or washing with products that contain benzoyl peroxide, salicylic acid, or ethyl lactate. Once resolved, topical therapy may need to be continued on a maintenance basis (two to three times a week) to prevent relapses. Tar-based products should be avoided in cats due to possible irritant or toxicity concerns. It is the author's experience that topical therapy, although often effective, fails due to lack of compliance by either the owner or the cat. Topical mupirocin ointment, metronidazole gel, glucocorticoids, or synthetic retinoid creams may be indicated in refractory cases. It is important to determine if persistent lesions are associated with pruritus or not. If so, underlying pruritic diseases such as food allergy and environmental allergies should be pursued. The diagnosis of "idiopathic feline acne" is a diagnosis of exclusion.

iii. Common findings include follicular keratosis and plugging, dilation of hair follicles with comedone formation, sebaceous gland duct dilation, epitrichial gland dilation, and in advanced cases, folliculitis, furunculosis, and pyogranulomatous dermatitis (Jazic et al., 2006).

16. Mast cell tumor (MCT). A canine MCT may enlarge after manipulation due to degranulation of the mast cells.

17. A 4-year-old neutered male Chesapeake Bay retriever presented for evaluation of hair loss affecting the caudal trunk and rear legs (**Figure 17a, b**). The alopecia began approximately 1–1.5 years ago and has progressed. The owners report that the patient is nonpruritic, has no other symptoms, and is current with all preventatives and vaccinations.

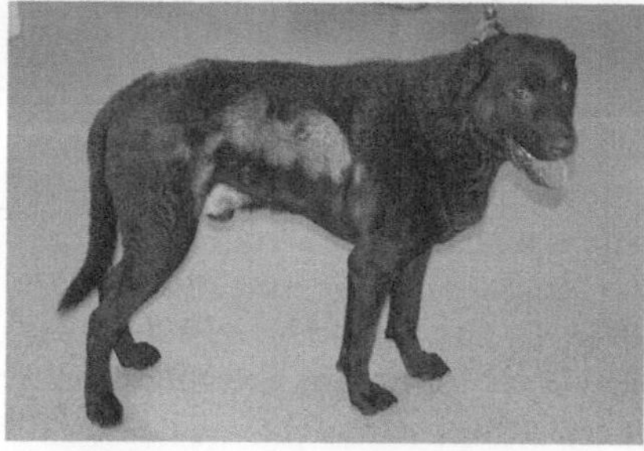
Figure 17a

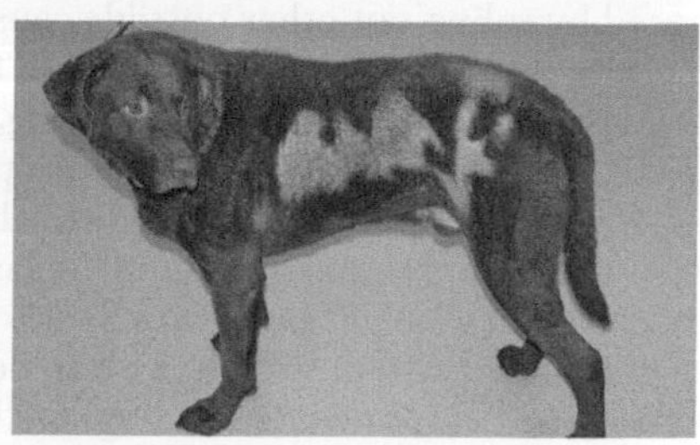
Figure 17b

i. What is the name of the condition that this patient has, how is it diagnosed, and how is it treated?
ii. What other breeds are known to have a similar condition?

18. Multiple circular, crusted lesions were found on the abdomen of a dog (**Figure 18a**) during examination. The owner reports that the lesions were small, red bumps a couple of days ago, and today there are these crusted lesions.

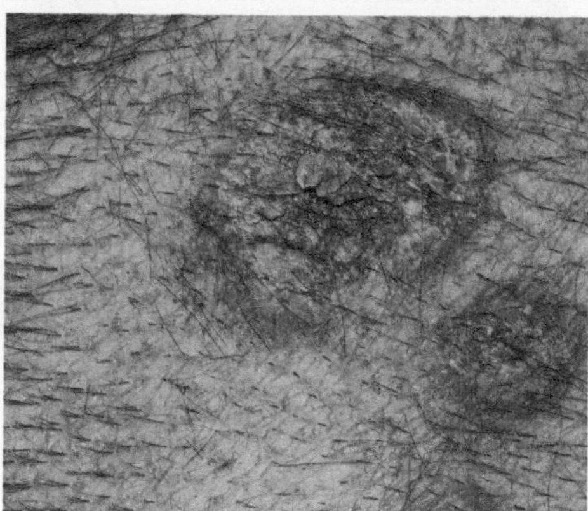
Figure 18a

i. What are these lesions called?
ii. What other skin disease(s) can this lesion be mistaken for clinically?
iii. What is superficial spreading pyoderma?

17. **i.** Adult-onset alopecia of the Chesapeake Bay retriever. This is considered a breed-specific hair-cycle disturbance. Noninflammatory alopecia is typically observed in adult dogs beginning some time between 1.5 and 4 years of age. Varying degrees of alopecia are seen affecting the axillae, ventrum, flanks, dorsum, and caudal rear legs that can resemble cyclic flank alopecia, but in this instance, the hair loss does not cycle and the lesions are always multifocal and not just confined to the flanks (Cerundolo et al., 2005). The condition is diagnosed by ruling out other possible causes for hair-cycle disturbance. Routine blood work and advanced endocrine testing (urinary cortisol to creatinine ratio [UCCR], thyroid function testing, low-dose dexamethasone suppression [LDDS] testing, and adrenocorticotropic hormone [ACTH] stimulation testing) fail to demonstrate abnormalities. Histopathology reveals follicular hyperkeratosis, atrophy, and occasional melanin clumping. At this time, therapeutic intervention with various drugs, neutroceuticals, and supplements have failed to provide consistent benefit. Benign neglect is appropriate as the condition is a cosmetic issue, and affected dogs are healthy otherwise.

ii. Similar but not identical conditions have been observed in the Irish water spaniel, Portuguese water dog, curly coated retriever, and greyhound.

18. **i.** This lesion is called an epidermal collarette and is representative of a superficial bacterial pyoderma. It results from the rupture of an intact pustule. After the pustule ruptures, a crust develops and spreads in a circular fashion creating a "collar of crust." There may or may not be a ring of erythema at the margin. As the lesion heals, the center often becomes hyperpigmented.

ii. Epidermal collarettes are commonly mistaken for "ringworm lesions" or dermatophytosis. Skin scrapings should be done to rule out demodicosis. If there are other dermatologic signs consistent with dermatophytosis, a fungal culture should be performed. Skin cytology should also be performed from the leading edge or from intact pustular lesions to verify the presence of bacteria prior to initiating therapy. The patient is best treated with a combination of topical and systemic antimicrobials, and treatment should continue for 1 week past clinical cure. If the patient does not respond to appropriate antibiotic therapy, then cytology should be repeated. If bacteria are observed on cytology, a culture should be taken to determine if the organism is resistant to the empirically chosen antibiotic. If bacteria are not present, then a skin biopsy is indicated to rule out other rare causes of these lesions (i.e., pemphigus foliaceus or epitheliotrophic lymphoma).

iii. Superficial spreading pyoderma is a unique form of superficial bacterial skin disease. It is characterized by large, rapidly expanding, coalescing epidermal collarettes with an erythematous and crusted leading edge (**Figure 18b**). What is unique about this clinical form of superficial pyoderma is the lack of pustules; lesions are extensive, and pustules are conspicuously absent. The Shetland sheepdog, Border collie, Australian shepherd, and collie have been reported to be predisposed to this superficial form of disease (Gortel, 2013).

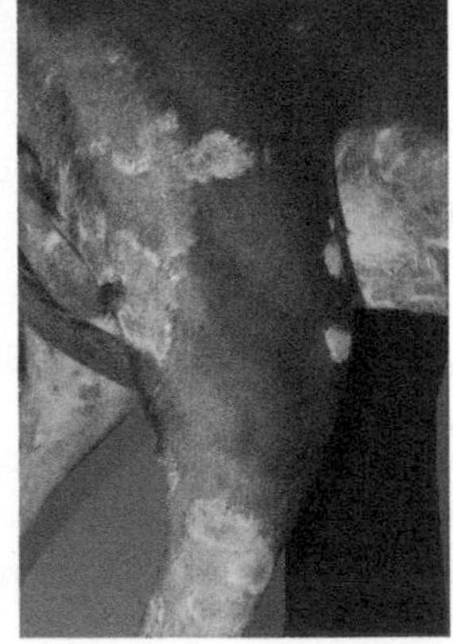

Figure 18b

19. A 9-month-old cat presented for a routine health examination after being adopted from an animal shelter. The unique coloring of the cat's hair coat especially impressed the owners, particularly the "white tips" on the ends of the hairs (**Figure 19a**). The owners reported the cat to be mildly pruritic. Flea combings were done, and an organism was found; several of the hairs with white tips were examined microscopically. The only other pet in the house was a dog, which was unaffected.

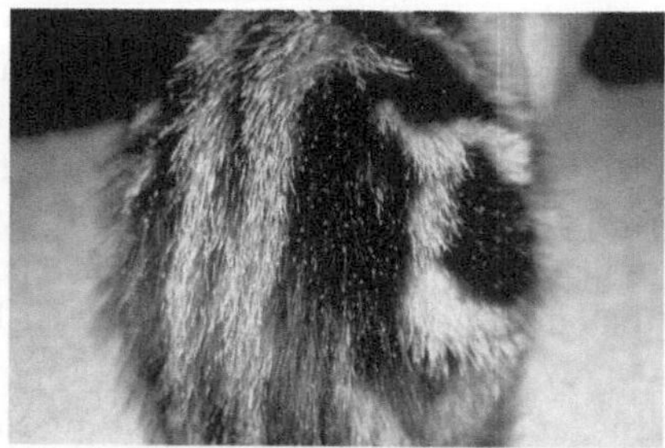

Figure 19a

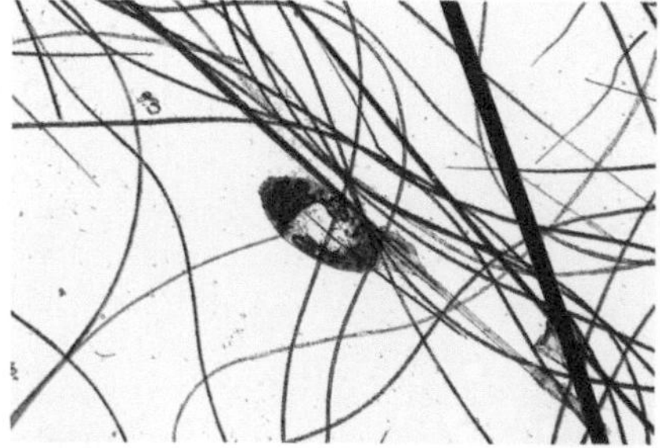

Figure 19b

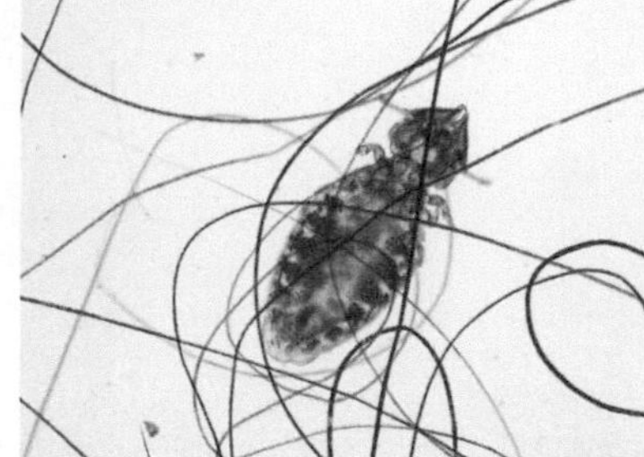

Figure 19c

i. A microscopic view of a "white tip" on the cat's coat is shown (**Figure 19b**) along with an organism (**Figure 19c**) found on flea combing of the hair coat.

What are these organisms, and how should the cat be treated?

ii. Three days after treating the cat, the owner calls. Both of her children have been diagnosed with what the cat has. The owner is very agitated that she was not warned about the zoonotic implications of her cat's infestation.

What are the zoonotic implications with respect to this owner's household?

19. **i.** The images show a louse egg or "nit" cemented to a hair shaft and an adult louse. This cat has pediculosis as a result of an infestation with *Felicola subrostratus*. The cat should be bathed to help mechanically remove as many of the lice and eggs as possible prior to treatment. Some authors report that removal of louse nits can be facilitated with a rinse of a 1:4 dilution of household white vinegar in water, which may aid in loosening their attachment to the hair. Following mechanical removal and allowing the cat to dry, the patient should be treated with a routine flea control product labeled for use in cats. Products suitable for this purpose include those containing fipronil, selamectin, or imidocloprid. As nits are more resistant to therapy, a second dose should be reapplied in 30 days per product instructions to ensure eradication. Additionally, topical isoxazolines may also be an effective treatment option in patients of appropriate age and weight. Treatment with ivermectin has been previously reported to be effective, but it is no longer recommended as safer alternatives exist. Although lice do not live long off their host, it is advisable that bedding be thoroughly washed at least once.

ii. Lice are host specific, and the children were not infested from the cat. In addition, the family's dog is not at risk.

20. A 6-year-old spayed female rat terrier who resides in the Midwest United States presented for paw licking and scratching in early October. The owner reports that these symptoms have occurred seasonally from late August through October since the dog was 3 years of age. The owner also believes that the issue this year is significantly worse and began earlier than in prior years. The patient receives monthly prescription adulticidal flea and heartworm preventatives. The owner has no other concerns other than their dog's licking and chewing. Physical exam reveals generalized erythema, axillary and inguinal alopecia, and interdigital salivary staining (**Figure 20a–e**). Impression cytology from the paws failed to reveal the presence of bacteria or yeast organisms.

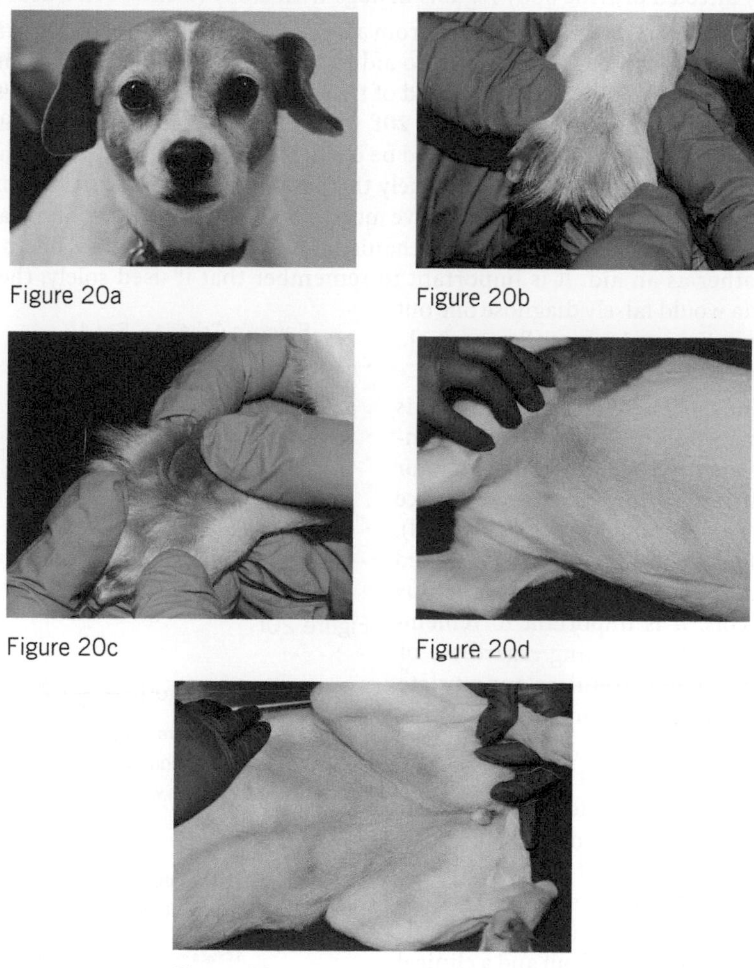

Figure 20a

Figure 20b

Figure 20c

Figure 20d

Figure 20e

i. What is the major dermatologic problem in this patient, and what is the diagnosis?

ii. What are Favrot's criteria, and how do they relate to this patient?

iii. What is the purpose of allergy testing this patient?

20. **i.** Pruritus as a result of canine atopic dermatitis. This is a classic presentation of atopy in the dog. The diagnosis of atopy is a clinical one that is made by ruling out other skin conditions that resemble or having overlapping symptoms of atopy (e.g., food allergy, *Malassezia* dermatitis, etc.), and through the interpretation of historical and clinical features. The initial clinical feature in most cases of canine atopic dermatitis is pruritus that can be manifested as scratching, rubbing, chewing, excessive grooming, licking, scooting, and/or head shaking. Seasonality of symptoms is dependent on the allergens involved, such as weeds (seasonal) or dust mites (nonseasonal). The face, ears, perianal area, paws, along with the inguinal and axillary regions are the most commonly affected pruritic body regions in dogs with atopy (Hensel et al., 2015).

ii. Favort's criteria were developed from a large case series of atopic dogs and are a set of benchmarks developed to aid in the clinical diagnosis of canine atopic dermatitis. They are composed of two criteria sets with varying levels of specificity and sensitivity (**Figure 20f**, **g**). Neither data set is superior, and the one that suits the user best should be used. If the data set with the higher specificity is used, then it is more likely the patient has atopy versus the one with higher sensitivity, which will have more false positives. These criteria are not intended to be used as a sole mechanism for making a diagnosis of atopy but rather as an aid. It is important to remember that if used solely, these criteria would falsely diagnose one out of every five to six dogs (Favrot et al., 2010).

iii. The purpose of allergy testing this patient would be twofold: (1) potentially identify offending allergens for the purpose of implementing avoidance measures (although rarely beneficial), or (2) identify allergens to be included in allergen-specific immunotherapy protocols. It is important to remember that allergy testing regardless of method is not useful or appropriate to be used as a screening test. Patients with atopy can have negative results, and patients without atopy may have positive results. Additionally, positive results do not confirm a diagnosis of atopy in a suspect patient. Allergy tests (intradermal of serologic) should only be performed once other conditions have been ruled out and a clinical diagnosis of atopy has been established (Deboer and Hillier, 2001).

Favrot's Criteria – Set 1

- Age of onset < 3years of age
- Patient lives mostly indoors
- Pruritus is Corticosteroid-responsive
- Chronic or recurrent yeast infections
- Affected front feet
- Affected ear pinnae
- Non-affected ear margins
- Non-affected dorso-lumbar area

5 Criteria met: Sensitivity 85.4%; Specificity 79.1%

6 Criteria met: Sensitivity 58.2%; Specificity 88.5%

Figure 20f

Favrot's Criteria – Set 2

- Age of onset < 3years of age
- Patient lives mostly indoor
- Non-lesional pruritus was first symptom
- Affected front feet
- Affected ear pinnae
- Non-affected ear margins
- Non-affected dorso-lumbar area

5 Criteria met: Sensitivity 77.2%; Specificity 83%

6 Criteria met: Sensitivity 42%; Specificity 93.7%

Figure 20g

21. A 4-year-old male castrated Labrador retriever presented for exercise intolerance, weight gain, hair loss, and excessive shedding (**Figure 21a**). In addition, the owner reported the dog has "lost his obedience training" and sleeps all of the time. Physical examination reveals a heart rate of 65 beats per minute, the dog's face has a tragic expression, and large clumps of hair are easily epilated from the hair coat.

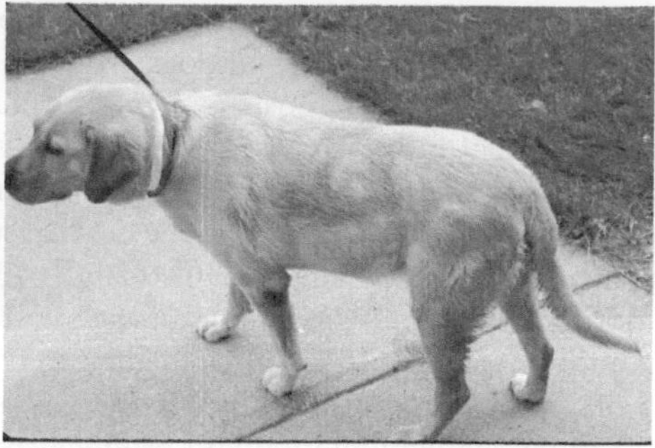
Figure 21a

i. What is the most likely cause of the dog's clinical signs, and what diagnostic tests should be performed?

ii. What breeds are overrepresented for this condition?

22. A 5-year-old spayed female Cavalier King Charles spaniel presented for evaluation of progressive hearing loss that had been noted over the last 2–3 months. During this time, no other behavioral changes had been observed by the owner. On examination, the patient was observed to be bright, alert, and responsive with a fairly unremarkable general physical exam. Neurologic examination was also mostly unremarkable with the exception of decreased reactivity to sudden loud noises. Otoscopic exam revealed the following in the right ear (**Figure 22a**) with a similar finding observed in the left.

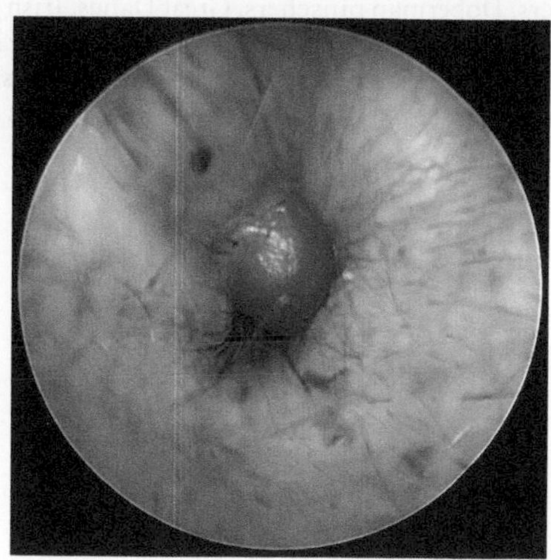
Figure 22a

i. What is the diagnosis?

ii. What other clinical signs have been observed in patients affected with this condition?

iii. How is the condition treated?

iv. What test can be done to assess a dog's ability to hear?

21. i. Canine hypothyroidism. The most common causes of naturally acquired hypothyroidism in dogs are lymphocytic thyroiditis and idiopathic thyroid atrophy. Diagnosis of hypothyroidism is normally straightforward if the patient is appropriately worked up with all recommended blood work including a complete blood count, serum chemistry panel, urinalysis, and full thyroid testing. In this patient, the clinical suspicion is high; therefore, thyroid testing (tT4, fT4 by equilibrium dialysis [ED], and thyroid-stimulating hormone [TSH]) would be an appropriate first diagnostic. Evaluation of a therapeutic thyroid hormone supplementation trial without blood work supporting a diagnosis of hypothyroidism is inappropriate and unreliable since thyroid hormone supplementation will produce changes in attitude, activity, obesity, and hair growth in nonhypothyroid dogs. Furthermore, the administration of a thyroid hormone supplement to euthyroid dogs is not without risk; complications from iatrogenic hyperthyroidism can occur. Measurement of fT4 concentrations by equilibrium dialysis is the most accurate single test, but this test can be expensive and is not always available. In general, a single measurement of tT4 is a good screening test but is rarely diagnostic by itself as the serum level can be artificially decreased by several factors. The author recommends evaluating a combination of tT4, fT4, and TSH concentrations when hypothyroidism is suspected. This dog was diagnosed with hypothyroidism.

ii. Hypothyroidism may affect any breed of dog, but those reported to have an increased occurrence of the disease include golden retrievers, Labrador retrievers, Doberman pinschers, Great Danes, Irish wolfhounds, boxers, English bulldogs, Newfoundlands, Malamutes, Brittany spaniels, cocker spaniels, beagles, Irish setters, English setters, old English sheepdogs, Doberman pinschers, dalmatians, and German shorthair pointers (Graham et al., 2007; Miller et al., 2013b).

22. i. Primary secretory otitis media. The condition is characterized by a buildup of sterile mucous within the middle ear. The Cavalier King Charles spaniel appears to be overrepresented for the condition, but it has also been observed in a dachshund, shih tzu, and other brachycephalic breeds such as the boxer (Cole, 2012). The condition is diagnosed by observing a large, opaque, or gray-green, bulging pars flaccida on otoscopic examination, which is seen in **Figure 22a**. However, it is worth noting that the presence of a flat, normal appearing pars flaccida on otoscopic exam does not rule out the possibility of the condition and that further radiographic imaging such as a computed tomography (CT) scan or magnetic resonance imaging (MRI) may be needed to confirm the diagnosis (Cole et al., 2015).

ii. No clinical sign is known to be pathognomonic for the condition, but one or more of the following have been reported to be observed in Cavalier King Charles spaniels diagnosed with primary secretory otitis media: head and neck pain, spontaneous vocalization, guarded or abnormal neck carriage, ataxia, facial paralysis, nystagmus, head tilt, seizures, ear pruritus without otits externa, otitis externa, hearing loss, fatigue, difficulties or pain while eating, "air scratching" (scratching behavior directed at the head/neck region without making actual contact), and abnormal yawning.

iii. At this time, the current treatment standard for managing the condition involves performing a myringotomy into the caudal ventral portion of the pars tensa and flushing the bulla to remove the buildup of mucous. Post-flushing the patient is often prescribed with a short, tapering course of glucocorticoids (0.5–1 mg/kg; prednisone or a derivative) to decrease swelling and inflammation associated with the procedure. As the exact pathogenesis of the condition is unknown, and no prospective studies have shown possible treatment options to prevent mucous accumulation, repeat myringotomies may be needed as symptoms recur in patients.

iv. Brainstem auditory-evoked response or BAER testing. BAER is a far-field recording of the neuroelectrical events of cranial nerve VIII and brainstem pathways in response to sound (Cole, 2012).

23. Essential fatty acid (EFA) supplementation is commonly recommended for the management of various inflammatory and dermatologic disorders in dogs and cats.

i. What is the difference between omega-3 and omega-6 fatty acids?

ii. What organs may be affected by the anti-inflammatory effects of omega-3 fatty acid supplementation?

iii. How have EFAs been utilized in the management of dermatologic conditions?

iv. What relationship do omega-6 fatty acids have to barrier function of the skin?

24. The following images (**Figure 24a**, **b**) show two mites that are found in association with dogs that presented for a compliant of dermatitis

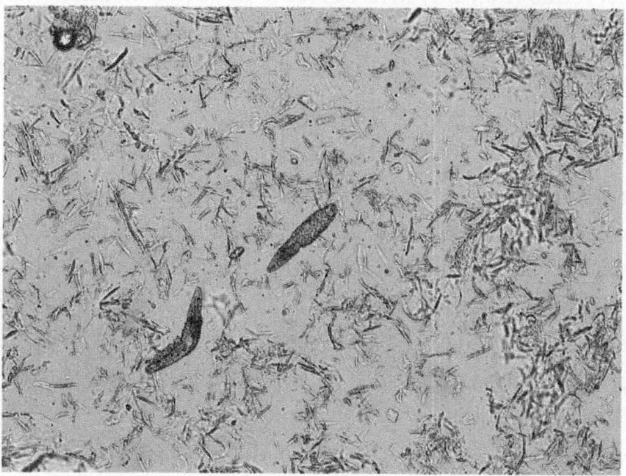

Figure 24a

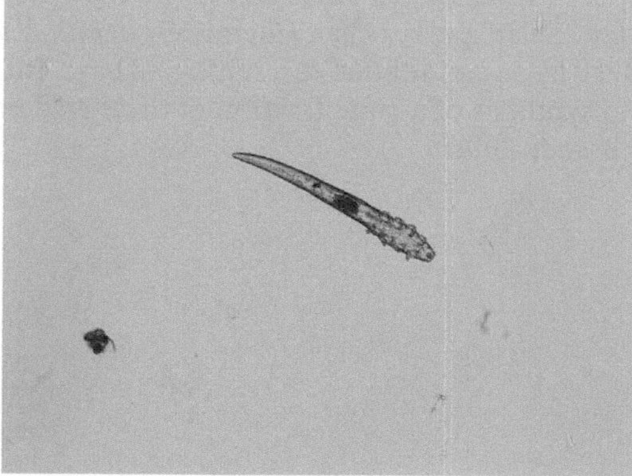

Figure 24b

What is the name of each parasite, and how does their clinical presentation differ?

23. **i.** Omega-3 and omega-6 fatty acids are considered essential because they are required for normal tissue function but cannot be synthesized. They are classified based on the length of the hydrocarbon chain, number of double bonds present, and location of the first double bond relative to the methyl (omega) end of the chain. Omega-3 fatty acids (i.e., docosahexaenoic acid [DHA] and eicosapentaenoic acid [EPA]) are found in cold-water fish, nuts, and flaxseed. Omega-6 fatty acids (linoleic acid [LA]) are predominantly derived from vegetables and seed oils (safflower, sunflower, corn or soybean oil). It is important to remember that these two types of fatty acids do not metabolically interconvert. Both of these fatty acids are a component of the phospholipid bilayer that compromise cell membranes, and dietary intake can alter the composition of the cell membrane. Omega-3 and omega-6 fatty acids compete for metabolic enyzmes that are activated in the arachodonic acid inflammatory cascade. Omega-6 fatty acids typically form pro-inflammatory mediators such as series 4 leukotrienes (i.e., B4) and series 2 prostaglandins (i.e., E2). Omega-3 fatty acids tend to form less pro-inflammatory mediators such as series 3 prostaglandins (i.e., E3) and series 5 leukotrienes (i.e., B5) (Lenox, 2016).

ii. Those organ systems affected by omega-3 EFA supplementation include skin, kidneys, GI tract, neural tissues, heart, blood, and bones (Bauer, 2011).

iii. EFA administration has been evaluated in dogs and cats with a wide range of cutaneous disorders from pruritic dermatoses (i.e., atopy) to immune-mediated conditions such as symmetric lupoid onychodystrophy. Various dosing regimens have been recommended, including 180 mg of EPA and 120 mg of DHA per 4.55 kg of body weight (BW), 700 mg of EPA and DHA per 10 kg of BW, or 125 mg (DHA and EPA) $\times$ BW $(kg)^{0.75}$ (Bauer, 2011; Bauer 2016; Logas and Kunkle, 1994).

iv. The epidermal barrier of the skin is composed of keratinocytes embedded in a lipid matrix. The epidermal water barrier function of the skin depends on content and quality of the lipid component. Ceramides comprise the largest fraction of strateum corneum lipids, which along with cholesterol and free fatty acids form the intercellular lipid lamellae. Chemically, ceramides are composed of a fatty acid linked by an amide bond to a sphingoid base. The omega-6 fatty acid LA is vital to synthesis of a large fraction of these epidermal ceramides (Meckfessel and Brandt, 2014).

24. The images show the two *Demodex* mite species that affect dogs. A prior third short-bodied mite commonly referred to as the unnamed species or *D. cornei* in the literature has been shown to actually represent a morphologic variant of *D. canis* (Sastre et al., 2012). **Figure 24a** depicts an image of *Demodex canis*, while **Figure 24b** shows the long-bodied mite known as *D. injai*. *D. canis* is the most common cause of demodicosis in the dog and is associated with juvenile and adult-onset disease. This is in contrast to *D. injai*, in which only adult-onset disease has been recognized at this time. Clinical signs of *D. canis* are extremely variable and include alopecia, erythema, scaling, papules, pustules, comedone formation, draining tracts, crusts, and lichenification with lesions occurring anywhere on the body. Both localized and generalized forms of the disease exist. *D. injai* infestations appear to more commonly affect the face and dorsal trunk with clinical signs consisting of alopecia, erythema, excessive oily exudate, a greasy hair coat, and pruritus. Pruritus is not a hallmark symptom of *D. canis* infestations unless lesions are complicated by a secondary bacterial infection. But, *D. injai* may be mild to moderately pruritic in the absence of secondary microbial overgrowth. Many breeds to date have been reported to be predisposed or overrepresented when it comes to *D. canis* (e.g., pit bull terriers, Doberman pinschers, English bulldogs, shar-pei dogs, etc.), while terriers and shih tzus appear to be predisposed to infestations with *D. injai*. With regard to diagnostics (skin scrape and trichogram), many mites including those of all life stages are usually observed and fairly easy to recover in the case of *D. canis*. With *D. injai,* mite numbers are usually much lower with fewer life stages observed, and the potential for negative results from sampling is higher.

25. What diagnostic test is shown in **Figure 25a**?

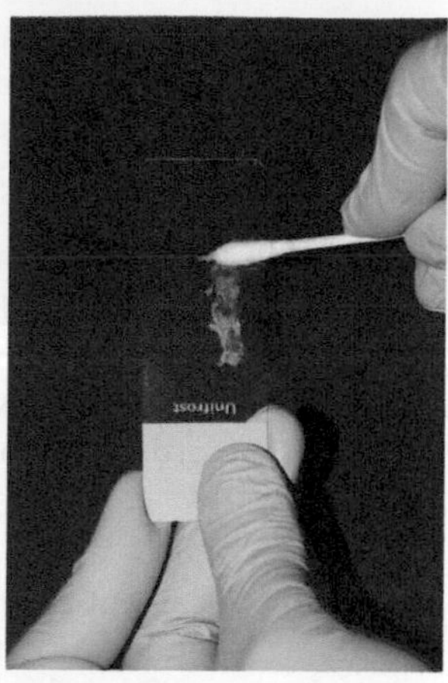

Figure 25a

26. The owners of an adult mixed breed dog with a history of chronic "nasal dermatitis" presented the dog for an emergency examination. Until now, the owners had refused all recommendations for diagnostic testing to determine the cause of the nasal lesions shown in **Figure 26a.** The depigmentation and crusting have been present for almost 2 years, and it did not seem to be problematic to the dog. The dog is presented today with the complaint of epistaxis. Further questioning of the owners reveals the epistaxis is a recent development and has happened on at least two other occasions, and the patient has no exposure to rodenticides. On physical examination, the dog is normal except for the skin of the nasal planum. There are no signs of petechial hemorrhage on any of the mucous membranes. Dermatologic examination reveals the presence of mild adherent crusting on the dorsum of the nose and bilateral ulceration of the nares. The blood appears to be coming from these ulcerative areas.

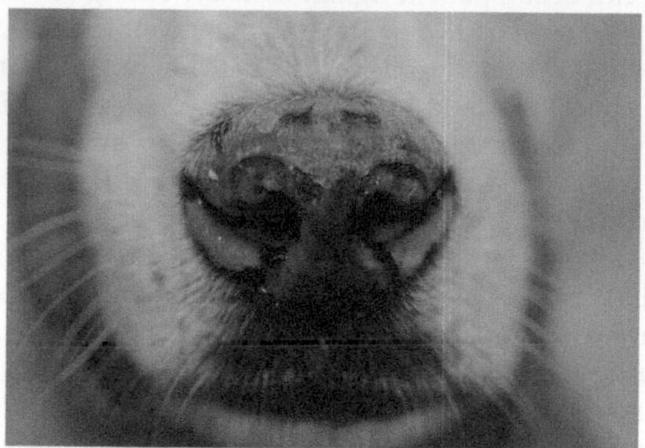
Figure 26a

i. What are the differential diagnoses? What must also be ruled out?

ii. What diagnostic tests should be performed on this patient?

25. **Figure 25a** demonstrates an ear swab cytology specimen being prepared. This sample is acquired by inserting a dry cotton-tipped swab into the ear canal to the level of the junction between the vertical and horizontal canals. The swab is then gently rotated, removed, and then rolled onto a glass slide to transfer the collected exudate onto the surface of the slide. Both ears should always be sampled when clinical disease is suspected, even if the canal is not grossly affected. The slide can then be heat-fixed as recommended by many dermatologists, which is believed to help material adhere to the slide, but this step has not been shown to be necessary (Toma et al., 2006). The sample is then stained with any standard Romanowsky stain variant (i.e., Diff-Quik) and examined microscopically.

26. **i.** The recurrent epistaxis may be due to the skin disease; however, an underlying coagulopathy must be ruled out. The depigmentation and symmetrical nature of the ulcerative nares and nasal crusting are most consistent with discoid lupus erythematosus. However, other differentials that must be considered include pemphigus erythematosus or foliaceus, mucocutaneous pyoderma, uveodermatologic syndrome, epitheliotrophic lymphoma, drug reaction, and leishmaniasis.

ii. Most conditions that affect the nasal planum present with similar lesions. Appropriate diagnosis of nasal planum disease requires understanding the conditions that can occur, patient signalment, and ruling out mucocutaneous pyoderma as a primary condition. The first diagnostic in this case should be a simple impression cytology from the ulcerated areas of the nasal planum. If intracellular coccoid-shaped bacteria are observed, the patient should be treated with an appropriate topical antimicrobial or systemic first-tier (e.g., cephalosporin) antibiotic. If the lesions fail to resolve with appropriate therapy for mucocutaneous pyoderma and/or bacteria are not observed on cytology, a biopsy of the area should be pursued for definitive diagnosis. A coagulopathogy should be ruled out before obtaining punch biopsy specimens from the affected areas. In this case, a mucosal bleeding time was normal, as was a platelet count. After determining the dog did not have a coagulopathy, skin biopsies were obtained under general anesthesia. Biopsy samples were obtained from the crusted and depigmented areas. To avoid excessive hemorrhage, biopsy specimens should not be taken from the center of the nose as there is a large vessel in this area. In this particular circumstance, the patient was diagnosed with discoid lupus erythematosus following histopathologic evaluation of acquired biopsies. The prognosis for this disease is good, and it can be successfully managed with a variety of drugs including glucocorticoids, tetracycline derivatives and niacinamide, cyclosporine, azathioprine, topical tacrolimus, and other immunosuppressive anti-inflammatory drugs.

27. Antihistamines are commonly used in veterinary dermatology as adjuvant therapy for the treatment of pruritus. Currently, both first- and second-generation antihistamines are used in clinical practice.

i. What is the primary mechanism of action of antihistamines?

ii. What is the primary difference between first- and second-generation antihistamines?

iii. What adverse events are associated with the use of antihistamines in small animal patients?

28. With the recent rise in extensively resistant staphylococcal infections in veterinary medicine, where there may be a complete absence of susceptibility to antimicrobials found on traditional screening panels, the natural tendency is to consider exploring the possible use of nonveterinary antimicrobials. However, many of these alternative agents are of critical importance to human medicine.

What drugs are considered third-tier, restriction-of-use antimicrobials and are not appropriate for infections in small animal patients?

29. A 2-year-old neutered male cat presented for a second opinion for hair loss around the base of the pinnae (**Figure 29a**). Previous skin scrapings, impression smears, and dermatophyte test medium (DTM) culture have all yielded negative results. The cat is not described as being pruritic by the owner and has no history of prior ear infections. The cat is otherwise reported to be healthy, up to date with vaccinations, and current with monthly preventative antiparasitics. Physical examination only reveals mild symmetric noninflammatory alopecia of the temporal region between the base of the pinnae and eyes, while otoscopic evaluation was unremarkable.

What should the owner be told?

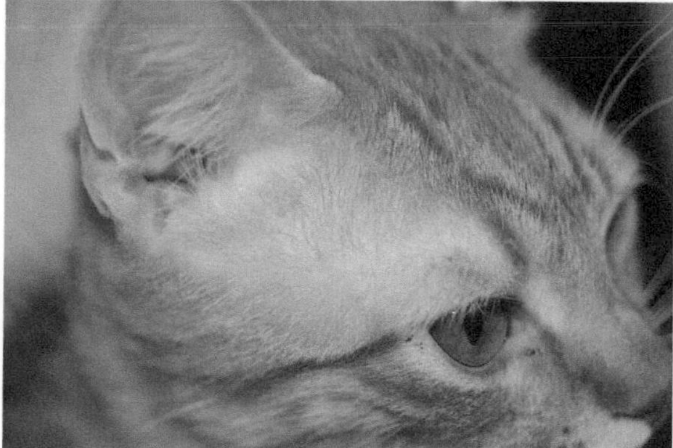

Figure 29a

27. **i.** Antihistamines are classified as H1 and H2 receptor antagonists; the latter includes drugs such as cimetidine, ranitidine, and famotidine. Antihistamine drugs are considered competitive inhibitors and are most effective if used before histamine binds to receptor sites.

ii. Second-generation antihistamines do not readily cross the blood-brain barrier. Therefore, they are associated with less sedation compared to first-generation antihistamines. Second-generation antihistamines also do not have antimuscarinic properties.

iii. The most common adverse events encountered with use of first-generation antihistamines are sedation and restlessness or excitement. These drugs can also cause antimuscarinic anticholinergic (atropine-like) issues. Animals may have a dry mouth leading to dental disease and halitosis. This may also lead to an increase in water consumption. Coughing due to a dry respiratory tract may also occur. Some animals become constipated or have diarrhea, have decreased appetite, and can develop abdominal bloating. Overdoses of second-generation antihistamines can cause life-threatening cardiac episodes. These drugs should not be used concurrently with ketoconazole, itraconazole, or erythromycin or other drugs that are metabolized via the liver.

28. Drugs that should be considered "off-limits" for bacterial pyodermas are linezolid, the glycopeptides (vancomycin, teicoplanin, and telavancin), anti-methicillin-resistant *Staphylococcus aureus* (MRSA) cephalosporins (ceftobiprole and ceftaroline), tigecycline, and any potentially new compounds specifically developed as an anti-MRSA drug for humans in the future. It cannot be stressed enough that the use of these drugs should be strongly discouraged (Hillier et al., 2014; Morris et al., 2017).

29. This is called feline preauricular alopecia, and it is a physiologic, not pathologic, condition. This area is not always noticeable in some cats, but in those with short or less dense coats, it may appear as complete alopecia. When owners ask about this condition, they should be informed that it is normal, with further diagnostics being completely unnecessary, and that no therapy is known to cosmetically improve the appearance. When inflammation, excessive scale, papules, pustules, or crusts are present in this region, then further diagnostic tests are indicated, and other diseases (including those manifesting with pruritus) should be suspected.

30. A 2-year-old spayed female English Springer spaniel presented for evaluation of red spots on the belly that were first noted after a morning hike with the owner along a creek. The patient has no prior history of skin issues, is given monthly flea/tick and heartworm prevention, and has no other clinical symptoms. Physical examination reveals multiple annular macules with a pinpoint central hemorrhagic center, a blanched edematous zone, and an outer erythemic rim along the inguinal and axillary regions (**Figure 30a, b**).

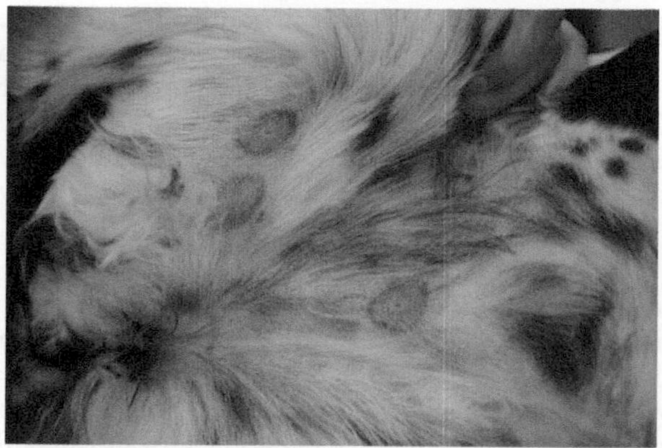

Figure 30a

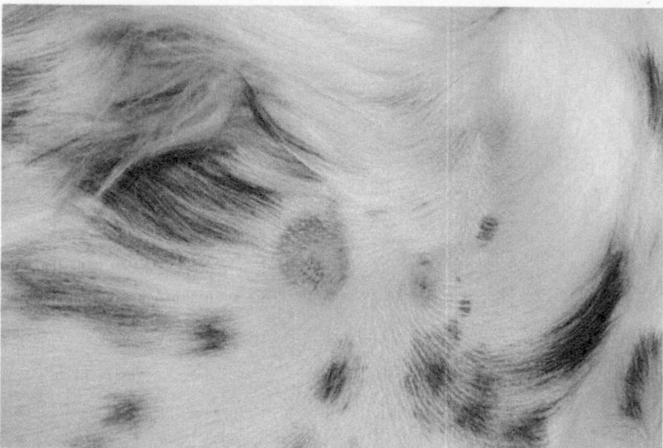

Figure 30b

i. What is the diagnosis for this patient's lesions?

ii. What is the life cycle and environmental niche of the likely causative agent?

31. What are the general functions of the skin and hair?

30. **i.** These lesions are characteristic of fly-bite dermatitis caused by *Simulium* spp. (i.e., black flies, buffalo gnats, or sandflies). These biting flies are an issue during the spring/early summer and are most active during the morning and evening. Bites tend to occur on sparsely haired or hairless regions such as the glaborous skin of the inguinal and axillary regions and occasionally along the head, ears, and distal legs. These flies can occur in swarms, which can overwhelm a patient and lead to anaphylaxis secondary to numerous bites.
ii. Adults lay eggs on stones or vegetation just below the water's surface. The eggs hatch following several days to several months. The larvae then attach to substrate in fast-moving water where they undergo four to nine larval stages over one to several months before pupating. The pupae then hatch in several days to weeks with adults living for 28 days or more (Hill et al., 2010). The length of the life cycle is dependent on the water temperature, fly species, and availability of food. The mature adults are strong fliers and can travel a significant distance from running water sources.

31. The general functions of the skin and hair include the following: act as an enclosing barrier, protect the body against the environment, thermoregulate/insulate, provide storage (e.g., electrolytes, water, vitamins, fats), act as indicators (physical identity, sexual identity, and social communication), provide immune regulation, protect against UV radiation, provide camouflage, enable sensory perception, produce vitamin D, and are a source of cells for wound healing.

32. A 3-year-old domestic shorthair (DSH) cat presented for acute onset of intense pruritus of the back half of its body. Physical examination revealed well-demarcated areas of alopecia along the caudoventral abdomen and caudomedial aspects of the rear legs (**Figure 32a, b**). The cat was very sensitive to touch anywhere along the caudal half of its body. The owner reported that the cat has no access to other animals and lives on the upper floor in an apartment complex but does occasionally sit on the outdoor patio. The owner moved into this apartment 5 months ago, and the pruritus began within roughly 2 months after the move. Skin scrapings were negative for mites, and flea combing did not reveal any live fleas or flea feces.

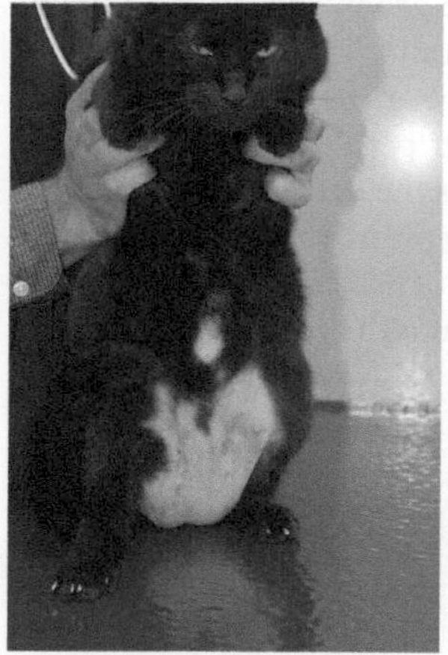
Figure 32a

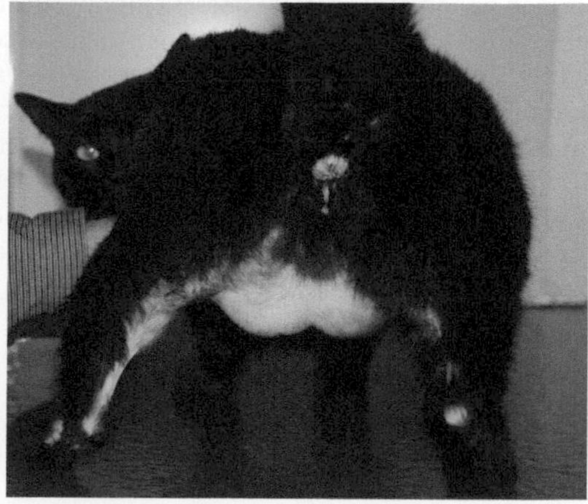
Figure 32b

i. Based on the physical examination findings and clinical suspicion, what condition do you initially elect to treat?
ii. How can you explain your treatment plan to the owner?

32. i. Flea allergy dermatitis.
ii. Some owners find it hard to believe that fleas are the underlying cause when no fleas are found on physical examination. Knowledge of the flea life cycle may help. A host is required for food and protection; fleas spend their entire adult life on their host. Eggs are laid on the animal and fall into the environment where they go through several larval stages and then one pupal stage. Fleas can remain in the pupal stage for an extended period of time. If the owners' apartment had previously housed animals that were infested with fleas, the cat may have provided the right stimuli (temperature, vibrations, carbon dioxide) to cause emergence of the adult fleas, leading to the current clinical presentation when an allergic reaction develops secondary to injection of flea salivary antigen as adults feed. Cats possess highly effective grooming skills and may remove most ectoparasites that cause them discomfort. This explains why in many flea-allergic cats, fleas are not recovered/seen at the time of examination or by the owner when at home with his or her pet. The reaction of this cat to touching along the back further demonstrates the extreme pruritus and discomfort fleas can cause. A fecal float may help confirm the clinical suspicion in some cases, but response to implementation of flea control medications combined with environmental cleaning for several months will help to confirm the diagnosis.

33. A 3-year-old castrated male Maltese dog presented for progressive matting, odor, bleeding sores, and lethargy. The owner reported that the lesions began as focal areas of hair loss a couple months ago, which had rapidly progressed over the last 3 weeks. Examination of the skin revealed marked generalized erythema, diffuse scaling and crusting with multiple serosanguineous to hemorrhagic punctate draining tracts (**Figure 33a–d**). The patient was also noted to have pain upon manipulation with a generalized lymphadenomegaly. An impression smear from one of the draining lesions revealed full fields of neutrophils, macrophages, and red blood cells along with large numbers of adult *D. canis* mites and intracellular coccoid-shaped bacteria. A clinical diagnosis of generalized demodicosis and secondary pyoderma was made.

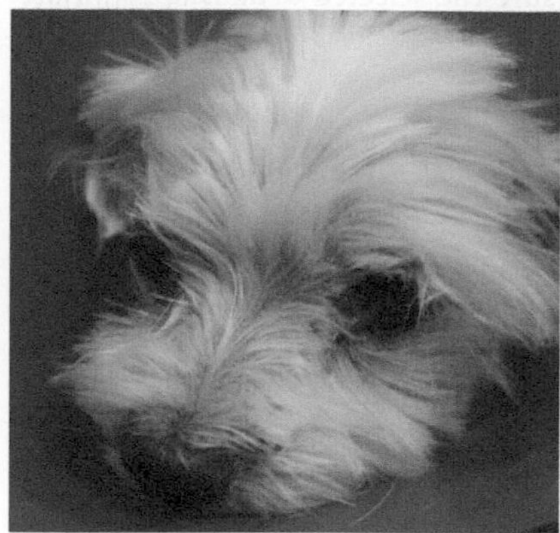

Figure 33a

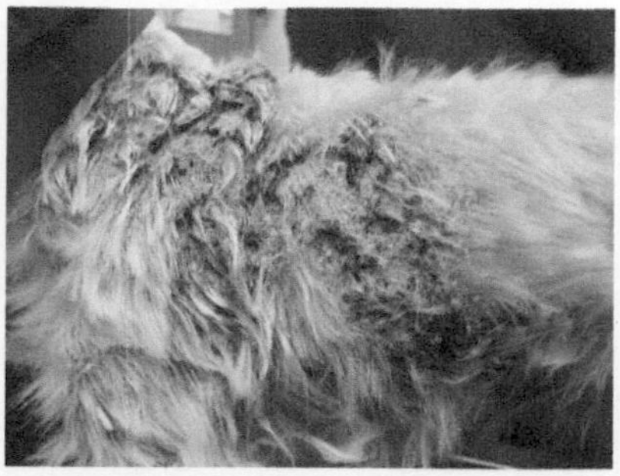

Figure 33b

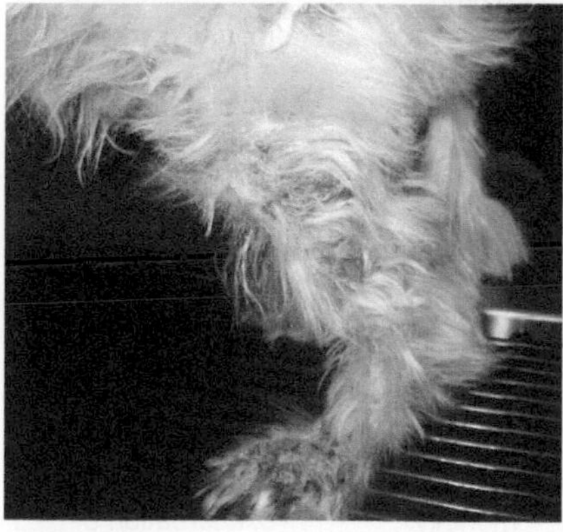

Figure 33c

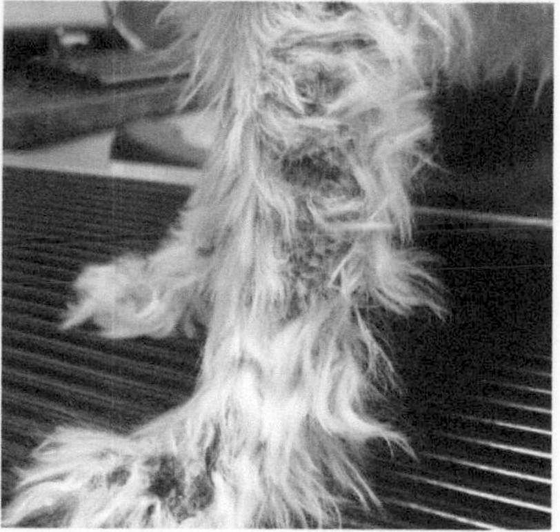

Figure 33d

i. This case is an example of a patient with what type of pyoderma, and how does this affect therapy?

ii. What are the possible mite-specific treatment options for this patient?

iii. How should this patient be monitored, and when can you consider ending this patient's mite-specific therapy?

33. i. Deep pyoderma. In deep pyoderma, the infection breaks through the follicular wall creating furuculosis, which results in draining tracts and pain, the hallmarks of deep pyoderma. Patients are often febrile and have a regional lymphadenopathy (also seen with demodicosis). Treatment duration in cases of deep pyoderma normally requires a minimum of 4–6 weeks of systemic antimicrobial therapy. Many cases will be greatly improved in 2 weeks, but therapy should ideally last for 14 days past clinical resolution (Beco et al., 2013). It is important that palpation of lesions should occur during rechecks, as they will heal superficially prior to resolution of the deeper component, which can still be felt. Because therapy in these cases is prolonged, it is recommended that bacterial culture and sensitivity be acquired prior to initiation of systemic antimicrobial therapy to ensure the selected drug is appropriate and effective.

Drug	Route of administration	Dosage	Adverse events
Amitraz	Topical	0.025% solution applied q2weeks	Vomiting/diarrhea, sedation, lethargy, bradycardia, hyperglycemia
Ivermectin	Oral	0.4 – 0.6mg/kg q24hrs	Lethargy, mydriasis, ataxia, coma, death
Moxidectin	Topical (spot-on in combination with imidacloprid)	Labeled size applied weekly	Local inflammation
Moxidectin	Oral	0.2-0.5mg/kg q24hrs	Lethargy, mydriasis, ataxia, coma, death
Milbemycin	Oral	0.5 – 2mg/kg q24hrs	Lethargy, ataxia
Doramectin	Injectable	0.6 mg/kg s.c. weekly	Lethargy, mydriasis, ataxia, coma, death
Fluralaner	Oral	Labeled size administered every 3 mos.	Vomiting, diarrhea, lethargy, possible exacerbation of neurological symptoms
Afoxolaner	Oral	Labeled size administered monthly	Vomiting, diarrhea, lethargy, possible exacerbation of neurological symptoms
Sarolaner	Oral	Labeled size administered monthly	Vomiting, diarrhea, lethargy, possible exacerbation of neurological symptoms
Lotilaner	Oral	Labeled size administered monthly	Vomiting, diarrhea, lethargy, possible exacerbation of neurological symptoms

Figure 33e

ii. To date, many different treatment options for demodicosis have been reported. Therapy has traditionally involved the application of topical amitraz or the off-label use of systemic macrocyclic lactones (e.g., ivermectin, moxidectin, doramectin, milbemycin) at elevated dosages. Recently, the isoxazoline class of antiparasitics (e.g., afoxolaner, flurolaner, sarolaner, lotilaner) marketed for flea and tick prevention has drawn considerable interest for their potential as a therapeutic option in the management of canine demodicosis. Results of recent investigations would suggest that therapy with isoxazolines at their labeled dosing for flea prevention may offer an effective and attractive alternative therapeutic option for patients affected with demodicosis. **Figure 33e** provides a list of possible treatment options. Different countries have various licensing requirements, so all options may not be able to be used or available in all locations.

iii. When mite-specific therapy is required, patients should be reevaluated on a monthly basis, and clinical findings as well as skin scraping results from previously scraped body locations (mite numbers, life stages, and viability) should be compared with those of prior visits. As long as clinical and parasitologic improvement is observed, treatment is continued. Mite-specific therapy should ideally continue for 1 month past two consecutive negative skin scrapes (no mites of any life stage, live or dead) taken a month apart to minimize the chance of recurrence. If no improvement is seen within 4–8 weeks of initiating therapy, owner compliance should be questioned or a change in the treatment protocol recommended. Additionally, underlying internal illness should be investigated (particularly in cases of adult-onset disease).

34. **Figure 34a** shows a Derm-Duet fungal culture plate 7 days post-inoculation with a sample taken from a patient suspected of having dermatophytosis. **Figure 34b** is a microscopic image from a sample acquired from the growth on the culture plate.

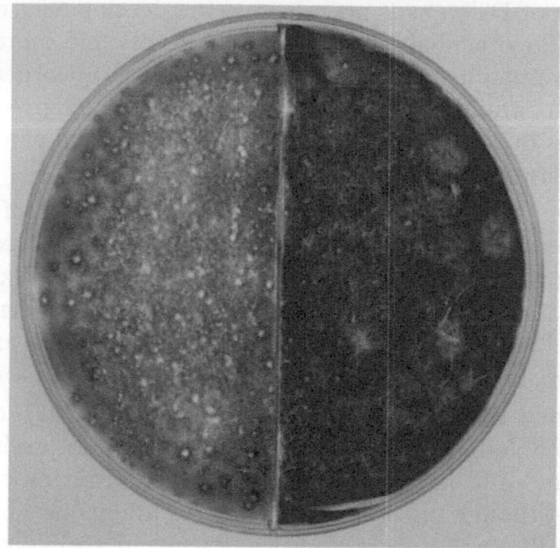

Figure 34a

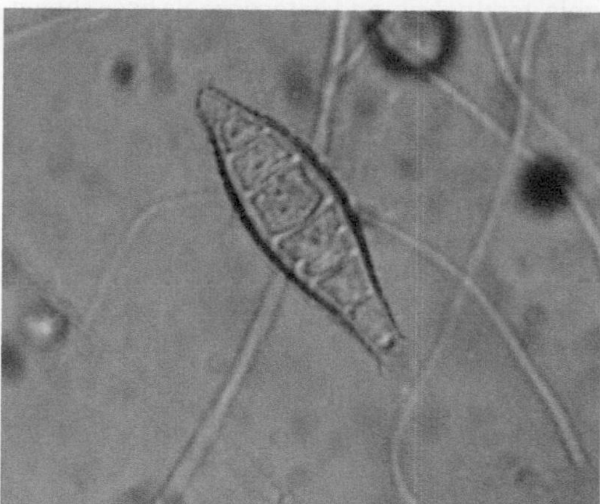

Figure 34b

i. What media compose the two halves of this culture plate?

ii. What is the diagnosis, and what are the identifying characteristics from both the culture plate and the microscopic image?

iii. What topical whole-body treatments for this condition have been consistently demonstrated to be effective?

34. **i.** A Derm-Duet plate consists of two halves. One half is dermatophyte test medium (DTM), which is composed of Sabouraud's dextrose agar with cycloheximide, gentamicin, and chlortetracycline as antimicrobials to inhibit contaminant growth. DTM also contains phenol red as a pH indicator that creates the red color change to the media. Some dermatologists do not like the routine use of DTM, as it may depress the development of identifying macroconidia. The other half of this plate consists of rapid sporulating media (RSM). RSM is similar to DTM but contains chloramphenicol gentamicin, and cycloheximide for antimicrobial inhibition of contaminant growth along with bromothymol as the color-changing pH indicator. Bromothymol changes the media from yellow to a shade of blue-green.

ii. *Microsporum canis.* The culture plate has diffuse growth of white to buff colonies that has a marked media color change associated with colony growth. The observed growth on the plate also has a "cottony" to wool-like appearance. On microscopic examination, a macroconidia is present that has a characteristic spindle or "boat-like" shape with thick echinulate walls and a terminal knob. The macroconidia of *M. canis* tend to consist of six or more cells.

iii. A large review of current literature (Moriello et al., 2017) concluded the most effective whole-body treatments at this time include products that contain lime sulfur, enilconazole, and miconazole-chlorhexidine combination formulations. Although miconazole-only formulations have been shown to be effective, studies indicate it performs best when in a 1:1 combination with chlorhexidine. Chlorhexidine when used as a monotherapy has been shown to be poorly effective and should not be recommended. Although products utilizing climbazole, terbinafine, and ketoconazole have shown promise, more *in vivo* studies are needed before they should be routinely recommended over the proven active agents.

35. The owner reports that for the last 3 years, this 5-year-old castrated male English bulldog has had recurrent hair loss every winter over both sides (**Figure 35a**). The hair coat regrows in the spring, but by fall, the alopecic pattern shown starts to develop. The dog is reported to be nonpruritic, while skin scrapings and dermatophyte cultures are consistently negative. Thyroid function tests, low-dose dexamethasone suppression test, and ACTH stimulation test are normal. The lesions do not respond to oral antibiotics, and the owner practices preventative flea control.

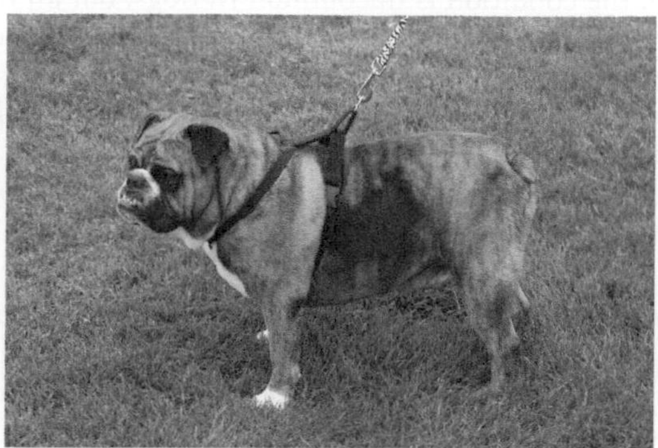

Figure 35a

i. What is the most likely diagnosis, and how is it treated?
ii. What is the cause of this syndrome?
iii. What histological findings characterize this disease?

36. A concerned owner presents his dog due to the rapid appearance of black spots and color change along its ventral abdomen. The affected area is shown in **Figure 36a**.

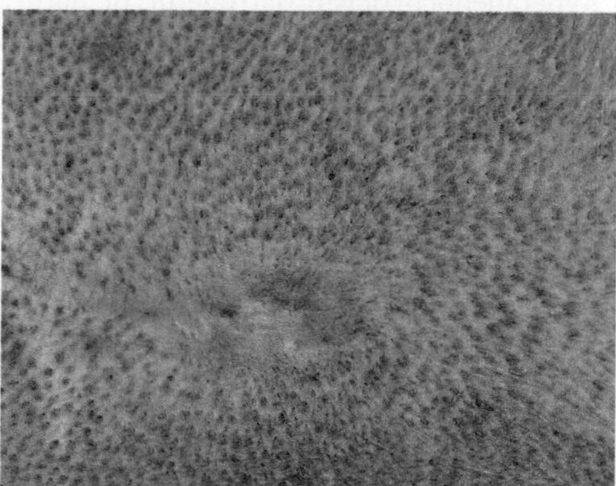

Figure 36a

i. What is the proper term for the lesion shown?
ii. What conditions are known to cause these lesions?

35. i. Canine recurrent flank alopecia (also known as seasonal flank alopecia or cyclic flank alopecia). The condition is characterized by episodes of rapid, symmetrical hair loss, most often affecting the flank or thoracolumbar region. Alopecic areas are noninflamed, well-demarcated, and hyperpigmented. Episodes of alopecia may occur sporadically once or twice, or regularly each year. With annual recurring episodes, a progressive amount and duration of hair loss may be seen that can become permanent. In areas of the world that do not experience much seasonal change, hair loss may be more consistently present. Overall, the condition is uncommon in dogs, but an increased incidence is seen in boxers, Airedale terriers, bulldogs, and Schnauzers. This is entirely a cosmetic disease, where benign neglect or observation is reasonable. Many dogs experience spontaneous hair regrowth several months after initial onset of alopecia. Prognosis is unpredictable due to variability in recurrence and spontaneous resolution. Anecdotally, some dogs may respond to melatonin administration. Oral melatonin at 3–6 mg PO q8–12h for 1–3 months is preferred.

ii. The etiology of canine recurrent flank alopecia is currently unknown. The high incidence in some breeds and occurrence within familial lines suggest a possible genetic predisposition. In addition, other observations suggest the photoperiod may be involved, and thus the proposed association with melatonin.

iii. Compatible histological findings include follicular atrophy and marked infundibular hyperkeratosis. The hair follicles have a characteristic dysplastic appearance, which has been described as a "witches foot" or being "octopus- or jellyfish-like" in appearance. Increased melanin within the epidermis, hair follicle, and sebaceous glands is also common (Müntener et al., 2012).

36. i. Numerous comedones ("blackheads") are present on the ventral abdomen.

ii. The most common reasons for the sudden occurrence of comedones are demodicosis and hyperadenocorticism (iatrogenic or naturally occurring). Other conditions associated with comedone formation include feline acne, chin pyoderma, dermatophytosis, Schnauzer comedone syndrome, vitamin-A responsive dermatosis, color dilution alopecia, and follicular or ectodermal dysplasias.

37. A 10-year-old spayed female Scottish terrier treated for lymphoma developed mild to moderate pruritus, erythema, and excessive scaling over the last several months (**Figure 37a**). The lesions shown were present extensively over the dorsum (**Figure 37b**). Skin scrapings revealed large numbers of mites and eggs per high-power field (**Figure 37c**).

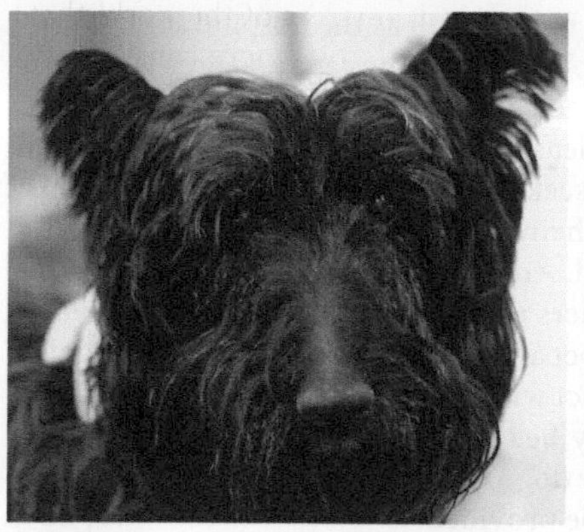
Figure 37a

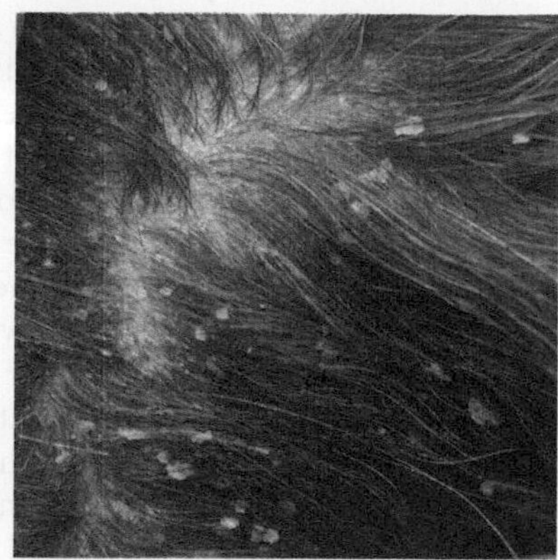
Figure 37b

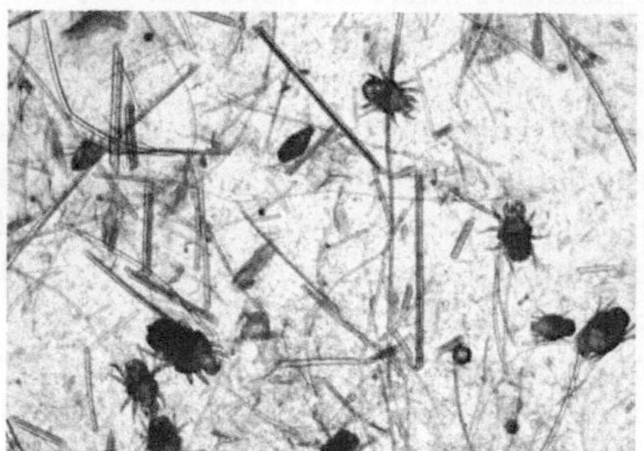
Figure 37c

i. What is the diagnosis?
ii. What recommendations will you make to your staff and other dogs who have come in contact with this patient while hospitalized for the day to receive her chemotherapy?

38. Pyoderma is a common clinical condition encountered in small animal medicine. When discussing clinical presentations of this superficial bacterial infection, the distinctions of relapse, recurrence, or resistance are important to make with respect to diagnostic workup and treatment recommendations.

What is meant by each term, and what are common primary causes for recurrent pyoderma in dogs and cats?

37. **i.** Cheyletiella infestation. This is a severe infestation; it is uncommon to find large numbers of mites and eggs per field.

ii. This is a highly contagious disease and presents a risk to other dogs and cats housed in the area that day. In this case, the risk is increased due to the large number of mites. Mites can live in the environment for short periods of time, and they are very mobile. Transmission may occur via direct contact, environmental exposure, or through a fomite such as the hospital staff. If possible, the dog should be moved to an isolated area. The cage and area where the dog was housed should be grossly cleaned and treated with an environmental insecticide labeled as effective against fleas. Technical staff need to be informed of the zoonotic risk and instructed to seek medical attention if they develop a pruritic rash. All staff should change their uniforms and laboratory coats and place them in a plastic bag until washed. Anyone handling the dog should wear gloves and disposable gowns. The owners need to be informed of the risk and educated about the treatment of their pet and other pets at home. Additionally, all dogs that may have come into contact with this patient while at the hospital should be verified to be on a monthly flea preventative that is known to be efficacious against the parasite. If any dog that came in contact is not on an appropriate preventative, one should be provided.

38. Relapse refers to instances where the infection was not treated appropriately or for a long enough time to resolve the infection. Relapse pyodermas are those where clinical signs/lesions reappear within days (<1 week) of therapy being stopped and are most often encountered in clinical practice when systemic antimicrobials are used for too short of a duration (<14 days). Recurrent pyodermas are those that fully resolve with appropriate therapy but recur within weeks to months of treatment cessation. In this case, the animal has an underlying primary condition that is predisposing the individual to development of a secondary infection that is not being appropriately managed. In these circumstances, the condition will continue to occur until the primary cause is resolved or appropriately managed. In the case of resistance, the patient's infection fails to improve with empiric therapy, and subsequent recheck examinations continue to document the existence of an active infection. Resistance can be inherent or acquired with the best-known example being that of methicillin resistance observed with *Staphylococcus* spp. Primary causes associated with recurrent pyoderma include demodicosis, allergic hypersensitivities (flea allergy dermatitis, atopic dermatitis, cutaneous adverse food reactions), ectoparasites (i.e., cheyletiellosis, fleas), endocrinopathies (Cushing disease, hypothyroidism, diabetes), keratinization disorders, follicular dysplasia, autoimmune conditions (sebaceous adenitits), and neoplasia.

39. A 6-year-old mixed breed dog presented for a complaint of constant paw licking that began 2 months ago. Prior to this, the patient had no history of skin or ear issues. The paws were observed to be alopecic, swollen, severely erythemic with hyperkeratotic pads and areas of self-trauma (**Figure 39a**). The claws were broken and slightly misshapen while patchy hypotrichosis and erythema of the distal and caudomedial aspects of the rear legs were also noted. Further questioning of the owner revealed the patient is kenneled outdoors in a dirt/mulch run with free access to the backyard during the day and walked twice daily. The patient also receives a monthly flea and tick preventative (afoxolaner).

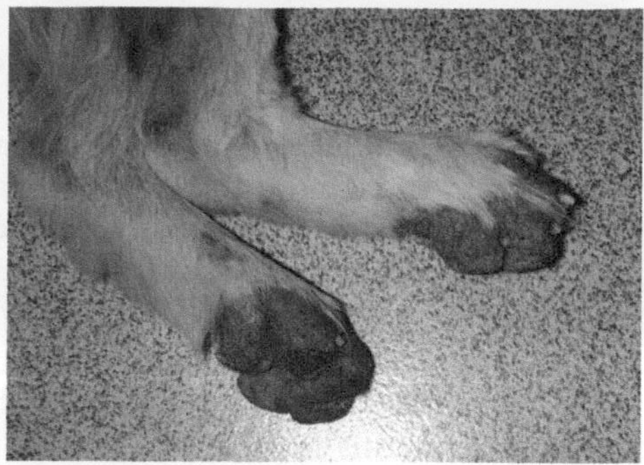
Figure 39a

i. What are the differential diagnoses for this patient, and what diagnostic tests should be performed?

ii. What is the primary differential for this patient, and why are the claws affected?

iii. What other conditions in the dog may present with significant hyperkeratosis of the paw pads?

40. A 5-month-old kitten that was recently adopted from an animal shelter presented for a 1-week history of scratching at their ears and excessive head shaking. Upon examination, there was granular dark brown to black debris present in both ear canals. A mite was found on the examination of an ear swab (**Figure 40a**).

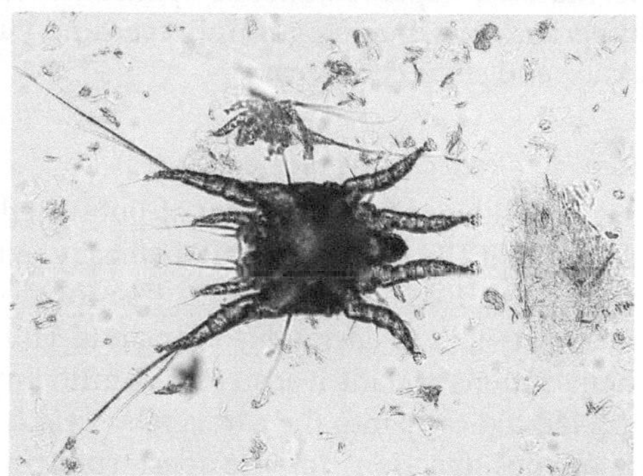
Figure 40a

i. What is the diagnosis?

ii. What are the recommended treatment options?

iii. How long can this parasite survive off the host in the environment?

39. i. Demodicosis, contact dermatitis, hookworm dermatitis, *pelodera* dermatitis, and bacterial or *Malassezia* podermatitis secondary to an allergic hypersensitivity. Skin scrapings and trichograms should be performed to rule out *Demodex* and *Pelodera*. Impression smears and/or cytological scrapings of material from the claw bed and interdigital areas should be performed to look for bacterial and/or *Malassezia* infection. Fecal floatation should be performed to look for hookworm ova. Biopsy and dermatohistopathology may also be performed if more basic diagnostics fail to yield expected findings.

ii. Hookworm dermatitis is the primary differential based on this patient's history, signalment, and exam findings. Although an allergic hypersensitivity or contact dermatitis are solid possibilities, the age and nature of onset along with a lack of change in environment or habits make these less likely given this patient's presentation. In addition, the monthly use of afoxolaner makes *Demodex* unlikely. Given this patient is housed outdoors in a dirt/mulch-bedded kennel, both hookworm and *pelodera* dermatitis are viable differentials that would produce similar clinical symptoms. However, as this patient had significant paw pad hyperkeratosis, hookworm dermatitis is the more likely differential. The claw changes are likely secondary to the severe digital inflammation that can cause the claws to grow more rapidly resulting in more friable claws that break or have a deformed appearance. Another possibility is that the patient could have chewed the claws off, which can be seen in dogs with marked pedal pruritus, but usually there is evidence of self-trauma to the claw in these cases.

iii. Besides hookworm dermatitis, conditions known to cause significant paw pad hyperkeratosis include canine distemper, leishmaniasis, zinc-responsive dermatosis, hepatocutaneous syndrome, idiopathic or familial nasodigital hyperkeratosis, pemphigus (foliaceus and vulgaris), systemic lupus erythematosus, and cutaneous horn.

40. i. *Otodectes cynotis* (ear mites).

ii. An evidence-based review of published treatment studies recently concluded that the best evidence of efficacy existed with the topical use of selamectin or a 10% imidacloprid + 1% moxidectin combination product applied once or twice, 30 days apart (Yang and Huang, 2016). Other published treatment options include ivermectin or milbemycin containing otic formulations applied topically into the ear canals, weekly oral ivermectin, ivermectin subcutaneous injections 14 days apart, spot-on application fipronil applied topically to the skin or into the ear canals, doramectin subcutaneous injection, a neomycin/thiabendazole/dexamethasone containing ear medication, or topical application of an isoxazoline approved for use in cats. Prior to treatment, the ear canals should be thoroughly cleaned to remove debris, if present. Any secondary bacterial or yeast ear infection should be addressed, and all those in contact with the animals should be treated to prevent acquisition of the mite, which is spread through direct contact.

iii. *O. cynotis* can survive off the host in the environment for up to 12 days if optimal temperature and relative humidity conditions are present.

41. Ivermectin is commonly used in veterinary dermatology for the treatment of various parasitic diseases, specifically generalized canine demodicosis. The most commonly recommended dose range for this medication in the treatment of canine demodicosis is 0.4–0.6 mg/kg PO q24h, which is slowly worked up to over the course of 5–7 days.

i. Calculate the initial daily dosing scheme in milliliters (mL) of ivermectin using a 1% solution of ivermectin (commercially available oral and injectable solution) for a 20 kg dog.

ii. What other commercially available avermectin has been shown to be effective in the management of canine demodicosis?

42. A 4-month-old coonhound puppy presented for evaluation of acute-onset pruritus. Flea combing collected the following from the hair coat of the patient (**Figure 42a**).

i. What is the parasite present?

ii. Roughly how many species have been documented, and which ones are most medically relevant to small animal practice?

iii. What infectious diseases is this parasite known to transmit?

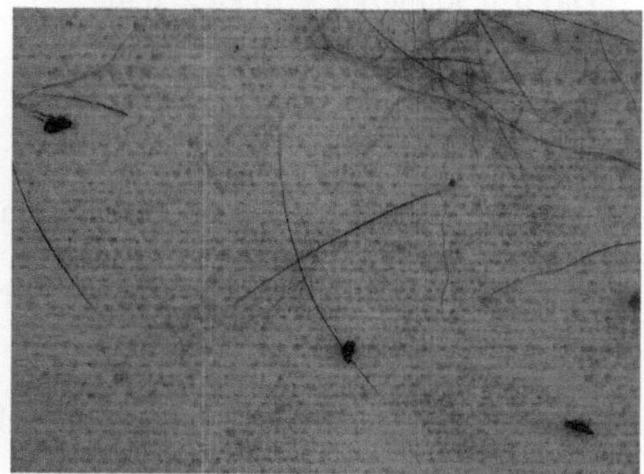
Figure 42a

43. A 3-year-old female German shepherd presented for evaluation of an enlarging mass in the perivulvar region. The mass was first noted several months ago but has recently become concerning to the owner as a blood-tinged discharge from the mass has been observed. The patient comes from a single dog household with free access to roam a large farm. Review of the patient's medical records shows that she is up to date on vaccinations and receives monthly flea, tick, and heartworm prevention. Physical examination reveals a 2 cm diameter cauliflower-like mass present along the right perivulvar fold. Based on examination, you question the owner further, who informs you that there are some stray dogs in the region. At this time, you elect to perform a fine-needle aspiration of the mass, results of which are shown in **Figure 43a**.

What is your diagnosis and treatment recommendations?

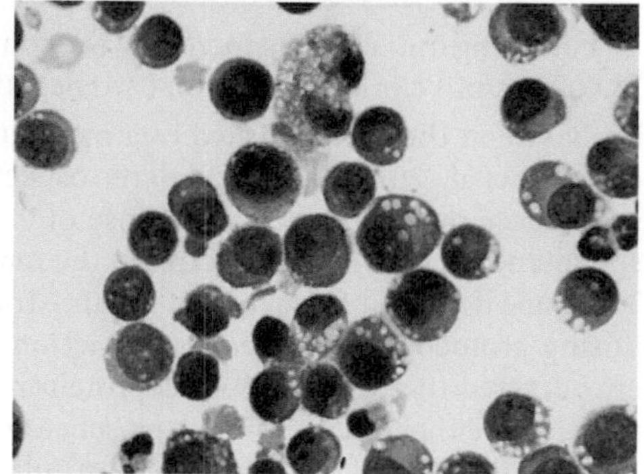
Figure 43a

41. i. This product is available as a 1% solution both orally and as an injectable. (Note: 1% solution = 1 g/100 mL = 1000 mg/100 mL = 10 mg/mL.)

First, calculate the number of milligrams of ivermectin needed for each day's dose:

Day 1: 0.05 mg/kg × 20 kg = 1 mg

Day 2: 0.10 mg/kg × 20 kg = 2 mg

Day 3: 0.15 mg/kg × 20 kg = 3 mg

Day 4: 0.20 mg/kg × 20 kg = 4 mg

Day 5: 0.30 mg/kg × 20 kg = 6 mg

Day 6: 0.40 mg/kg × 20 kg = 8 mg

Day 7: 0.50 mg/kg × 20 kg = 10 mg

Note: The author prefers not to exceed 0.5 mg/kg PO q24h when treating dogs with generalized demodicosis. If no adverse reactions were encountered in the patient during this initial dosing scheme, the final day 7 dosage becomes the continued daily recommended dose.

Next, calculate the milliliters required to achieve each day's target dose:

Day 1: 1 mg ÷ 10 mg/mL = 0.1 mL

Day 2: 2 mg ÷ 10 mg/mL = 0.2 mL

Day 3: 3 mg ÷ 10 mg/mL = 0.3 mL

Day 4: 4 mg ÷ 10 mg/mL = 0.4 mL

Day 5: 6 mg ÷ 10 mg/mL = 0.6 mL

Day 6: 8 mg ÷ 10 mg/mL = 0.8 mL

Day 7: 10 mg ÷ 10 mg/mL = 1.0 mL

Following initial dosing increases, the continued daily dose would be 1.0 mL PO q24h until clinical resolution (two negative scrapes 4 weeks apart).

ii. Based on the last published treatment guidelines for demodicosis in dogs (Mueller et al., 2012a) and a recent retrospective study (Hutt et al., 2015), there is evidence that doramectin at a dose of 0.6 mg/kg administered via weekly subcutaneous injection is effective in the management of canine demodicosis. The same dose and frequency of administration have also been used for oral dosing protocols. Similar adverse reactions to that of ivermectin have been encountered in dogs with P-glycoprotein mutations. As a result, it is recommended to either test dogs for the presence of this genetic mutation or gradually increase the dose of doramectin in a similar manner to the recommendation for ivermectin.

42. **i.** *Ctenocephalides felis*; the adult cat flea.

ii. Greater than 2,200 species and subspecies of fleas are known throughout the world. Although dogs and cats could act as a transient host for almost any flea species, those that are seen with enough regularity to be of medical importance are *Ctenocephalides felis felis* (cat flea), *C. canis* (dog flea), *Pulex irritans* (human flea), *Echidnophaga gallinacea* (poultry sticktight flea), *Spilopsyllus cuniculi* (rabbit flea), and *Tunga penetrans* (sand flea) (Blagburn and Dryden, 2009).

iii. Besides causing severe anemia secondary to blood loss in young and debilitated animals or flea allergy dermatitis in dogs and cats, the flea may act as the intermediate host for *Dipylidium caninum* (flea tapeworm) and *Hymenolepis nana* (dwarf tapeworm). The most serious infectious disease that fleas may spread is *Yersina pestis* (plague). Additional infectious diseases they may spread are *Rickettsia typhi* (murine typhus), *R. felis* (flea-borne spotted fever), *R. prowazekii* (rural epidemic typhus), *Bartonella henselae* (cat scratch fever), *B. clarridgeiae*, *B. quintana* (trench fever), *Mycoplasma* spp., and *Leishmania* spp. (Bitam et al., 2010; Ferreira et al., 2009).

43. Canine transmissible venereal tumor (TVT). The image shows a population of round cells that have a round nucleus, prominent nucleolus, abundant basophilic cytoplasm without granules, and numerous punctate intracytoplasmic vacuoles (hallmark of this round cell tumor). This tumor is transmitted to damaged mucosal surfaces during coitus, or social behaviors such as sniffing and licking. The tumor is commonly seen in free-roaming, sexually intact dogs and typically occurs on the external genitalia, face, or nasal region. Therapeutic options include surgery, radiation therapy, or chemotherapy. To date, the best and most consistent treatment response has been observed with single-agent chemotherapy utilizing vincristine.

44. A 2-year-old spayed female Australian shepherd presented for evaluation of a slowly enlarging "bump" on her head. The owner reports that they first appreciated the mass about a year ago and at that time it was about the size of a pea. The owner does not think the lesion bothers the patient, but it is concerning to them as it has continued to slowly grow since it was first noted. Physical examination reveals a firm, raised 2 cm diameter nodule that is nonpainful on palpation located along the dorsal midline just caudal to the eyes (**Figure 44a**). You elect to start with a fine-needle aspiration of the mass. Upon manipulation during aspiration, the mass ruptures exposing material that is consistent with hair and keratosebaceous debris (**Figure 44b**).

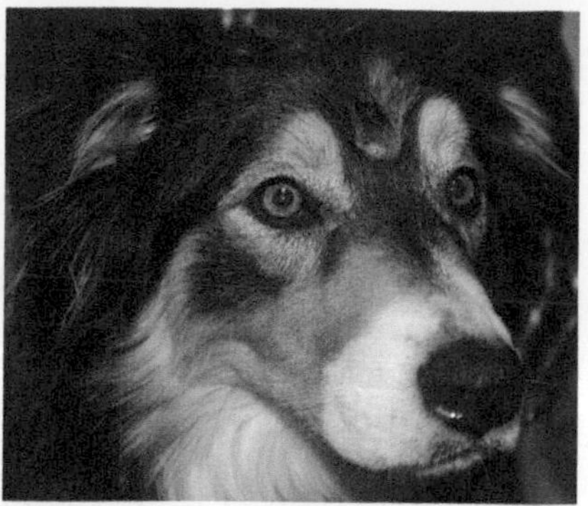
Figure 44a

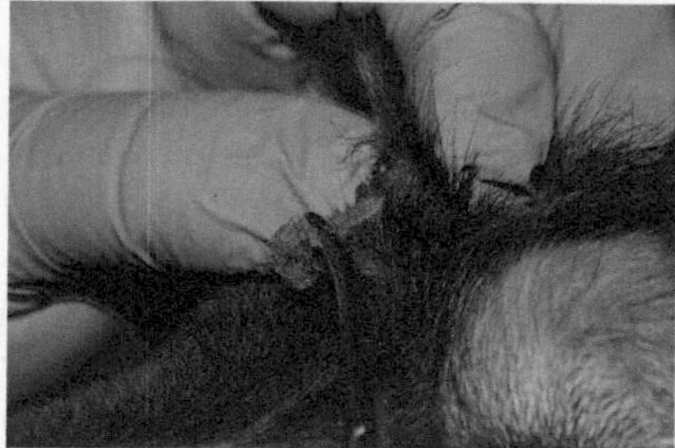
Figure 44b

What is your diagnosis and treatment recommendation for the owner?

45. A 3-year-old spayed female indoor cat presented for emergency examination. Approximately 3 days after spending the night locked outside on the family's screened-in porch, the cat developed acute facial pruritus and presented with the lesions shown in **Figure 45a**. Similar lesions were seen on the cat's ear tips. The cat was otherwise healthy with no history of prior skin issues. Skin scrapings were negative, while impression smears of the nose revealed an inflammatory exudate composed of predominantly eosinophils and lesser numbers of neutrophils, lymphocytes, and mast cells.

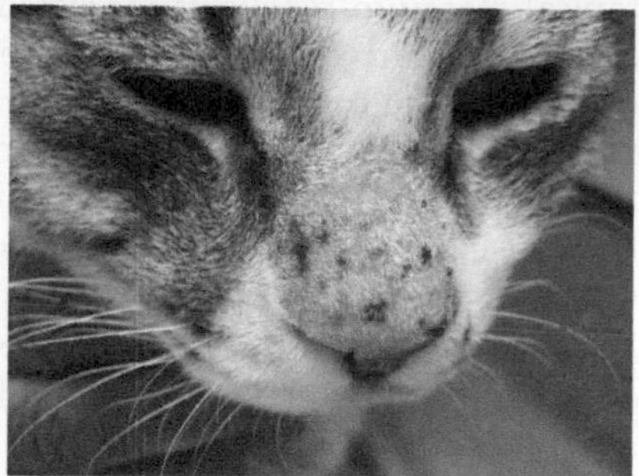
Figure 45a

i. What are possible differential diagnoses for the cat's presentation, and based on the information provided, what is the most likely diagnosis?

ii. If the owners decline a skin biopsy, how can the likely disease be confirmed, and what are the treatment recommendations?

iii. What is expected on a skin biopsy specimen from this cat?

44. Dermoid cyst. This is a rare congenital abnormality that occurs typically as a solitary nodule or multiple nodules along the dorsal midline. The wall of the cyst undergoes epidermal differentiation and contains well-developed hair follicles and glands. Manipulation of these cysts can cause rupture that may result in a granulomatous foreign-body–like reaction if the material is released into the subcutaneous tissues. A variant of this condition known as dermoid sinus or pilonidal sinus is seen in Rhodesian ridgebacks, where the exact mode of inheritance is still unknown (Appelgrein et al., 2016). The preferred method of treatment for these lesions is surgical excision.

45. i. Differential diagnoses would include flea allergy dermatitis (FAD), cutaneous adverse food reaction (CAFR), atopy, dermatophytosis, demodicosis (*D. gatoi*), pemphigus foliaceous, and mosquito-bite hypersensitivity. The most likely diagnosis is mosquito-bite hypersensitivity. The clinical lesions and history are characteristic of the disease. The rapid development of the lesions after spending the night outside (most screened porches are not insect proof) and the marked eosinophilia seen on cytological examination of impression smears are highly supportive of the diagnosis. Although not present in this patient, lesions have also been reported to involve the footpads.

ii. This disease is seasonal and coincides with mosquito activity. Confining the cat indoors for 5–7 days and watching for lesion resolution can confirm the diagnosis; the other differential diagnoses will not respond to this therapy. Keeping the cat indoors can also prevent recurrences. Application of repellent products such as permethrins and pyrethroids can be toxic to cats, and only products labeled as safe for use in cats should be used. Additionally, topical mosquito repellents marketed for human use such as N,N-diethyl-meta-toluamide (DEET) should not be used in cats. To speed up resolution of pruritus and inflammation, oral or injectable glucocorticoids may also be required. This cat was treated with oral methylprednisolone (4 mg PO q24h for 14 days), and the lesions resolved within 10 days. The lesions were observed to recur if the cat spent excessive time on the family's screened porch in the evening when mosquitoes were present.

iii. Histological findings most compatible with this syndrome include an eosinophilic perivascular to diffuse dermatitis with eosinophilic folliculitis and furunculosis, which may be suggestive of insect stings compared to other allergic causes. Flame figures are also commonly observed. It is important to understand that these findings are not necessarily diagnostic for the condition but may help eliminate other differential diagnoses.

46. A 2-year-old castrated male DSH presented for a 9-month history of recurrent otitis externa of the left ear only. The owner reports that they adopted the cat 10 months ago from a local shelter and at that time the patient was diagnosed with ear mites and treated with topical selamectin, which they have continued monthly for flea and heartworm prevention. Review of the patient's records reveals that the cat is current on recommended vaccinations, and further questioning reveals no history of upper respiratory issues. General physical examination and otoscopic examination of the right ear are unremarkable. Otoscopic exam of the left ear reveals the presence of a marked mucopurulent exudate and what is shown in **Figure 46a**.

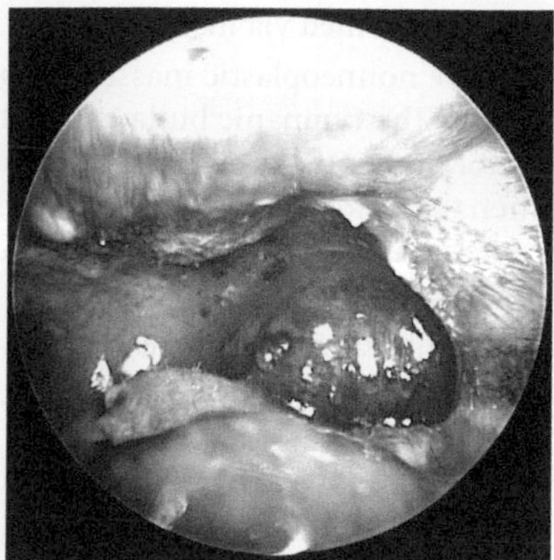

Figure 46a

i. What is the most likely diagnosis for this patient?

ii. Where do these growths originate?

iii. What treatment options should be provided to the owner?

iv. What are the most common neoplasms that affect the ear canals of dogs and cats?

47. The periocular region of an otherwise healthy 20-week-old puppy presented because of nonpruritic alopecia is shown (**Figure 47a**). Mites were found on trichogram (**Figure 47b**). Skin scrapes and trichograms from other areas of the body were negative for mites.

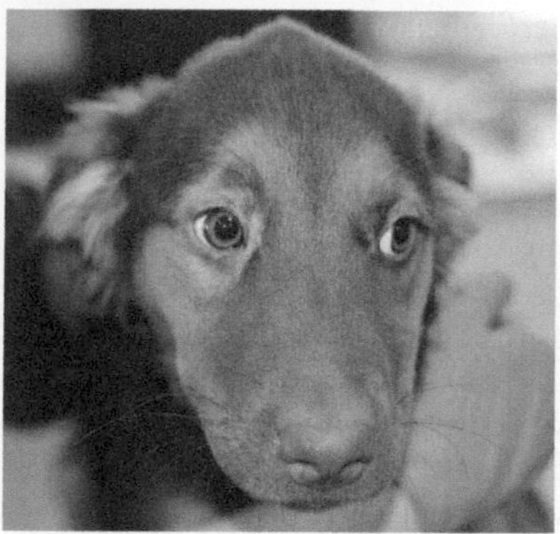

Figure 47a

i. What is the diagnosis?

ii. How are patients with localized or generalized disease typically defined?

iii. What are the treatment options for this patient?

iv. The owner of this puppy is interested in breeding her. What are the current recommendations regarding breeding?

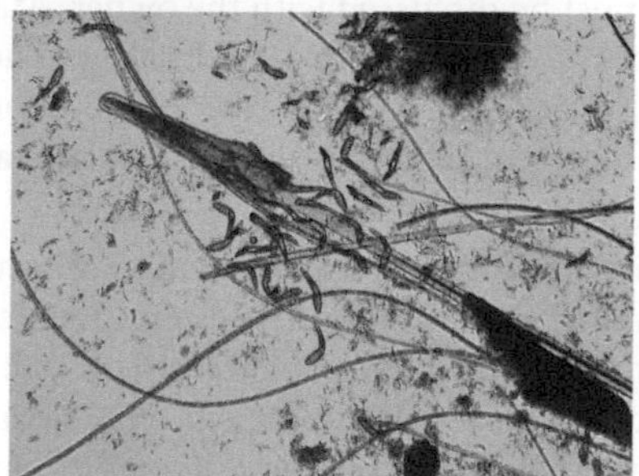

Figure 47b

46. i. Feline inflammatory polyp. Given the patient's young age, chronicity of the problem, character of the exudate, and presence of an erythemic polypoid mass occluding the external canal, this is the most likely diagnosis, which can be confirmed via histopathology of the mass.

ii. These nonneoplastic masses are presumed to originate from the epithelial lining of the tympanic bulla or auditory tube. When they originate from the auditory tube, the growths may invade the tympanic cavity or nasopharynx. When the nasopharynx is involved, clinical signs such as nasal discharge, stertorous breathing, sneezing, dysphagia, or dyspnea may be observed (Greci and Mortellaro, 2016).

iii. At this time, there are two main treatment options for the removal of inflammatory polyps. The first is a minimally invasive technique known as traction avulsion (i.e., "grip and rip"). This procedure requires minimal specialized equipment or skill and is performed by grabbing the mass as close to the base as possible with grasping forceps and twisting in a single direction while applying slow, even traction trying to detach the mass from the origin in a single piece (**Figure 46b**). After removal, a short tapering course of systemic anti-inflammatory glucocorticoids (prednisolone or methylprednisone) is started along with topical ear medication based on cytologic findings. The other method is a traditional open surgical method known as a ventral bulla osteotomy (VBO). A VBO allows full exploration of both chambers created by the septum in the middle ear of a cat and is thought to lead to less recurrence. However, a VBO is associated with greater adverse risk and costs that must be discussed with the owner. At this time, prospective, randomized, comparative clinical trials are lacking to help determine which is the best approach. The author prefers to reserve VBO for cases where inflammatory polyps recur in a short period of time following traction avulsion or when traction avulsion is not considered feasible.

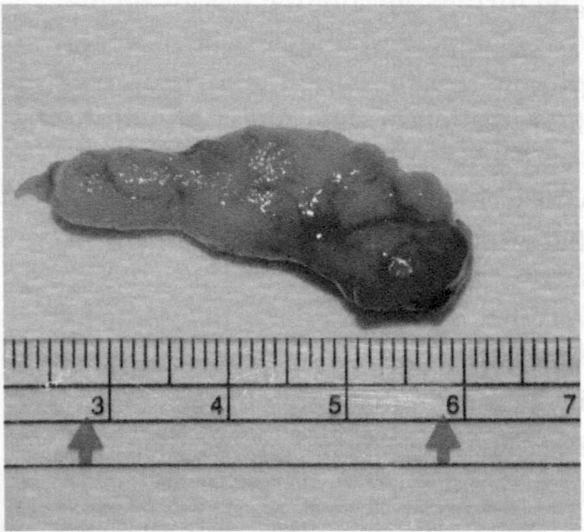

Figure 46b

iv. The most common malignant and concerning tumors of the canine and feline ear are squamous cell carcinoma and ceruminous gland adenocarcinoma. Other neoplastic diseases that may affect the region include plasmacytoma, basal cell tumors, fibroma, hemangiopericytoma, ceruminous/sebaceous adenoma, hemangioma/hemangiosarcoma, melanocytoma, mast cell tumor, lymphoma, histiocytic tumors, and leiomyosarcoma/rhadomyoma (Sula, 2012). A general rule of thumb derived from retrospective studies is that aural tumors in cats tend to be more biologically aggressive and more likely to be malignant compared to those observed in dogs.

47. i. Localized, juvenile-onset demodicosis. It is important to remember that demodicosis by itself is rarely pruritic, with pruritus becoming more variably severe when a secondary pyoderma is present.

ii. Demodicosis is typically described as localized or generalized. Although there are no uniformly accepted criteria for differentiating one form from the other, generalized demodicosis usually involves an entire body region, more than two paws, the ear canals, or more than six lesions. Localized disease has been described as no more than four lesions with a diameter of up to 2.5 cm and mites cannot be demonstrated in nonaffected regions (Mueller et al., 2012a). Localized disease most commonly occurs in young dogs, affecting the face and extremities. Localized demodicosis has a good prognosis with many cases experiencing spontaneous resolution without mite-specific therapy; progression to generalized disease is rare. Topical antiseptic and/or antimicrobial therapy may be indicated to prevent or treat secondary bacterial infections. Generalized demodicosis is a severe and potentially life-threatening condition with spontaneous remission being highly unlikely. The author recommends that all cases of generalized demodicosis regardless of age of onset be treated with mite-specific therapy. Also, almost all dogs with generalized disease have a secondary pyoderma, which requires treatment with topical antibacterial shampoos or systemic antibiotics based on extent and severity.

iii. The best course of treatment is difficult to determine in cases of localized demodicosis. Conservative treatment would involve a "watch and wait" approach, as many cases undergo spontaneous resolution. With this puppy being otherwise healthy and being unable to demonstrate mites elsewhere, this would be an appropriate treatment approach. Topical therapy with an antimicrobial agent, such as mupirocin ointment or benzoyl peroxide gel, may be prescribed if needed for secondary bacterial infection. The owners should be informed that lesions likely will worsen before they improve. If more lesions develop, a more aggressive treatment approach can be used, utilizing mite-specific therapies. However, dogs that require or use mite-specific therapy should not be bred and should be spayed or neutered.

iv. Although the exact genetic and pathologic mechanisms of canine demodicosis are not completely understood, it is likely that the disease is the result of one or more genetic traits. This concept is supported by observations of strong breed predispositions and the fact that selective breeding programs have decreased the incidence of the condition (Mueller et al., 2012a). Ideally, all dogs with demodicosis should be eliminated from breeding pools, but this is not always a realistic option. As a result, it is currently recommended that any dog requiring mite-specific therapy or with generalized disease be spayed or neutered. In this particular case, if the owner wishes to potentially breed this animal, then it should not be treated with mite-specific therapy and monitored to make sure it undergoes spontaneous resolution. If it does not, or if mite-specific therapy is instituted or required for clinical resolution, this patient should not be bred but instead spayed.

48. What is the pinnal-pedal reflex? How is it performed, and what do positive results indicate?

49. A photomicrograph of normal dog skin is shown in **Figure 49a**.

i. What are the three major layers of the skin and the layers of the epidermis?

ii. What adnexal structures are produced in the skin?

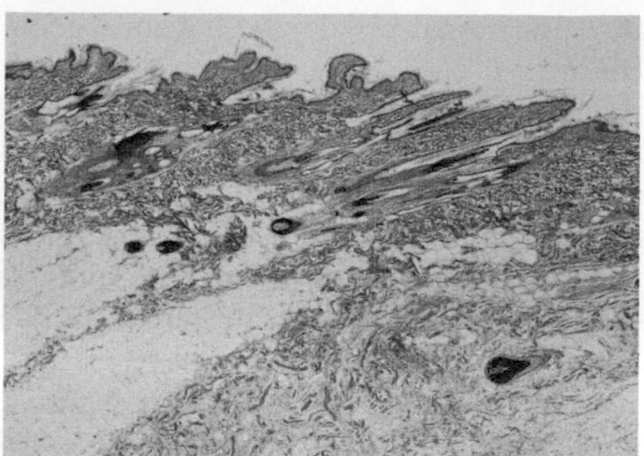
Figure 49a

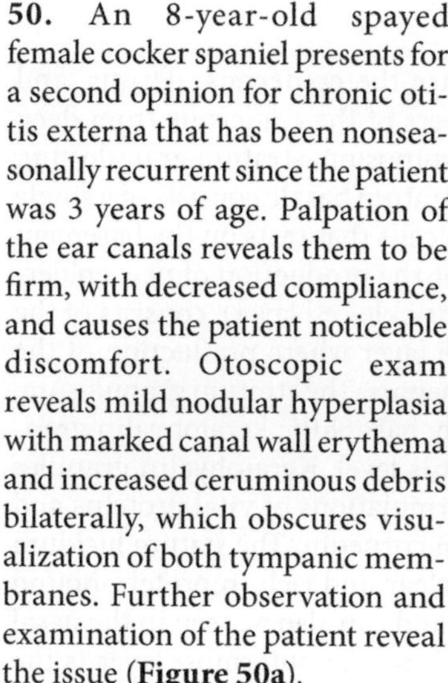

50. An 8-year-old spayed female cocker spaniel presents for a second opinion for chronic otitis externa that has been nonseasonally recurrent since the patient was 3 years of age. Palpation of the ear canals reveals them to be firm, with decreased compliance, and causes the patient noticeable discomfort. Otoscopic exam reveals mild nodular hyperplasia with marked canal wall erythema and increased ceruminous debris bilaterally, which obscures visualization of both tympanic membranes. Further observation and examination of the patient reveal the issue (**Figure 50a**).

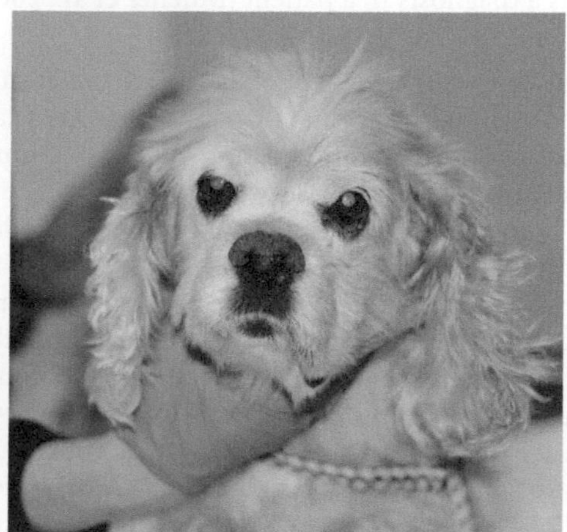
Figure 50a

i. What complication to chronic otitis should you be concerned with given these findings?

ii. What other etiologies can cause the issue observed in **Figure 50a**?

iii. What advanced diagnostic should be recommended for this patient given her history to further evaluate your concerns?

iv. What are considered primary versus predisposing causes of otitis externa?

48. The pinnal-pedal reflex is a nonspecific test for scabies infestation in dogs. The test is performed by vigorously rubbing or scratching the edge of the pinna and is considered positive if the dog's hind leg attempts to make a scratching movement. A study evaluating the usefulness of the pinnal-pedal reflex evaluated 588 dogs with nonresponsive or recurrent pruritic skin disease. In this study, 55 of the dogs were diagnosed with scabies and had a positive pinnal-pedal reflex 82% of the time. These findings resulted in a specificity of 93.8% and sensitivity of 81.8% for the pinnal-pedal reflex, while the positive predictive value was 0.57 and negative predictive value was 0.98. Taken all together, what these results indicate is that a positive pinnal-pedal reflex is as likely to indicate an allergic hypersensitivity as it is scabies, while the finding of a negative reflex would make scabies less likely. This test is a piece of the much larger clinical picture and should not be used as a definitive test to confirm or exclude scabies as a diagnosis in a patient (Mueller et al., 2001).

49. i. The three major layers of the skin are the epidermis, dermis, and hypodermis (subcutis or panniculus). The layers of the epidermis from deep to superficial are the stratum basale, stratum spinosum, stratum granulosum, stratum lucidum, and stratum corneum. The stratum basale consists of a single layer of active germinal columnar or cuboidal cells that rests on the basement membrane. This layer of cells is responsible for the production of new epidermal cells. The stratum spinosum (spinous or prickle cell layer), consists of the daughter cells from the basal layer and is the layer where production of the fully differentiated keratinocyte cytoskeleton begins. The stratum granulosum, or granular layer, gets it name from the deeply basophilic keratohyalin granules that are variably present and visible at this level. Keratohyalin granules are synthesized within this layer and are accumulations of vital proteins and lipids required for construction of the stratum corneum. The statum lucidum or "clear layer" contains cells, which are anuclear and rich in protein-bound lipids. This layer is best developed in footpads and can also be seen in the nasal planum. It is not seen in other areas of the skin. The outermost layer is the stratum corneum, which is the skin layer in contact with the environment. It is the fully cornified layer and is made of flattened, anuclear, densely packed, terminally differentiated keratinocytes.

ii. The skin produces hairs and hair follicles, sebaceous glands, sweat glands, specialized glands (i.e., anal sacs, tail gland, glands of the external ear canal, and circumanal glands), claws, and the horny layer of the skin.

50. **i.** Otitis media. The patient has facial nerve paralysis that can be observed by the patient's facial asymmetry due to the left lip and ear dropping along with the widened palpebral fissure in **Figure 50a**. The most common cause of otitis media in the dog is a secondary extension of otitis externa through the tympanic membrane, which can also act as a perpetuating factor in chronic ear disease. Facial nerve paralysis can occur in cases of otitis media as a result of the nerve being briefly exposed to the middle ear cavity as it travels through the facial canal, which is incomplete as it opens briefly near the oval/vestibular window. Lesions to this portion of the nerve will produce the following clinical signs: facial drooping, inability to move the ear and lip, an enlarged palpebral fissure, absent spontaneous or provoked blinking, absent abduction of the nostril during respiration, deviation of the nose due to unopposed muscle tone, and neurogenic keratoconjunctivitis and dry nose (Garosi et al., 2012). In addition to facial nerve paralysis, Horner syndrome and vestibular syndrome are other neurologic conditions that can occur secondary to otitis media.

ii. Causes of facial nerve paralysis include otitis media, middle ear neoplasia (benign and malignant), intracranial neoplasia, trauma, hypothyroidism, polyneuropathies, iatrogenic (surgical complications), and idiopathic, which is the most common cause.

iii. Pending normal blood work, thyroid parameters, and the ability to eliminate trauma based on history and physical exam findings, a CT scan should be performed to further evaluate the middle ear structures. CT scan is the preferred cross-sectional imaging modality for evaluating cases for otitis media as it provides better boney detail, can be performed more quickly, and is more cost effective compared to an MRI. Additionally, CT scan was more reliable than other imaging modalities such as ultrasound, as determined by recent studies (Classen et al., 2016).

iv. Primary causes of otitis are those that can directly induce otitis externa by themselves. Examples of primary causes are parasites (*Otodectes*, *Demodex*, *Otobius megnini*), foreign bodies, allergic hypersensitivities, keratinization disorders, endocrinopathies, neoplasia, and autoimmune conditions. Predisposing factors are issues that increase the risk of developing otitis externa if the individual patient has a primary condition, but in and of themselves do not directly lead to a problem. Examples of predisposing factors include ear conformation (pendulous versus erect, canal length), behavior (swimming), grooming and treatment habits (hair plucking, excessive cleaning, altering microflora), breed (i.e., shar-pei and their narrow aural canal openings), and geographic environment (tropical versus temperate).

51. A 3-year-old neutered male Labrador retriever with a previous diagnosis of atopic dermatitis presented for increased pedal pruritus over the past 2 weeks. Prior to this, the patient was reported to be well controlled with daily oclacitinib maleate. Examination revealed interdigital erythema and salivary staining affecting all four paws. Impression smears with clear acetate tape were acquired from the affected interdigital region and stained with a Romanowsky-type stain. The cytology results are shown in **Figure 51a**.

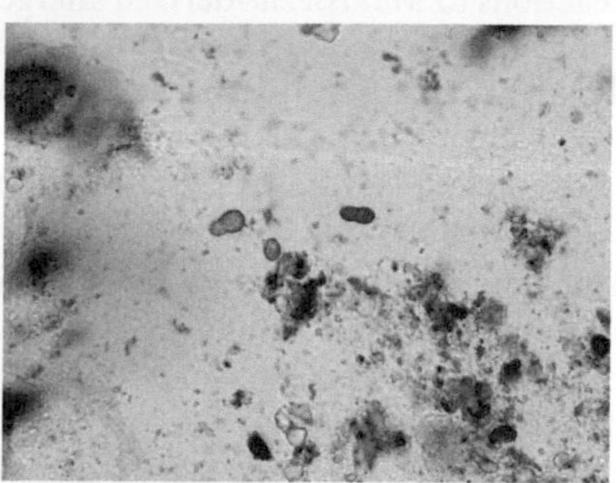
Figure 51a

i. What is the name of the organism found on cytology?

ii. What relevance does this organism have with respect to the patient's current presentation?

iii. What will cause a well-controlled atopic patient to have an increase in pruritus?

52. What procedure is being demonstrated (**Figure 52a**) on this 2-year-old neutered male pit bull that presented for hair loss, erythema, and scaling with waxing and waning crusting over the dorsal muzzle for the past 3 months?

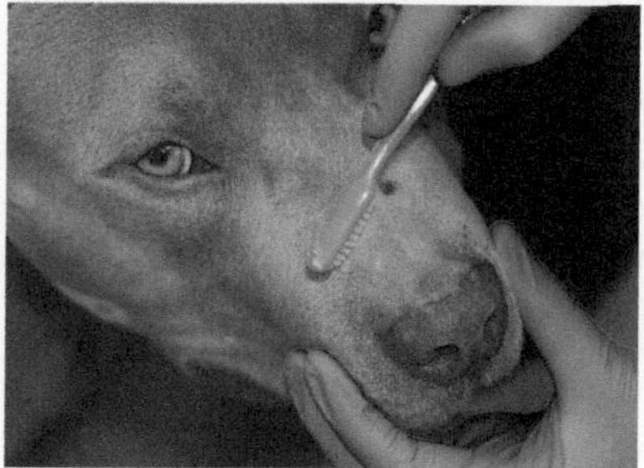
Figure 52a

53. A 5-year-old castrated male mixed breed dog presented for examination. The owners were complaining about the skin changing color and turning purple along the medial thigh and inguinal region of the dog (**Figure 53a**).

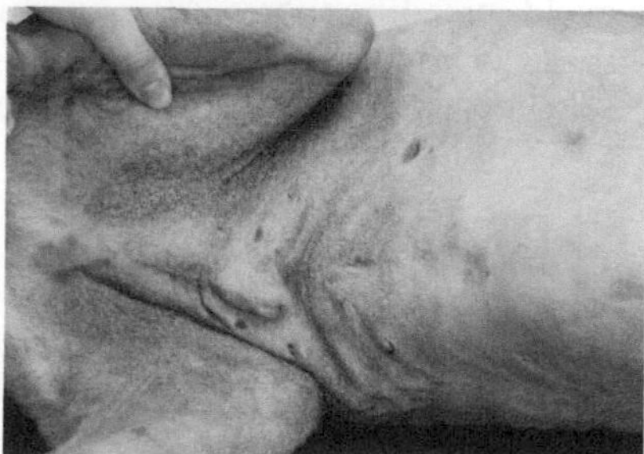
Figure 53a

i. What dermatologic abnormality is depicted?

ii. What causes should be considered, what is the most likely cause, and what should the owner be asked?

iii. What diagnostic tests are indicated?

51. **i.** *Malassezia pachydermatis.*

ii. Canine atopic dermatitis is the most frequent cause for *Malassezia* dermatitis in dogs, and atopic patients as a group have been shown to have higher skin populations of *M. pachydermatis* than nonatopic patients. In addition, studies have demonstrated both immediate-type and delayed-type hypersensitivity reactions to *Malassezia*-derived allergens in some dogs with atopic dermatitis, indicating a role for the yeast in the pathogenesis of atopy (Oldenhoff et al., 2014). Therefore, besides acting simply as an opportunistic pathogen, it may also act as a flare factor for dogs that have developed a hypersensitivity. Finally, skin infections (bacterial and yeast) are a common reason why pruritus and lesions acutely worsen in canine patients with atopy.

iii. Common reasons for a well-controlled atopic patient to experience increased pruritus include the following: improper medication administration or varying allergen exposure, which may be encountered throughout a year or season; development of a secondary infection such as pyoderma, *Malassezia* dermatitis, or otitis externa; acquisition of a contagious ectoparasite (*S. scabiei* or *Cheyletiella* spp.) or flea infestation; and the simultaneous occurrence of a cutaneous adverse food reaction or contact allergy in a patient with atopic dermatitis.

52. This is an example of a toothbrush (Mackenzie) fungal culture technique, which is the favored method for obtaining a sample for dermatophyte culture in companion animals. This technique allows sampling of much larger areas and decreases the chance of missing an active infection. It also prevents the clinician from having to find the proverbial "needle in a haystack" for direct microscopic examination or hair plucking for fungal culture. The technique is performed using an inexpensive, individually wrapped human toothbrush, and combing over regions of suspected infection. These brushes are mycologically sterile in their original wrapping and should only be used once (**Figure 52b**). Unaffected areas should be brushed prior to lesional areas in an attempt to avoid spreading spores. After brushing, hairs and/or scale should be visible within the bristles. The bristles are then lightly and repeatedly pressed onto the surface of DTM culture media (**Figure 52c**). It is important to note that the

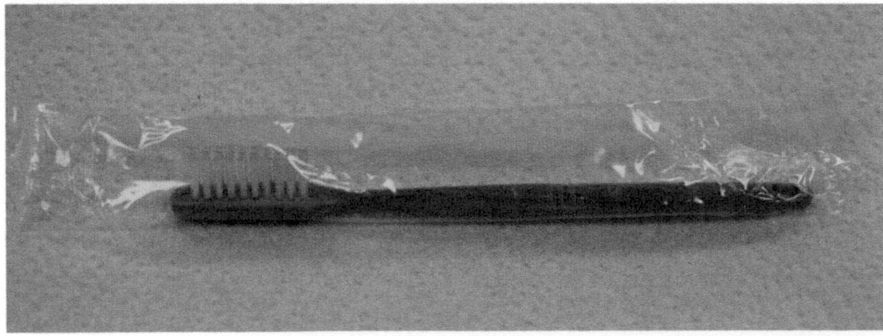

Figure 52b

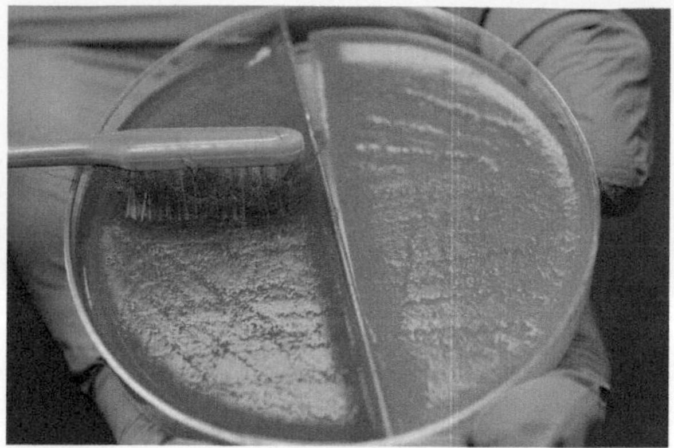

Figure 52c

toothbrush technique requires culture medium be in plate form (as opposed to tube/slantform) to facilitate inoculation of the media. Care must also be taken not to press the bristles too firmly into the media. It is unnecessary with this technique to leave or implant hairs into the media. This technique is also helpful for screening asymptomatic carriers and sampling patients undergoing therapy (Moriello and DeBoer, 2012).

53. **i.** Hyperpigmentation of the skin.

ii. Owner concerns over pigmentary changes to the skin is a common reason for patients to be presented to their veterinarian. Hyperpigmentation may be hereditary, acquired (post-inflammatory or endocrine related), or associated with viruses (papillomavirus) and tumors (vascular, glandular, melanomas, basal cell). The most common cause for hyperpigmentation of the skin is inflammation. Post-inflammatory hyperpigmentation may occur with or subsequent to demodicosis, sarcoptic mange, pyoderma, *Malassezia* dermatitis, dermatophytosis, friction, or chronic generalized inflammation seen with hypersensitivity disorders. The owner should be asked if this dog has any other clinical signs of skin disease. In particular, questions should focus on whether or not the dog is showing signs of pruritus. Atopic dermatitis is one of the most common causes of hyperpigmentation in the axillary, inguinal, and medial thigh regions.

iii. Skin scrapings and impression smears of the skin to rule out parasitic and secondary infectious causes. Although there is no specific treatment for hyperpigmentation, treatment of secondary infections often results in a marked cosmetic improvement. However, complete resolution is only possible when the primary cause for the secondary infections is adequately addressed. It is important to note that some cases may never completely resolve even when all of the causes have been managed.

54. A 15-year-old indoor-only spayed female DSH cat presented for progressive, generalized hair loss. The cat had no previous diagnosis of skin disease and based on her medical record had only been seen for routine vaccination throughout the years. The cat is not noted to be grooming more or having issues with hairballs. The owner did note the patient had a decreased appetite and has been slightly more lethargic. Evaluation of the medical record revealed a 1 kg weight loss since her last presentation. No other changes in behaviors or litter box usage were reported. Physical examination revealed moderate generalized hypotrichosis with mild to moderate scale accumulation. No other gross abnormalities were noted during examination. A skin scraping was performed from along the cat's dorsal thorax (**Figure 54a**).

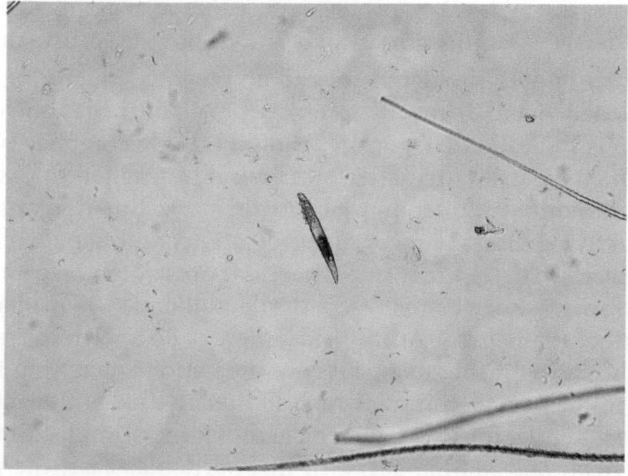

Figure 54a

i. What is the organism?
ii. What is the difference between this skin disease in cats versus dogs?
iii. How should the condition be managed?

55. What are the major classes of compounds used for flea control, and what are their modes of action?

54. i. *Demodex cati.*

ii. To date, there is no evidence that cats have a disease process similar to canine juvenile-onset demodicosis. In cats, three mite species are reported: *D. gatoi*, *D. cati*, and an unnamed third species (Ferreira et al., 2015). *D. gatoi* is considered to be contagious, unlike all other forms of demodicosis causing a pruritic dermatosis in cats. It is the more prevalent form of feline demodicosis and occurs with geographic variance. *D. cati* is more similar to *D. canis* in its presentation causing alopecia, erythema, scaling, and crusting. Identification of *D. cati* should strongly raise concern about underlying systemic illness, although it can occur as a ceruminous otitis in otherwise healthy individuals. It is often reported in association with feline leukemia virus (FeLV) and feline immunodeficiency virus (FIV), diabetes mellitus, hyperadrenocorticism, and neoplasia. The third unnamed species resembles *D. gatoi* but is larger. No specific clinical presentation has been well described at this time in association with the yet unnamed species.

iii. When *D. cati* mites are identified, and an obvious underlying cause (i.e., excessive glucocorticoid administration) is not identified, thorough medical evaluation is indicated. Diagnostics should include complete blood count (CBC), serum chemistries, urinalysis, retroviral testing, and possibly radiographs and abdominal ultrasound when other first-line diagnostics fail to reveal an underlying disease process. Identification of the concurrent systemic illness and initiation of treatment are a necessary part of management. Unless the underlying disease can be managed, the demodicosis will probably only be controlled rather than cured. At this time, there is no approved treatment for feline demodicosis with therapeutic recommendations including ivermectin, doramectin, milbemycin, amitraz (which should be used with caution in cats due to higher potential for toxicity), topical moxidectin/imidacloprid and fluralaner (Matricoti and Maina, 2017). In this particular case, the patient was eventually determined to have large cell intestinal lymphoma.

55. Neonicotinoids (imidacloprid, nitenpyram, dinotefuran) act as agonists at insect postsynaptic nicotinic acetylcholine receptors and result in rapid inhibition, paralysis, and death of adult fleas. Phenylpyrazoles (fipronil) inhibit γ-aminobutyric acid (GABA)-gated chloride channels causing excessive neuronal stimulation, paralysis, and death of adult fleas. Macrocyclic lactones (selamectin) bind to receptors on glutamate-gated chloride channels leading to flaccid paralysis and death. Semicarbazones (metaflumizone) work by blocking voltage-gated dependent sodium channels leading to the blockage of nerve impulses causing paralysis and death. Pyrethyroids (permethrin, deltamethrin, flumethrin) affect voltage-dependent sodium channels of neurons resulting in hyperexcitation of nerve cells causing paralysis. Oxadiazines (indoxacarb) block voltage-gated dependent sodium channels inhibiting neural activity leading to paralysis similar to semicarbazones. Spinosyns (spinosad, spinetoram) stimulate nicotinic acetylcholine receptors similar to neonicotinoids but at a different site that still causes inhibition and paralysis. They also bind to GABA sites that likely contribute to their mechanism of action. Isoxazolines (fluralaner, afoxolaner, sarolaner, lotilaner) work by inhibiting insect GABA-gated chloride channels (different site from other known inhibitors of this pathway) resulting in hyperexcitation and death (Blagburn and Dryden, 2009; Halos et al., 2014; Rufener et al., 2017).

56. A 5-year-old neutered male Jack Russell terrier presented for a second opinion for chronic skin issues and mild lethargy. The patient's clinical symptoms began about 1 year ago and were first appreciated as mild hair loss that proceeded to pustule and crust formation. Physical examination shows alopecia, erythema, papule, pustule and crust formation affecting the head, pinnae (convex and concave), ventral abdomen, and distal extremities (**Figure 56a**). The patient was also mildly febrile at the time of presentation.

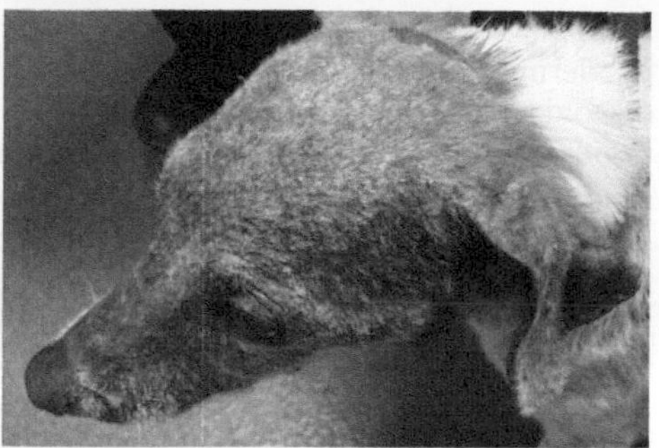

Figure 56a

i. What are your initial differentials for this patient, and what initial diagnostics should be pursued?

ii. Further questioning of the owner reveals that the patient had a biopsy taken a couple of months ago at which time he was diagnosed with pemphigus foliaceus. The patient was prescribed oral prednisone but did not tolerate it and symptoms worsened, so it was tapered and discontinued a couple of weeks prior to presentation. At this time, the owner allows you to reacquire skin scraping, trichogram, and skin cytology samples. Skin scraping and trichogram samples were negative, but cytology samples reveal the presence of septated, nonpigmented fungal hyphae. Given these results, you elect to collect a fungal culture via toothbrush technique. The microscopic results of a sample taken from observed fungal growth with color change on a DTM culture plate are shown in **Figure 56b, c**.

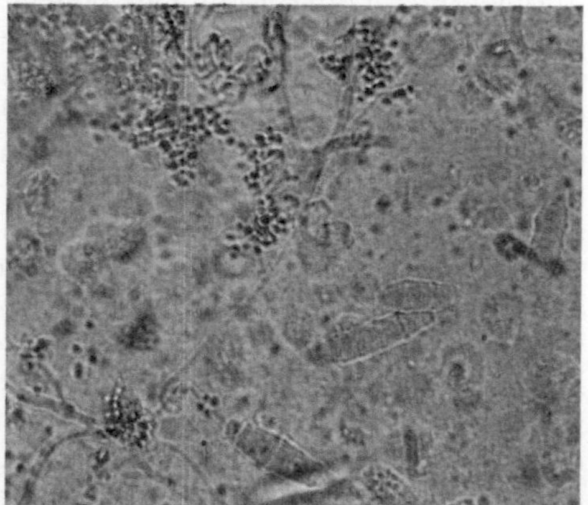

Figure 56b

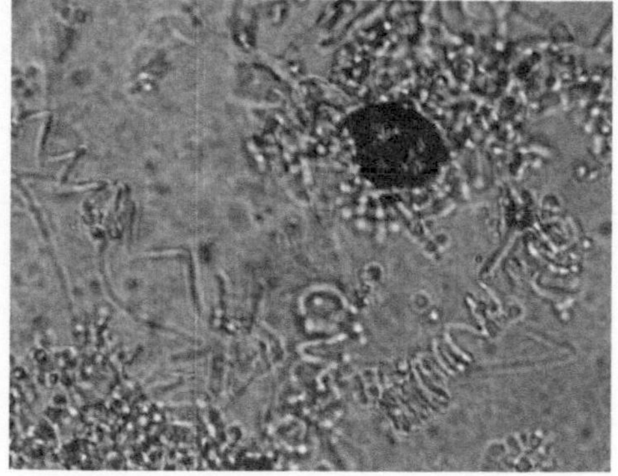

Figure 56c

What is your diagnosis, and how does this correlate to the dog's prior histopathology diagnosis?

56. i. Differentials based on clinical lesions and presentation should include pyoderma, dermatophytosis, demodicosis, pemphigus foliaceus, systemic and discoid lupus erythematosus, leishmaniosis (geographic regions where condition is endemic), or adverse drug eruption. Initial diagnostics in a patient presenting with alopecia, papules, pustules, and crusts, regardless of the severity, should always consist of skin scraping, trichogram, and cytology. The information these basic diagnostic tests provide is invaluable in determining which further diagnostics or possible treatments should be pursued. Additionally, in many instances, these basic, inexpensive tests provide a diagnosis.

ii. Dermatophytosis caused by *Trichophyton mentagrophytes. T. mentagrophytes* colonies produce abundant small, round microconidia; rare thin-walled, smooth, cigar-shaped macroconidia, and occasionally, spiral-shaped hyphae (spring-like). All three features are present in the microscopic images shown from the sampled culture growth. This patient has a rare clinical presentation of dermatophytosis known as canine acantholytic dermatophytosis. This form of the disease associated with *T. mentagrophytes* both clinically and histologically resembles pemphigus foliaceus. Acantholytic keratinocytes arise from the loss of cohesion between keratinocytes as a result of autoantibody attack against desmosome proteins. This process is the histologic hallmark finding in the pemphigus complex of diseases. However, the formation of these cells can also occur with several other inflammatory conditions, most notably, superficial bacterial folliculitis and dermatophytosis. In these cases, proteolytic or hydrolytic enzymes disrupt the cellular adhesion resulting in acantholysis (Peters et al., 2007). As a result of this potential overlap in clinical presentation, all cases suspected to have pemphigus foliaceus should be screened via cytology and culture to ensure lesion formation is not the result of an infectious etiology prior to initiating immunosuppressive therapy.

57. A 3-year-old female German shorthaired pointer presented for progressive pruritus and hair loss that was first noted several weeks ago. The patient has no prior history of skin or ear issues before the current presentation. The patient is an outdoor dog and lives on a farm where she is kenneled at night. The owner notes her kennel is bedded with straw to help insulate and keep her warm at night. Physical examination revealed erythema, excoriations alopecia, and crusts along the ventral thorax/abdomen, lateral rear legs, and palmar/plantar aspects of the paws (**Figure 57a**). A skin impression was performed that revealed paired intracellular coccoid-shaped bacteria. A skin scrape was also performed and revealed what is shown in **Figure 57b**.

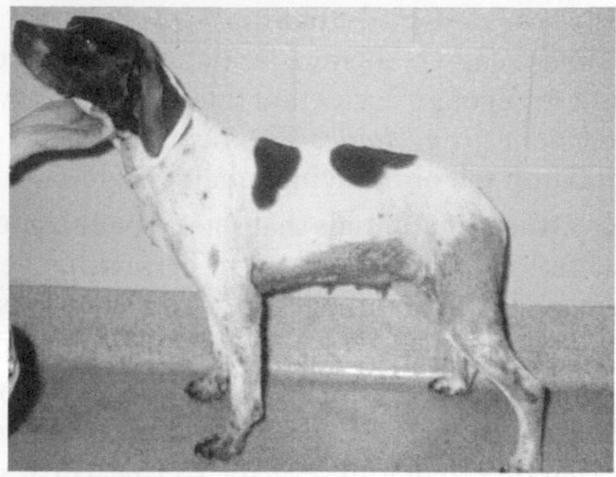

Figure 57a

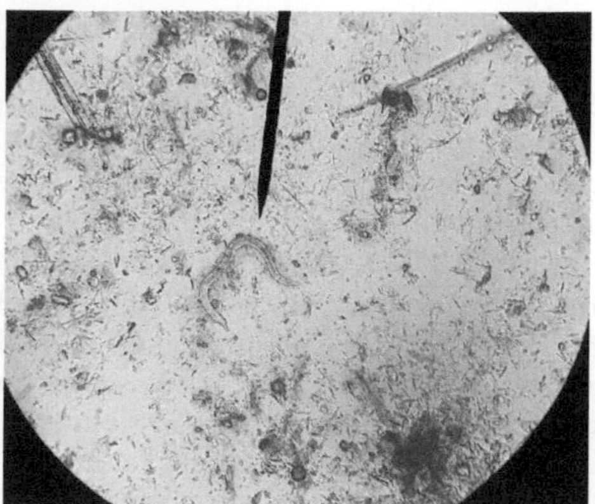

Figure 57b

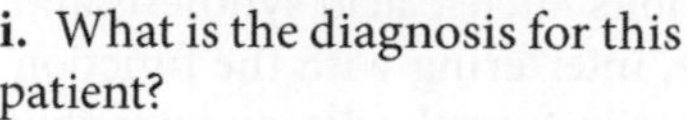

i. What is the diagnosis for this patient?

ii. What other differentials should be considered for a patient with this presentation?

iii. What should this patient's therapeutic plan consist of?

58. A kitten was born dead to a queen treated with griseofulvin for dermatophytosis during the first trimester of her pregnancy.

i. What is the most likely cause of the kitten's death?

ii. What is the mechanism of action of griseofulvin?

iii. How is the drug absorbed and delivered to the skin?

57. **i.** *Pelodera* dermatitis (i.e., rhabditic mange or "barn-itch"). This is a pruritic and erythemic dermatosis that occurs secondary to dirty conditions as a result of an accidental infestation of larvae from the free-living nematode *Pelodera strongyloides*. The nematode has a direct life cycle that is completed in damp soil or decaying organic material such as straw or hay.
ii. Other differentials that should be considered in patients with a similar presentation include hookworm dermatitis, demodicosis, sarcoptic mange, and secondary bacterial or *Malassezia* infections.
iii. Treatment for this patient requires cleaning the environment and spraying an insecticide to kill remaining larvae. The patient's secondary bacterial infection should be treated topically or with concurrent systemic antimicrobials based on extent and severity. Ivermectin at similar doses used in the management of sarcoptic mange are recommended to kill larvae. A short-term course of glucocorticoids may be helpful to relieve pruritus. The infestation is self-limiting, and future episodes can be prevented with improved sanitary efforts.

58. **i.** The kitten likely died as a result of a griseofulvin-induced birth defect. Griseofulvin is a known teratogen and should not be administered to pregnant cats. Pregnant queens cannot be safely treated with any of the commonly used systemic antifungal agents. Topical therapy with lime sulfur (sponge-on dips twice weekly) is recommended as a safe alternative therapy.
ii. Griseofulvin is a fungistatic antifungal drug produced by *Penicillium griseofulvum*. It works by inhibition of cell wall synthesis, nucleic acid synthesis, and mitotis. It is primarily active against growing organisms, but it may keep dormant cells from dividing. Griseofulvin inhibits nucleic acid synthesis and cell mitosis by arresting division at metaphase, interfering with the function of spindle microtubules, morphogenetic changes in fungal cells, and possibly with chitin synthesis.
iii. Griseofulvin is not well absorbed from the gastrointestinal tract and should be administered with a fatty meal to enhance absorption. Since particle size also affects absorption of the drug, it is formulated in microsize and ultramicrosize formulations. The drug can be detected in the stratum corneum within 8 hours to 3 days of administration. The highest concentrations are in the stratum corneum. The drug is delivered to the stratum corneum by diffusion, sweating, and transepidermal fluid loss. It is deposited in keratin precursor cells and remains there throughout the differentiation process. Griseofulvin concentrations drop rapidly after discontinuation of therapy, as it is not tightly bound to keratin.

59. An owner presents with his 2-year-old castrated male DSH for evaluation of patchy hair loss affecting the ears and face. The owner reports that they first observed hair loss starting 3 weeks prior to presentation and adopted the patient 2 months ago from a shelter. On physical exam, multifocal, circular patches of alopecia with associated scaling and crusting are present along both ears, the cranial aspect of the head, and ventral cervical region. You elect to perform a trichogram and cytology via skin impression. The trichogram reveals normal hairs and no significant findings. On skin, numerous organisms similar to that shown in **Figure 59a** are observed.

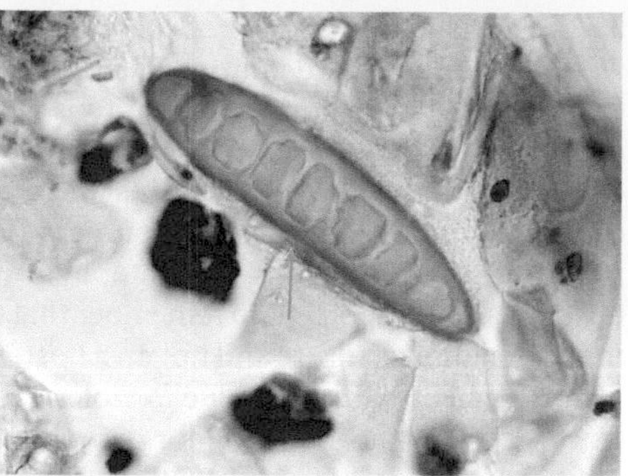
Figure 59a

What is present on cytology, and what is its significance to the patient's clinical presentation?

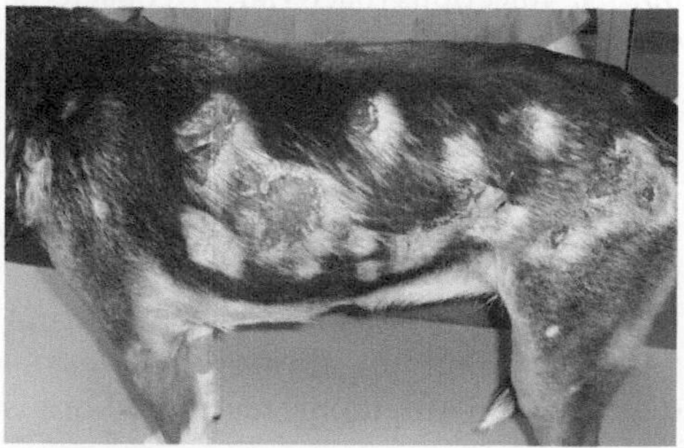
Figure 60a

60. A 4-year-old spayed female beagle presented for evaluation of rapidly developing nodules that rupture and drain an oily yellow-brown to serosanguineous material (**Figure 60a, b**). The lesions were painful upon palpation, and the dog was depressed, febrile, and had a mild generalized lymphadenopathy.

i. What are the differential diagnoses for this patient?

ii. What diagnostics should be pursued to diagnose this patient's condition?

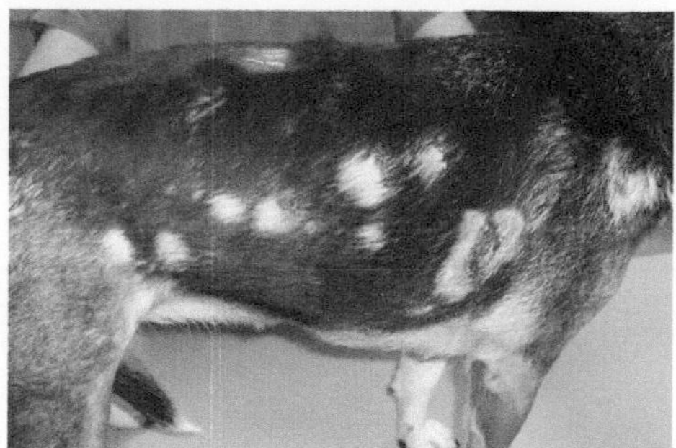
Figure 60b

59. This is a *Bipolaris/Drechslera/Curvularia* spp. conidia (gene analysis would be needed for definitive identification). These species are dematiaceus (pigmented) fungi that are ubiquitous in nature and associated with plant debris and soil and rarely disease in small animal patients. In this particular case, this is an insignificant finding and is a contaminant on the patient's skin acquired from the patient's environment. These spores when present are occasionally misinterpreted as dermatophyte species macroconidia by untrained observers. It is important to remember that dermatophyte species only produce macroconidia in culture and not on a host. Additionally, dermatophyte species fungal elements will stain blue to violet with normal Diff-Quik variant stains. In this case, as the suspicion for dermatophytosis is high, a fungal culture or polymerase chain reaction (PCR) for dermatophyte species should be recommended as no confirmatory evidence was found on initial diagnostics.

60. i. Infectious (bacterial, mycobacteria, and fungal), cutaneous drug reaction, neoplasia, sterile nodular panniculitis, sterile granuolma/pyogranuloma syndrome, foreign-body reaction, adult-onset juvenile cellulitis, and systemic lupus erythematosus.
ii. Diagnostics that should be performed in this patient are cytology, fine-needle aspiration, skin biopsy with dermatohistopathology including special stains, tissue culture for bacterial (aerobic and anaerobic bacteria, mycobacteria) and fungal organisms, a CBC, serum chemistries, and urinalysis, along with dimorphic fungal titers (e.g., *Blastomyces*, *Histoplasma*, *Coccidioides*) depending on geographic region and/or history of travel.

61. A 7-year-old castrated male DSH cat presented for evaluation of growing "pigmented masses" on the inside of his pinnae that the owner fears is melanoma. The patient has no history of prior skin or ear disease and is not reported to be pruritic per the owner. The patient is current on vaccinations and has topical selamectin applied monthly for flea and tick prevention. On physical exam, multiple 2–5 mm diameter, blue-gray papules were noted along the concave aspect of the pinnae (**Figure 61a**) but were not found within the vertical or horizontal canals of either ear. The rest of the physical exam was unremarkable.

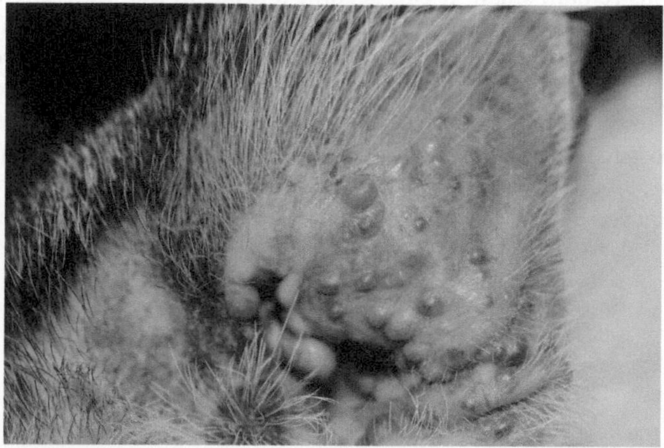

Figure 61a

i. What is the diagnosis?
ii. What is the preferred treatment option?

61. **i.** Feline ceruminous cystomatosis. This is an uncommon, nonneoplastic disorder seen in middle-aged to older cats (any age of cat can be affected). Clinically, lesions are striking and consist of multiple discrete to coalescing blue-gray or purple papules, vesicles, and/or nodules that when ruptured express a yellow/brown to black viscous fluid. As a result of the unique presentation, diagnosis is typically uncomplicated (early lesions may be mistaken for melanocytic or vascular tumors), but histopathology can be performed to confirm clinical suspicion (Sula, 2012).

ii. Ceruminous cystomatosis is normally an asymptomatic cosmetic condition when lesions remain small. It can become a problem that necessitates treatment when lesions enlarge and occlude the ear canal resulting in disruption of normal otic physiology and secondary otitis externa. The preferred treatment when lesions enlarge and cause problems is ablation of cysts via a carbon dioxide laser. However, surgical excision, cryotherapy, and chemical cautery have been proposed as alternative methods to address the condition. With appropriate therapy, long-term resolution is quite good, but more than one procedure may be required depending on the extent and severity of cysts at presentation.

62. A 3-year-old castrated cocker spaniel presented for a second opinion regarding a diagnosis of primary idiopathic seborrhea (**Figure 62a**). The owner is seeking a second opinion because the dog's scaling, crusting, and pruritus have been nonresponsive to topical antiseborrheic shampoo, systemic antimicrobials, and oral glucocorticoid therapy. Mild scaling and increased keratosebaceous debris were first noted by the owner roughly 9 months ago with a significant worsening of symptoms over the past 6 months. The dog is professionally groomed monthly, and there are three other dogs in the household who are also reported to be mildly pruritic over the last several weeks as well. The patient receives monthly heartworm prevention and is current on recommended vaccinations. Physical exam revealed moderate generalized erythema, increased adherent scale formation (**Figure 62b**), especially along the dorsum, and multifocal crust formation in the axillary regions (**Figure 62c**). Skin impression cytology from affected regions was unremarkable. Skin scrapings from along the dorsum and axillary regions revealed rare mites (**Figure 62d**).

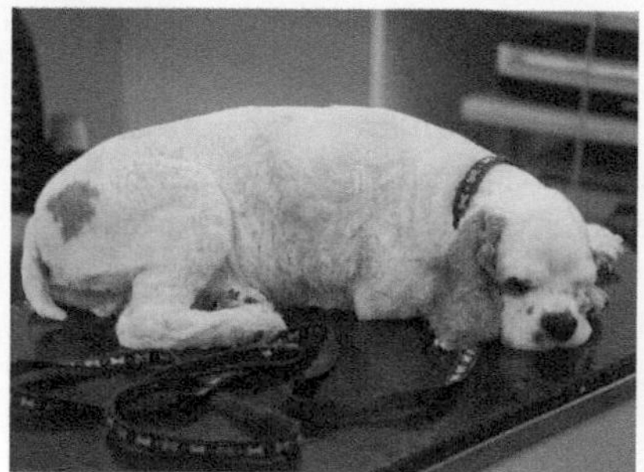

Figure 62a

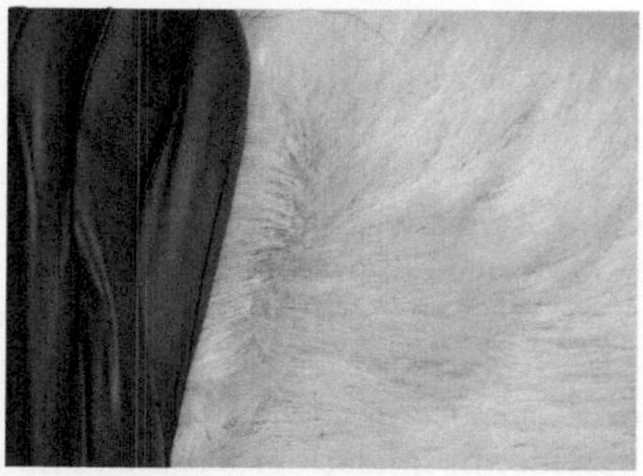

Figure 62b

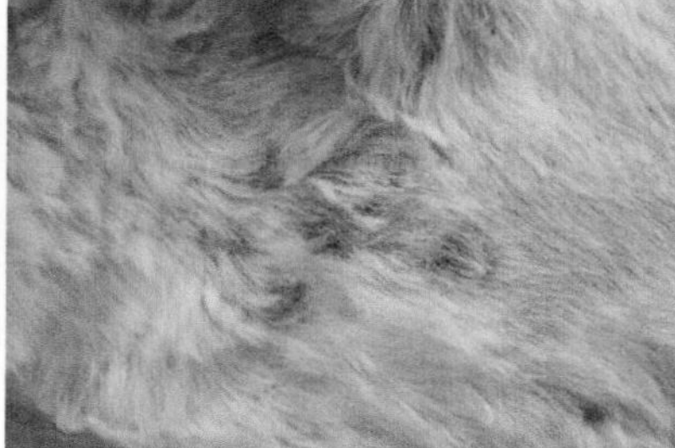

Figure 62c

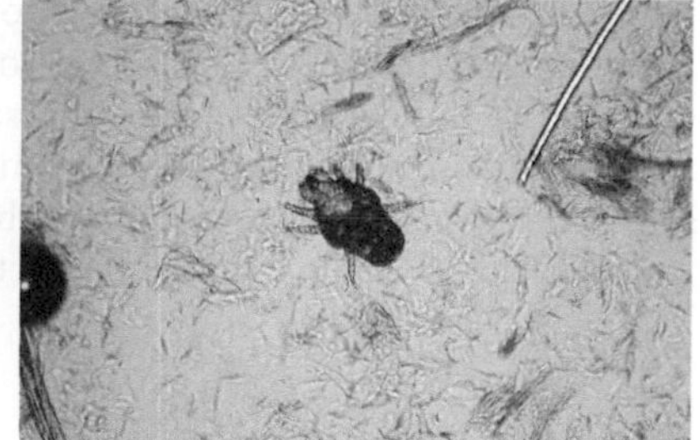

Figure 62d

i. What is the diagnosis?

ii. What is the life cycle of this mite?

iii. What are the treatment options and recommendations for this patient?

62. i. Cheyletiellosis. Cheyletiellosis is an uncommon contagious dermatosis caused by an infestation with the surface dwelling *Cheyletiella* spp. mite. It occurs in dogs, cats, and rabbits, and can cause a transient infestation in humans who have contact with pets carrying the mites. An increased incidence of the mite may be observed where routine flea prevention is not practiced or following exposure to high-volume housing situations. *C. yasguri* is the most commonly isolated species from dogs, while *C. blakei* and *C. parasitovorax* are isolated more commonly from cats and rabbits, respectively. Any breed can be affected, but there may be an increased frequency of occurrence in cocker spaniels.

ii. This mite lives in the superficial layers of the epidermis; it does not burrow. It lays its eggs on hair shafts, and the eggs are smaller and more loosely attached than louse eggs. This mite is an obligate parasite and only requires one host. The mite has a standard life cycle of egg, larva, nymph, and adult that can be completed in roughly 3 weeks. Larvae, nymphs, and adult male mites do not survive long off the host, while adult female mites are capable of surviving 10 days or more off the host.

iii. Currently, there are no licensed products specifically indicated for the treatment of cheyletiellosis. Therapeutic protocol and medication selection primarily depend on the species affected and clinician preference. Most acracidal flea preventative products and lime sulfur are effective as long as all in-contact animals are treated and conventional environmental decontamination is performed to prevent reinfestation. It is very important to treat for at least 6 weeks since the life cycle of the mite is 3 weeks. Treatments reported to be effective include topical pyrethrin sprays, weekly application of 2% lime sulfur dips, selamectin applied topically every 2–4 weeks for three doses, a topical moxidectin/imidacloprid combination product (AdvantageMulti or Advocate) applied at 2- to 4-week intervals for three doses, 0.25% fipronil spray 3 mL/kg applied as a pump spray to the body at 2-week intervals for three doses, ivermectin 0.2–0.3 mg/kg given via subcutaneous injection every 2 weeks, milbemycin 2 mg/kg orally given weekly, or one of the newer isoxazoline antiparasitics (afoxolaner, fluralaner, lotilaner, and sarolaner) at standard flea preventative dosages. The previous diagnosis of primary idiopathic seborrhea was incorrect; rather this was a case of secondary seborrhea that resolved after the dog was treated for cheyletiellosis with selamectin.

63. Numerous spot-on formulations have been developed and marketed over the years for the treatment and prevention of flea infestations. As a whole, reported adverse events for the majority of these products are infrequently encountered and fairly minor, including clinical symptoms such as lethargy, pruritus at the site of application, application site irritation, hypersalivation, hyperactivity, alopecia, and GI symptoms. However, recently there have been a series of documented cases where patients have developed an acantholytic pustular dermatitis consistent with probable drug-associated pemphigus foliaceus shortly after application of spot-on flea preventatives.

i. What spot-on flea preventative(s) has this clinical entity been associated with, and what were the clinical highlights of the case presentation(s)?

ii. What is meant by the terms *drug-induced* and *drug-triggered* when discussing cases of pemphigus foliaceus?

64. A 4-year-old spayed female mixed breed dog presented as an emergency with a skin lesion on its lateral right thigh. The owners left for dinner a few hours ago, and when they returned, the dog was biting and chewing at this lesion. The dog is extremely agitated with a 7 cm diameter circular plaque-like lesion on its lateral left thigh. The lesion is extremely painful, pruritic, and exudative (**Figure 64a, b**).

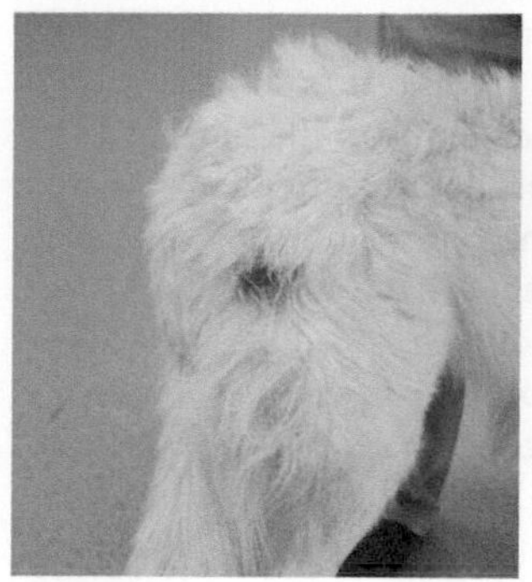

Figure 64a

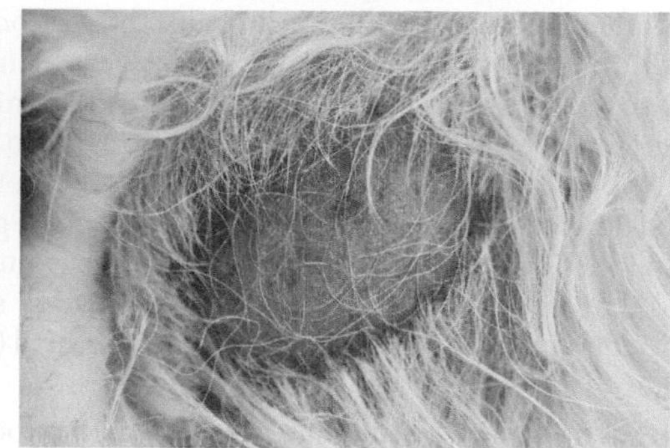

Figure 64b

i. What is the clinical diagnosis?

ii. What essential diagnostic should always be performed in this clinical condition prior to treatment?

iii. How should this lesion be treated?

65. With regard to the case of pyotraumatic dermatitis in **Question 64**:

i. Recurrent lesions of this type are commonly seen in what disease(s)?

ii. What other diseases can present as areas of chronic recurrent pyotraumatic dermatitis and are diagnosed via skin biopsy?

63. i. The first report involved ProMeris Duo (metaflumizone and amitraz) and described 22 dogs (Oberkirchner et al., 2011). In this report 8 dogs developed lesions only at the application site, while 14 dogs developed widespread lesions distant from the site of application. Overall, 14 dogs required immunosuppressive therapy for treatment of their lesions with outcome being poorer for those with lesions occurring at distant sites. This case series also suggested that large breed dogs (Labrador and golden retrievers) and female dogs were at an increased risk for developing this drug-associated variant of pemphigus foliceus. The number of applications prior to lesion development ranged from one to eight, and most patients showed lesion development within 14 days of application of the product. The second product linked to the development of pemphigus-like drug reactions was Certifect (fipronil, amitraz, and (S)-methoprene) (Bizikova et al., 2014). The case series described 21 dogs with similar findings to those of the dogs that had probable ProMeris Duo drug-associated pemphigus foliaceus. In this report, 6 dogs had local lesions while 15 displayed lesions at distant sites. The Certifect-associated disease was also observed more frequently in female and larger breed dogs similar to that described in the first report. The number of applications prior to disease development ranged from 1 to 15 (62% of the dogs developed lesions within the first two applications), and the majority of patients displayed lesion development within 14 days of the last application. Additionally, 18 dogs received some form of therapy and two dogs were euthanized as a result of their disease. The final product associated with this probable drug associated clinical entity is Vectra 3D (dinotefuran, pyriproxyfen, and permethrin) (Bizikova et al., 2015). In a case report, three dogs were described with similar clinical, histological, and immunological findings to those of the other two probable pesticide-associated pemphigus foliaceus adverse drug reactions. In the report, one dog displayed local lesions, while the other two exhibited the generalized form. In all three dogs, lesions developed after the first reported use of the product and within 10 days of application. All three dogs required some form of treatment with two obtaining clinical remission, while the third (generalized form) was euthanized as a result of treatment-related issues.

ii. Drug-induced pemphigus is used to describe cases where a drug is pharmacologically linked to the development of disease that mimics the naturally occurring variant, which undergoes remission with removal of the offending agent. In drug-triggered pemphigus, the drug acts as a "trigger" of the patient's latent genetic predisposition to develop disease, which remains active even after treatment with the offending agent is discontinued.

64. i. The lesion is most compatible with pyotraumatic dermatitis (acute moist dermatitis or "hot spots"). Pyotraumatic dermatitis is an acute, rapidly developing, erosive to ulcerative superficial bacterial infection that occurs secondary to self-inflicted trauma.

ii. An impression smear for cytologic evaluation should be acquired prior to treatment to verify the presence of bacteria. In cases of pyotraumatic dermatitis, large numbers of extra- and intracellular bacteria are present.

iii. The dog should be sedated, hair from around the area clipped, and the lesion cleaned with a mild antibacterial scrub. Topical drying agents (astringents) may be irritating and slow the healing of the wound, so their use should be avoided. Cleaning of the wound is a key step in treatment, and some dogs will no longer traumatize these areas after they have been clipped and cleaned. The daily application of a topical antibiotic ointment (i.e., mupiricin) may be used, but the author prefers early intervention with systemic antimicrobials, as many of these lesions are actually focal areas of deep pyoderma. Systemic antibiotics should be continued for 1 week past clinical improvement as resolution of the superficial lesions will occur prior that of the deeper component. Although the use of concurrent glucocorticoids in the treatment of bacterial pyoderma is contraindicated, the author prefers to use a short tapering course of methylprednisolone (0.5–1.0 mg/kg PO q24h for 3 days, then q48h for three doses) in severely pruritic cases to help prevent further self-trauma and provide temporary relief.

65. i. The most common causes of recurrent areas of pyotraumatic dermatitis are inappropriate therapy for the original lesions, unresolved bacterial pyoderma, and/or an unrecognized pruritic disease such as atopy, food allergy, and/or fleas. Recurrent facial "hot spots" due to atopy are common and may also be associated with otitis externa. Given the location of the lesion in **Figure 64a**, fleas/flea allergy should be investigated and addressed with consistent use of an adulticidal flea preventative.

ii. Areas of resolving calcinosis cutis and apocrine gland carcinomas can present as nonhealing areas of pyotraumatic dermatitis/folliculitis. Also, skin lesions associated with epitheliotrophic T-cell lymphoma may present as acute erosive, exudative, pruritic plaques in older dogs.

66. Dermatophytosis is an important infectious disease in small animal medicine that commonly affects both dogs and cats.

i. What dermatophyte species most commonly cause disease, and what are their main reservoirs in nature?

ii. What breeds have been proposed to be at an increased risk of this condition?

iii. What techniques have been described for use when culturing patients suspected to have dermatophytosis?

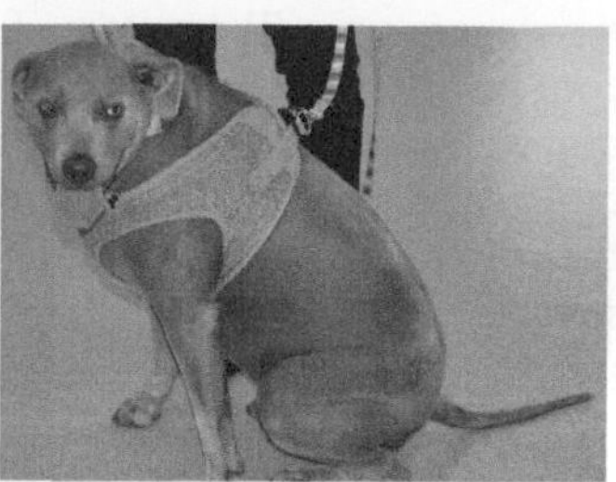

Figure 67a

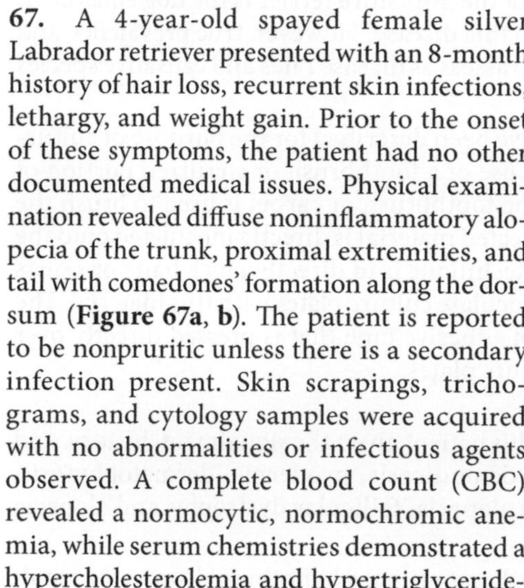

67. A 4-year-old spayed female silver Labrador retriever presented with an 8-month history of hair loss, recurrent skin infections, lethargy, and weight gain. Prior to the onset of these symptoms, the patient had no other documented medical issues. Physical examination revealed diffuse noninflammatory alopecia of the trunk, proximal extremities, and tail with comedones' formation along the dorsum (**Figure 67a, b**). The patient is reported to be nonpruritic unless there is a secondary infection present. Skin scrapings, trichograms, and cytology samples were acquired with no abnormalities or infectious agents observed. A complete blood count (CBC) revealed a normocytic, normochromic anemia, while serum chemistries demonstrated a hypercholesterolemia and hypertriglyceridemia. Urinalysis results were unremarkable. Given these findings, serum for a thyroid function panel was submitted, the results of which are shown.

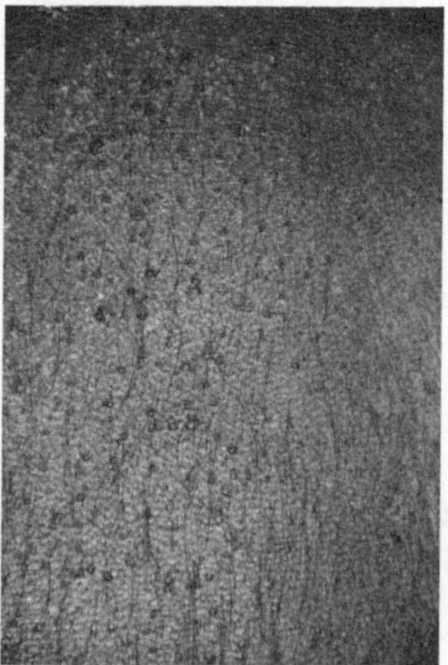

Figure 67b

Michigan State University—Thyroid Panel	Results	Normal
Total thyroxine (TT4)	8	15–67
Total triiodothyronine (TT3)	1.1	1.0–2.5
Free T4 by equilibrium dialysis (ED)	5	8–26
T4 autoantibody	5	0–20
T3 autoantibody	0	0–10
Thyroid-stimulating hormone	48	0–37
Thyroglobulin autoantibody %	7	<10

i. What are the primary differential diagnoses for this patient?

ii. What is your diagnosis in this case, and what are the primary reasons for this condition in the dog?

iii. What are reasons to observe a decreased total thyroxine in a patient?

66. i. Three dermatophyte species are routinely documented to cause disease in dogs and cats. They are *Microsporum canis, M. gypseum,* and *Trichophyton mentagrophytes.* The source of *M. canis* infections is typically a cat or fomite contaminated by cats. *M. gypseum* is a geophilic organism that is found in organic-laden soil with dogs and cats being exposed following digging in contaminated soil. *Trichophyton mentagrophytes* is associated with rodents or their nests, and disease is usually connected with exposure to one of these two sources.

ii. Persian cats have been proposed to be predisposed to dermatophytosis due to their overrepresentation in clinical studies and descriptions of subcutaneous dermatophytic infections predominantly in this breed. Likewise, similar observational studies have suggested that the Yorkshire terrier is the dog equivalent of the Persian cat when it comes to this disease. However, true prevalence and breed predisposition are difficult to assess as disease rates and causative species vary geographically.

iii. Three sampling techniques have been described for the purpose of culturing small animals. The first is the use of a toothbrush or sterilized portion of fabric/carpet. In this technique, the toothbrush or carpet is used to brush the suspected patient and then the collected material is directly inoculated onto the plate with the device. The second technique is to directly pluck hairs or crusts from the margins of lesions and inoculate culture plates with this material. The final technique is to use a piece of adhesive tape that is pressed directly over lesions and then pressed onto culture plates.

67. i. Primary differentials for this patient given the signalment, history, and physical findings should include demodicosis, pyoderma, dermatophytosis, an endocrinopathy, color dilution alopecia, follicular dystrophy, and alopecia areata.

ii. Hypothyroidism. Dogs primarily get primary hypothyroidism as the result of autoimmune lymphocytic thyroiditis or idiopathic thyroid atrophy.

iii. Although total thyroxine (tT4) can be used for screening patients for hypothyroidism, it should not be used as a confirmatory test. When total thyroxine levels are found to be low, it should be followed up with at least a free thyroxine (fT4) by ED and TSH level. The reason for this is many factors can cause total thyroxine levels to be measured low, such as breed (sighthounds, i.e., greyhounds have lower circulating levels), patient age, nonthyroidal illness (euthyroid sick syndrome), hypothyroidism, hyperadrenocorticism, drug administration (phenobarbital, glucocorticoids, sulfonamides, carprofen, clomipramin, furosemide), and analytical error.

68. A 5-year-old female miniature poodle presented with the complaint of anal licking and scooting. The owner reported that the problem started about 4 weeks ago after they returned from their winter vacation to Florida. Physical examination revealed salivary staining of the skin around the anus and a mildly erythematous perineal area. Rectal examination revealed mildly filled anal sacs that were difficult to express; the secretion was thick and tan in color.

i. What are the differential diagnoses?

ii. What is the immediate diagnostic and/or treatment plan?

69. A 5-year-old cat presented for hair loss and sores along the ventral abdomen (**Figure 69a**). The owner reports that the lesions have waxed and waned over the past 7 months but recently have worsened and are not going away. Physical examination was normal except for the skin. There was ventral abdominal and medial rear leg barbering alopecia with multiple, firm, raised, eroded plaques ranging in size from 5 mm to 1 cm present. The cat was the only animal in the household and was kept strictly indoors. The patient was treated monthly with flea and heartworm preventatives. Flea combing, skin scrapings, and fecal float were negative. Impression smears of the skin were acquired, the results of which are shown in **Figure 69b**.

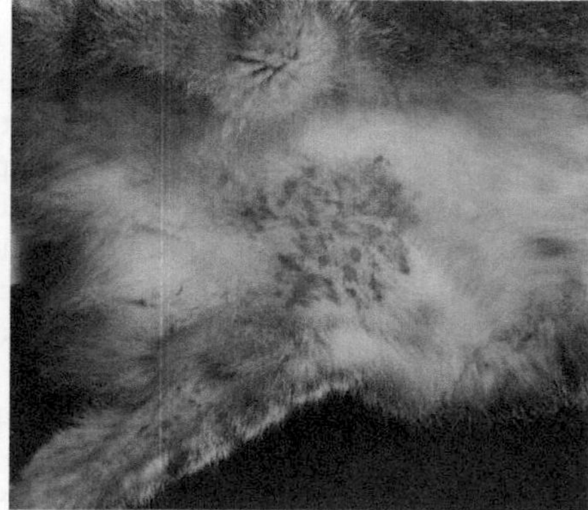

Figure 69a

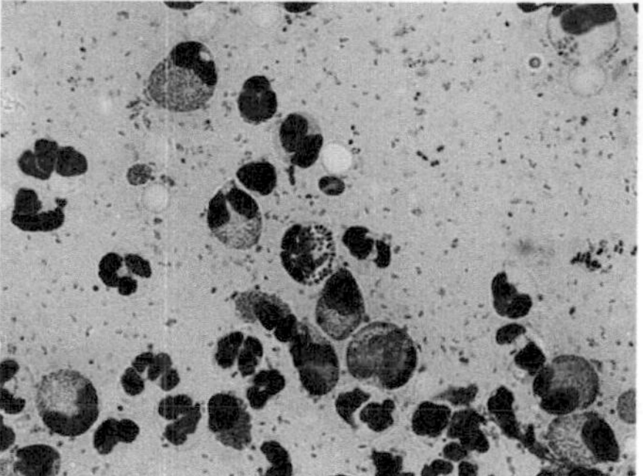

Figure 69b

i. What is the clinical term for this cat's skin issue? What differential diagnoses should be considered?

ii. What is the initial treatment plan?

68. i. Impacted anal sacs with or without secondary infection or pruritus ani resulting in secondary anal sac disease. Anal sac problems are more common in smaller breed dogs, especially obese dogs. Licking and scooting are suggestive of anal sac impactions or anal pruritus. It is possible that the dog became infested with fleas and subsequently tapeworms as a result of the trip to Florida. Tapeworm segments can be found on fecal examinations and/or on rectal examination. Many dogs with allergic skin disease (atopy, food allergy, contact allergy), vulvar fold dermatitis, vaginitis, tail-fold dermatitis, and prostate disease will develop pruritus ani. The resulting inflammation of the anal area causes the anal sac ducts to become narrowed leading to anal sac impactions, and possibly infection.

ii. Manual expression of the anal sacs is recommended. The secretion should be examined cytologically for evidence of infection. If there is evidence of infection, the anal sacs should be filled with an antimicrobial solution that contains a glucocorticoid. This should be repeated every 5–7 days. Alternatively, systemic antimicrobials can be administered for 14–21 days. In this case, flea control should be discussed with the owners, and prophylactic deworming for tapeworms should be considered. Surgical removal of the anal sacs will not resolve the anal pruritus if there is an underlying pruritic cause; however, this may be considered in dogs with chronic anal gland impactions for which an underlying cause cannot be identified/managed.

69. i. Eosinophilic plaques. This is one of the components of eosinophilic skin lesions (commonly referred to as the "eosinophilic granuloma complex") that also include eosinophilic granulomas and indolent ulcers. It is important to remember that this is not a specific dermatologic diagnosis but rather a clinical symptom/reaction pattern in the cat. These lesions are primarily encountered in cats as a result of a primary disease process such as dermatophytosis, flea allergy dermatitis, parasitic hypersensitivity (*Otodectes, Notoedres, Cheyletiella, Demodex gatoi*), cutaneous adverse food reaction, or environmental hypersensitivity (plant pollens, molds, house dust mites) (Buckley and Nuttal, 2012).

ii. Initial treatment in this case should consist of addressing the secondary pyoderma as evident by the presence of intracellular coccoid-shaped bacteria on cytology. Appropriate systemic options include a 21-day course of amoxicillin-clavulanate, cefpodoxime, or cefovecin. A tapering course of glucocorticoids (oral methylprednisolone) can also be administered to help alleviate pruritus and resolve the skin lesions. The addition of glucocorticoids may not be necessary in all situations and should be considered on a case-by-case basis, since many of these lesions (and others within the eosinophilic skin lesion group) will respond completely to antimicrobial therapy alone (Wildermuth et al., 2012). Following initial treatment, the patient should be reevaluated to determine the underlying cause of lesion development. This may consist of further flea control measures, a parasite elimination trial, diet elimination trial, or medical management/investigation of an environmental hypersensitivity. It is important to remember that repeat treatment with systemic glucocorticoids may be required to manage potential flares of the eosinophilic lesions during workup of the primary disease and that subsequent flares may not always affect the same area or present with the same manifestation.

70. A 10-year-old cat presented for sudden development of greasy seborrhea and excessive grooming resulting in alopecia (**Figure 70a**, **b**). Physical exam reveals a seborrheic unkempt hair coat, noninflammatory alopecia of the ventral abdomen, and no other cutaneous lesions. The cat has no previous history of skin disease. The owner reports that the cat seems restless, is drinking more, is using the litter box more, has a voracious appetite, and has lost weight.

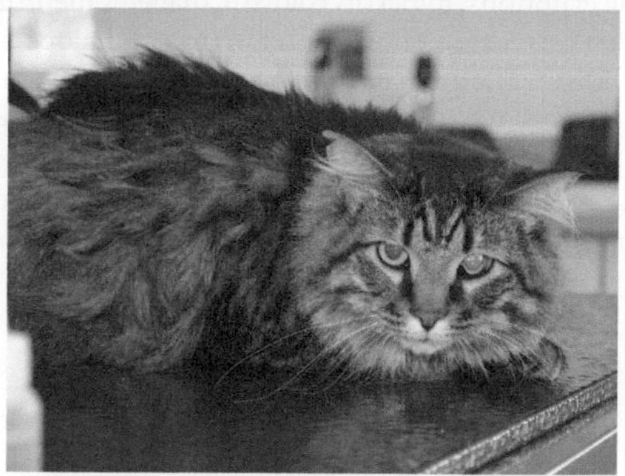

Figure 70a

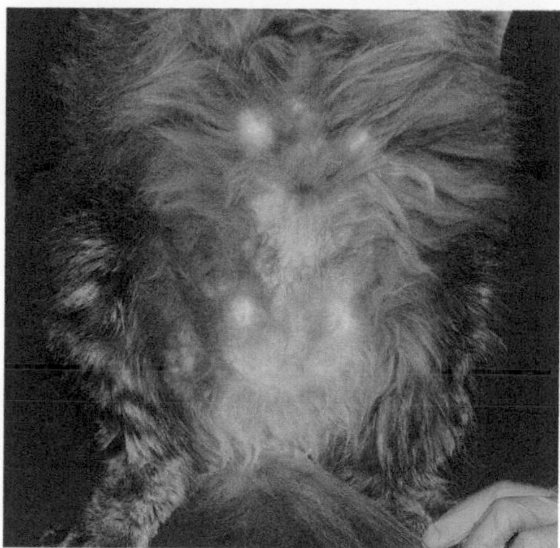

Figure 70b

i. What are your differential diagnoses for a cat with excessive barbering alopecia of the ventral abdomen?

ii. What possible etiology should be investigated in this patient?

iii. What unique dermatologic adverse event may be encountered during medical management of this cat's condition?

70. i. Differentials for excessive grooming resulting in alopecia of the ventral abdomen in a cat include FAD, cheyletiellosis, notoedric mange, *D. gatoi* infestation, lice, CAFR, environmental allergy, contact hypersensitivity, urinary tract infection, idiopathic cystitis, inflammatory bowel disease, arthritis, abdominal neoplasia, and psychogenic alopecia.

ii. Greasy seborrhea is very rare in the cat, and when it happens it should be considered a dermatologic sign of a systemic disease: liver, pancreatic, or intestinal disease, drug eruptions, hyperthyroidism, diabetes mellitus, FeLV or FIV, and neoplasia. This was a case of greasy seborrhea and alopecia secondary to feline hyperthyroidism. The greasy seborrhea seen in feline patients with these diseases is most likely due to poor grooming on the part of the cat and not a direct relationship between the disease and the skin.

iii. Severe facial pruritus has been associated with methimazole administration in cats and may occur in as high as 15% of cases where the medication is utilized (Voie et al., 2012).

71. You are presented with a 9-year-old spayed female shih tzu who has a historical diagnosis of seasonal atopy (fall) that is well managed with symptomatic use of antihistamines (cetirizine). The chief complaint today is an 8-month history of recurrent swollen paws that have been responsive to systemic antimicrobials (cefpodoxime) but upon discontinuation of therapy, clinical symptoms quickly recur. On physical exam, all four paws are noted to be affected similarly with hyperpigmentation, scaling, crusting, and comedones' formation, which was well demarcated (**Figure 71a, b**). The rest of the physical exam was unremarkable. Based on history and physical exam, a skin scrape and cytology were elected as initial diagnostics. Skin scrapings revealed what is shown in **Figure 71c**.

i. At this time, what is your diagnosis, and from a clinical perspective what is the significance of this with respect to the patient's medical workup?

ii. What conditions in the dog may present with lesions confined predominantly to the paws?

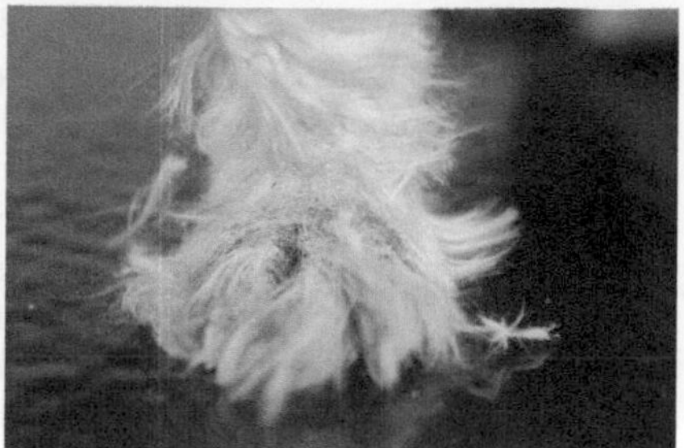

Figure 71a

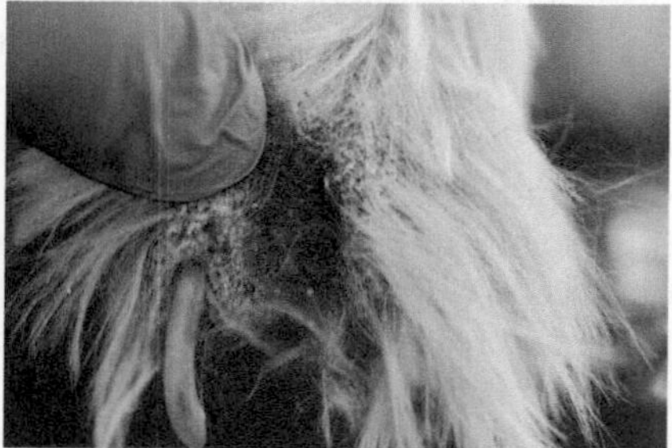

Figure 71b

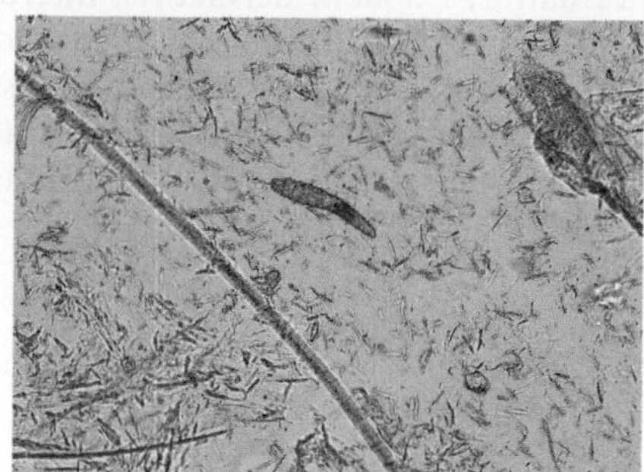

Figure 71c

71. i. Adult-onset generalized demodicosis. Adult-onset demodicosis is traditionally classified as disease that first appears after 18 months of age. However, some authors do not recognize the condition as "true" adult-onset unless clinical symptoms are first recognized after 4 years of age. Regardless, in cases of adult-onset disease, patients should be evaluated for underlying conditions that may be perpetuating immune suppression. Possible contributing conditions include malnutrition, endoparasitism, treatment with glucocorticoids, chemotherapy, neoplasia, hypothyroidism, diabetes, and hyperadrenocorticism. With such cases, a minimum diagnostic workup should consist of routine screening blood work (CBC and serum chemistries), urinalysis, thyroid testing, and potentially pituitary-adrenal axis evaluation and imaging based on clinical suspicions. It is important to remember that total thyroid hormone concentrations may be suppressed in these patients due to the presence of severe inflammatory disease (euthyroid sick syndrome). Despite diagnostic efforts, in many cases (>50%), an underlying condition cannot be documented at the time of diagnosis. These cases should be monitored carefully in the months following diagnosis as signs of systemic illness may later become evident. In adult-onset cases where an underlying cause cannot be found, the odds of curing the patient decrease, and lifelong therapy on a reduced dosing regimen of miticidal therapy may be required to control clinical symptoms.

ii. Conditions in the dog that may present with lesions first noted to affect or confined only to the paw include demodicosis, dermatophytosis, hookworm dermatitis, *Pelodera* dermatitis, interdigital follicular cysts, atopy, contact hypersensitivity, cutaneous adverse food reactions, canine distemper, pemphigus foliaceus or vulgaris, leishmaniasis, symmetric lupoid onychodystrophy, systemic lupus erythematosus, vasculitis, zinc-responsive dermatosis, hepatocutaneous syndrome, familial or idiopathic nasodigital hyperkeratosis.

72. A 2-year-old spayed female boxer presented for severe progressive pruritus that was first reported to begin roughly 2–3 months ago. A prior short-term course of prednisone using a tapering dose that started at 1 mg/kg was previously dispensed and provided negligible pruritus relief. The patient is otherwise healthy and is current with recommended vaccinations. Physical examination revealed generalized erythema with patchy alopecia and excoriations most prominently around the ears, axillary regions, and distal rear legs. Several impression smears were taken for cytology from lesional areas that revealed an absence of bacterial or fungal etiologic agents. Skin scrapings from the concave aspect of the left pinna and right axillary regions revealed **Figure 72a**, which were observed in multiple fields on both acquired samples.

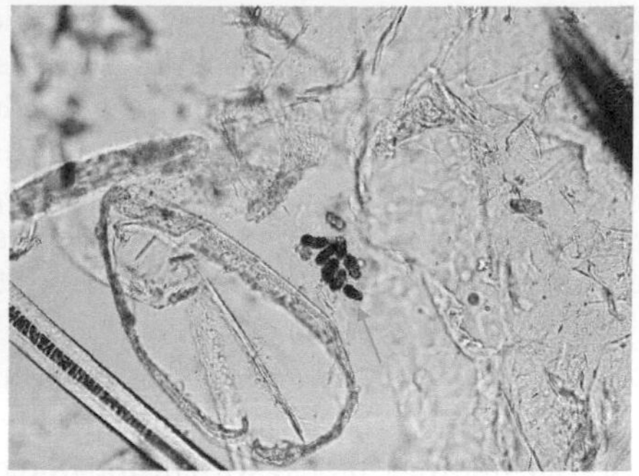
Figure 72a

i. What is present on the skin scraping samples, and what is the significance of this finding?

73. A 12-year-old spayed female miniature schnauzer presented for evaluation of a rapidly growing mass affecting the fourth digit on the right front paw, which has been causing non-weight-bearing lameness for the last several days (**Figure 73a**). The lesion was first observed as an ulcerated region near the digital pad roughly 6 weeks ago. An impression smear of the lesion revealed neutrophilic inflammation with extra- and intracellular coccoid-shaped bacteria. Fine-needle aspirate of the nodule revealed atypical spindle cells, and radiographs of the paw demonstrated a soft tissue mass without osseous involvement.

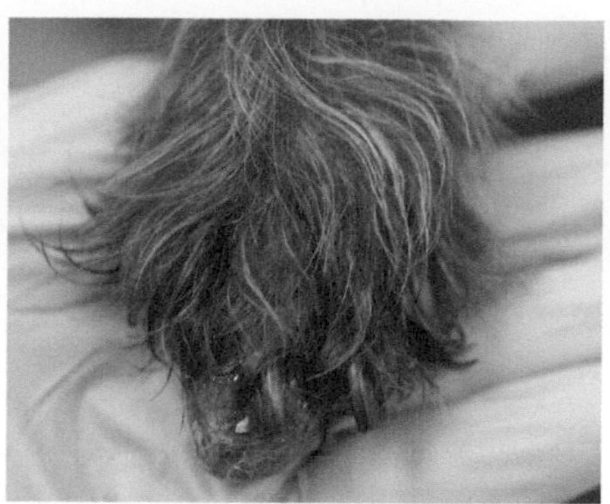
Figure 73a

i. What are the top differentials for a single affected digit or claw in the dog, and what recommendation should be made to this owner at this time?

ii. What tumors most commonly affect the claw bed of dogs?

iii. What conditions are most likely to simultaneously affect multiple claws in a dog?

72. i. The brown debris shown are scabies fecal pellets known as scybala. The presence of this material on a skin scrape sample from a scabies suspect should be viewed similar to finding an egg or adult mite. However, in circumstances where the clinician is inexperienced or unsure, additional samples should be acquired from the patient to see if *Sarcoptes* spp. eggs or adult mites can be recovered to confirm the diagnosis. If these life stages fail to be recovered with additional scrapings, the patient should still be treated for sarcoptic mange.

73. i. The top differentials for a single affected digit include trauma, neoplasia, or infection (bacterial or fungal). Given the rapid growth and fine-needle aspirate findings, biopsy with histopathology, three-view thoracic radiographs, and regional lymph node aspirates were recommended due to concern for a neoplastic process. In this particular case, toe amputation was elected because it had the potential to be curative with a single procedure since lymph node aspirates and thoracic radiographs were unremarkable.

ii. The most commonly observed tumors affecting the claw region of dogs are squamous cell carcinoma, malignant melanoma, osteosarcoma, various soft tissue sarcomas, and mast cell tumors. In this case, histopathology was consistent with a fibrosarcoma.

iii. Conditions in dogs that will affect multiple claws simultaneously include symmetric lupoid onychodystrophy, systemic lupus erythematosus, vasculitis, adverse drug eruption, nutritional deficiency, hepatocutaneous syndrome, and leishmaniasis.

74. A dog presented as an emergency with the complaint of acute rectal bleeding. The dog was noted by the owner to recently be licking the perianal region and scooting. Both behaviors were considered abnormal for the patient. Physical exam revealed a 5 mm diameter ulcerative, draining perianal lesion 1–2 cm lateral to the anus in the 4 o'clock position (**Figure 74a**).

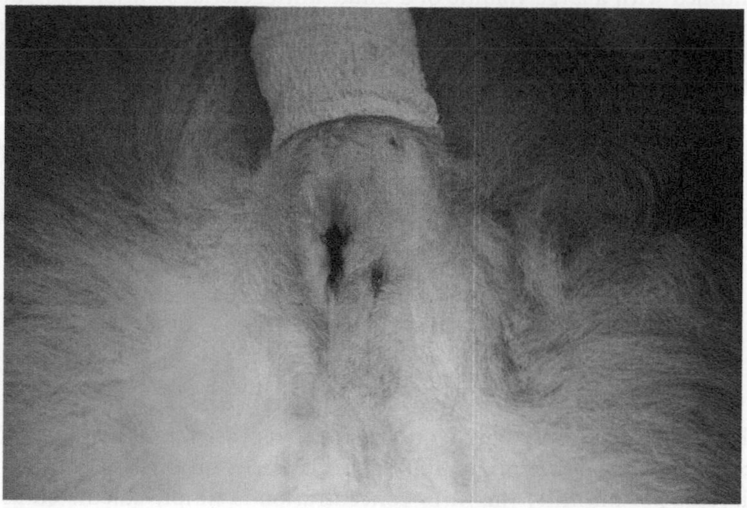

Figure 74a

i. What is the most likely diagnosis, and what are the other primary differentials for this lesion?

ii. How should the dog be treated?

75. How many milligrams per milliliter (mg/mL) of an active ingredient does a lotion, cream, ointment, or solution contain if it is labeled as containing a 0.3% concentration of that agent?

74. **i.** A ruptured anal sac abscess. Other differentials that should be considered would be anal sac neoplasia depending on the age of the patient and perianal fistulas.
ii. This is a chronic problem due to extensive perianal furunculosis and cellulitis. Under heavy sedation or general anesthesia, the areas should be cleaned and flushed with a large volume of a dilute antibacterial solution (povidone-iodine or chlorhexidine). Then an antibiotic/glucocorticoid ointment should be instilled. Appropriate broad-spectrum systemic antibiotics should be administered for 14 days along with analgesic therapy as needed.

75. This is a simple calculation that gives many people problems and can be thought about several different ways.

The first is that the basic formula to obtain the required milligrams of solute for any percentage of solution needed is mg/mL = % × 10.

So, mg = % × 10 × mL; using this formula to make a 0.3% solution:

$$\text{mg} = 0.3 \times 10 \times 1$$

$$\text{mg} = 3$$

The second is simply based on the idealized assumption that a 100% concentration equals 1 g/mL or 1000 mg/mL. Based on this assumption, the milligrams per milliliter (mg/mL) concentration is simply calculated as the fraction of 1,000.

So, a 0.3% solution would equal 0.003 × 1000 = 3 mg/mL

The third method for making this calculation is to simply move the decimal point one place to the right, which equals the milligrams per milliliter (mg/mL):

i.e. 0.3% = 3 mg/mL, 3.0% = 30 mg/mL, or 30.0% = 300 mg/mL

Regardless of the method used to make this determination, a 0.3% concentration is equivalent to 3 mg/mL.

76. A 4-year-old spayed female West Highland white terrier presented for a second opinion on nonresolving pustules. The patient has received cephalexin at a dosage of 20 mg/kg orally twice a day for the previous 14 days. The owners report no improvement has been observed in the last 2 weeks, and new "spots" have continued to occur. Based on the history, a sample for cytology was acquired and revealed numerous neutrophils with intra- and extracellular doublets of coccoid-shaped bacteria. Given cytology results, a resistant bacterial infection was suspected, and a culture from an intact lesion was performed. The results of the bacterial sensitivity report are shown.

Culture Summary

Animal ID	Specimen	Growth	Organism
001	Skin swab	Heavy, pure	*Staphylococcus pseudintermedius*

Antimicrobial	*S. pseudintermedius*
Amikacin	S
Ampicillin	R
Amoxi/Clav acid	R
Cefazolin	R
Cefpodoxime	R
Cephalexin	R
Chloramphenicol	S
Clindamycin	S
Doxycycline	S
Enrofloxacin	S
Marbofloxacin	S
Erythromycin	R
Oxacillin	R
Tetracycline	R
Trimethoprim/Sulfa	R

Abbreviations: S, susceptible; I, intermediate; R, resistant; NI, no interpretation.

i. What is a D-test?

ii. What antimicrobials are possible therapeutic options for this patient?

iii. What are potential adverse events associated with use of the available antimicrobials?

76. **i.** The D-test is a double disc diffusion test used by microbiology laboratories to identify inducible clindamycin resistance. The D-test is performed by placing erythromycin and clindamycin discs adjacent to each other. If a D-shaped zone of inhibition forms around the clindamycin disc, the bacterial isolate is interpreted as resistant to clindamycin (**Figure 76a**). Currently, this test is not routinely performed by veterinary diagnostic laboratories, and limited published data on investigations utilizing this test have shown a low rate of inducible clindamycin resistance among methicillin-resistant *Staphylococcus pseudintermedius* (MRSP) isolates, which is in contrast to MRSA isolates (Faires et al., 2009). Regardless, in the absence of this test, if a susceptibility report indicates erythromycin resistance but clindamycin susceptibility, clindamycin use should be avoided.

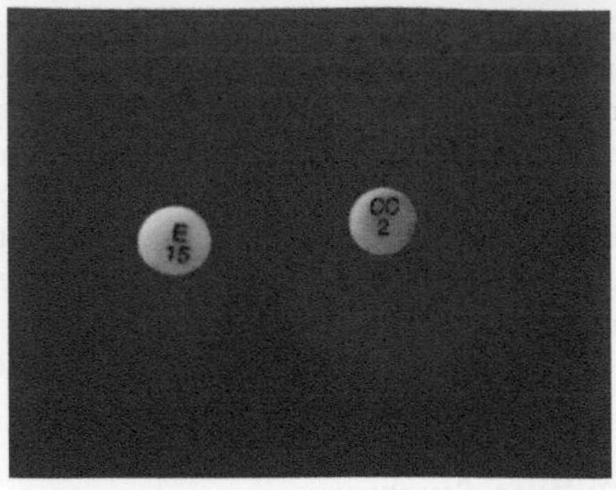

Figure 76a

ii. Given the presence of erythromycin resistance, clindamycin should be avoided in this case. Along these lines, resistance to tetracyclines is mediated through acquisition of tetracycline resistance genes that either confer ribosomal protection or encode for efflux pumps. Tetracycline is used as a class indicator, and in the presence of tetracycline resistance, doxycycline should be avoided even if results suggest it is susceptible. An exception to these guidelines would be the use of minocycline, which is not affected by the most common tetracycline resistance genes. *Staphylococcus* spp. possessing the tet(K) gene may retain susceptibility to minocycline even though they are resistant to other tetracyclines. A request for specific minocycline susceptibility testing should be done prior to utilizing this drug in patients. This leaves enrofloxacin, marbofloxacin, chloramphenicol, and amikacin as possible options for systemic therapy.

iii. *Enrofloxacin:* Vomiting, diarrhea, anorexia, elevated hepatic enzymes, and cartilage defects in young growing animals (use should be avoided in large to giant breed dogs under 18 months of age and all other dogs under 1 year of age). Rarely seizures, ataxia, and behavioral changes have been observed. *Marbofloxacin:* Similar to enrofloxacin, but generally tolerated better. *Chloramphenicol:* GI adverse events are most common with potentially 50% of patients experiencing vomiting, diarrhea, or anorexia. Reversible bone marrow suppression, hindlimb weakness, and increased hepatic enzymes are also reported (Short et al., 2014). *Amikacin:* Nephrotoxicity (higher-dose range, prior renal impairment, in patient not properly hydrated), vomiting and diarrhea, injection site reactions, and ototoxicity. In this case, marbofloxacin was chosen as it offered the best safety profile of the available options.

77. Superficial bacterial folliculitis (i.e., pyoderma) is a common clinical entity encountered in veterinary medicine. **Figure 77a, b** demonstrate two frequently observed lesions in patients affected by pyoderma.

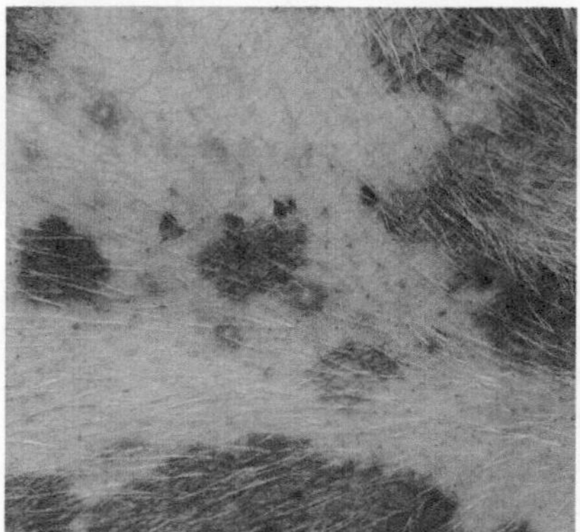
Figure 77a

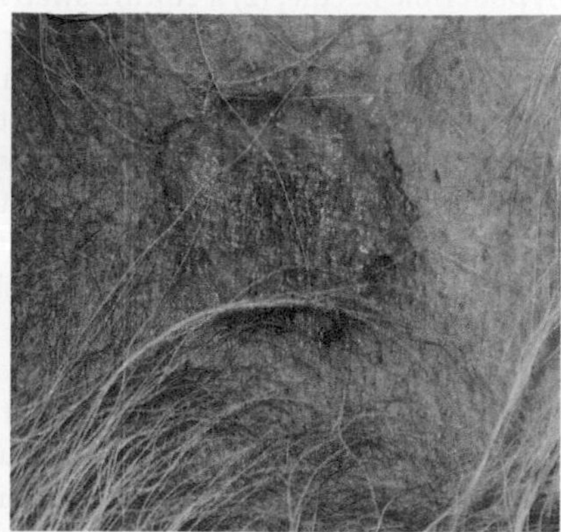
Figure 77b

i. What is the name of each lesion?

ii. If a resistant infection is suspected, how should each lesion be cultured?

78. This dog presented for evaluation of pruritus for the past 2 months (**Figure 78a, b**). Note the pattern of hair loss over the dorsum and rear legs. The patient had been previously treated with antimicrobials, which failed to provide benefit, while treatment with an appropriate dose and dosage of glucocorticoids only yielded partial pruritus relief. Skin scrapings were negative, and flea combing failed to yield any results.

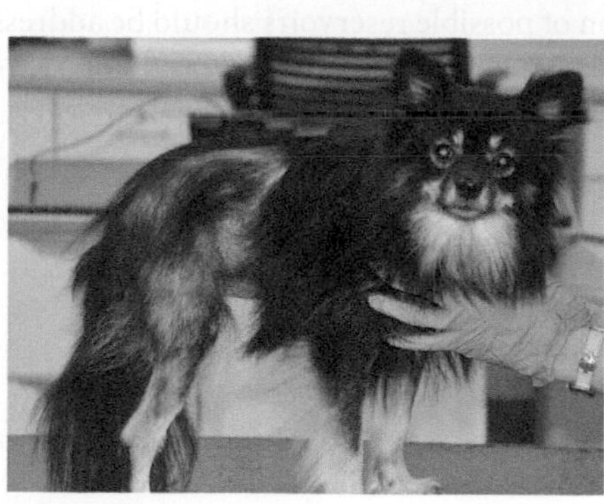
Figure 78a

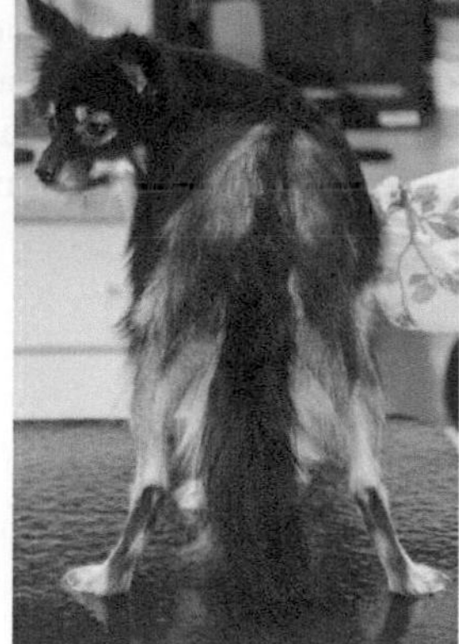
Figure 78b

i. What is the most likely diagnosis given the information provided?

ii. What is the treatment for this condition?

77. i. Figure 77a shows three pustules, while **Figure 77b** is an epidermal collarette.

ii. In the case of a pustule: (1) The pustule should first be lanced using a sterile hypodermic needle; (2) a culture swab is inserted into the ruptured pustule; (3) the culture swab is then placed in the transport system; (4) the acquired sample should then be submitted to a veterinary reference laboratory as subtle differences with respect to commonly isolated organisms do exist that can impact proper identification and susceptibility reports; and (5) finally, a cytology from the pustule should be acquired to ensure bacteria are present in the sampled lesion and that clinical findings correlate with culture results. The same general process is used to culture epidermal collarettes with the exception that instead of lancing the lesion, the leading edge (periperhal edge) is lightly lifted up to expose the exudative margin, and this area is sampled by rolling the culture swab along this boundary. Just like in the case of a pustule, cytology should be acquired post-culture sampling to ensure bacteria are present and that culture/clinical findings correlate. An alternative to this method for bacteriologic culture of an epidermal collarette has been described where a dry, sterile culture swab is simply rolled across the collarette three to four times, placed in the transport system, and submitted to a microbiology laboratory (White et al., 2005). This method was determined to be simple and reliable for the identification of *Staphylococcus pseudintermedius* when present.

78. i. Fleas or flea allergy dermatitis. This is a classic distribution for flea allergy in dogs. Flea allergy dermatitis is a hypersensitivity to allergens found within the saliva of the flea, and it is not uncommon to find a low number or absence of fleas in some animals.

ii. The management of flea infestations in dogs requires four critical components. First, the flea population on the affected pet must be controlled. Second, all pets in the household, even if they are not demonstrating clinical symptoms, need to be treated with adulticidal flea preventatives. Third, thorough environmental cleaning with identification of possible reservoirs should be addressed. Finally, identification and treatment of any secondary bacterial and/or yeast infections must also be performed.

79. Canine demodicosis is a common parasitic condition encountered in veterinary medicine.

What are the life stages of *Demodex* mites, how are they identified, and why should the numbers of each be monitored and recorded during therapy?

80. Three 6-month-old German shepherd littermates are shown in **Figure 80a**. Both male dogs were born with abnormal hair coats, which over the last several months have become more noticeably alopecic. Dermatologic examination revealed an absence of hair on the male puppies' forehead, ventrum, and proximal forelimbs. The female littermate's examination was unremarkable.

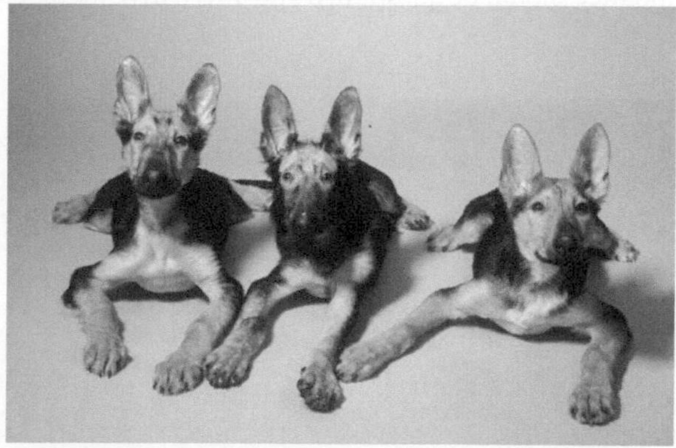

Figure 80a

i. What is this condition called?
ii. What will a skin biopsy be expected to show?
iii. What other ectodermal defect is often present in animals with this disorder?

81. What is the metal instrument shown in **Figure 81a**?

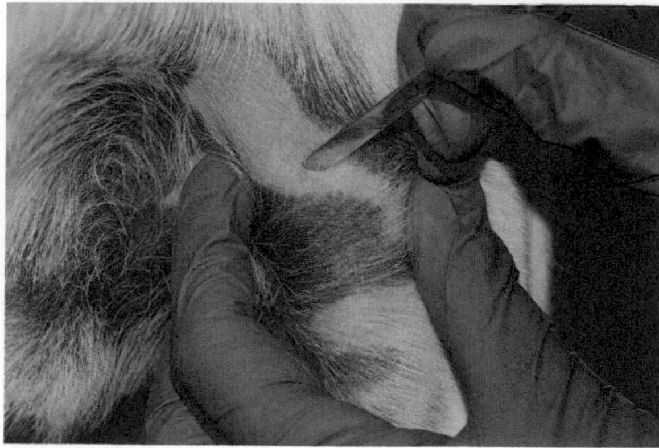

Figure 81a

79. Egg, larva, nymph, and adult. Eggs are usually fusiform or lemon shaped with a light-pink hue (**Figure 79a**). Eggs then hatch into six-legged larvae (**Figure 79b**), which eventually molt into eight-legged nymphs (**Figure 79c**) and finally eight-legged adults with more defined and fully developed cytoskeletal features (**Figure 79d**). It is important when monitoring dogs during therapy to record the sites sampled, number of mites per visual field, the proportion of immature versus adult life stages, and number of live versus dead mites so efficacy of therapy can be determined. As therapy progresses, the number of immature stages to adults should decrease, the proportion of dead mites should increase, and the overall number of mites should decrease. If for any reason at a reevaluation these trends are not being seen, the efficacy of the current therapy or owner compliance should be questioned and alternative therapeutic options considered.

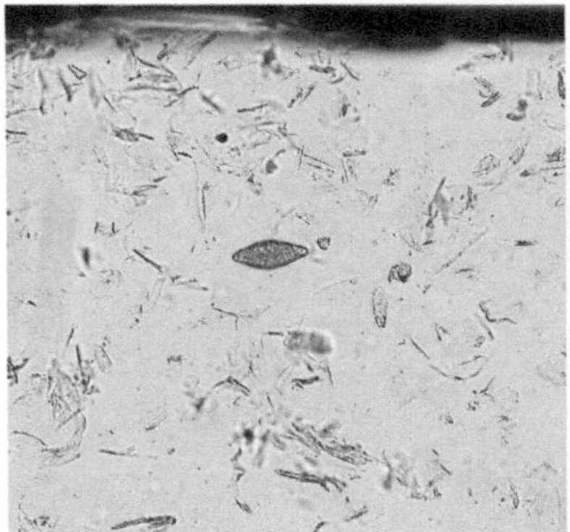

Figure 79a

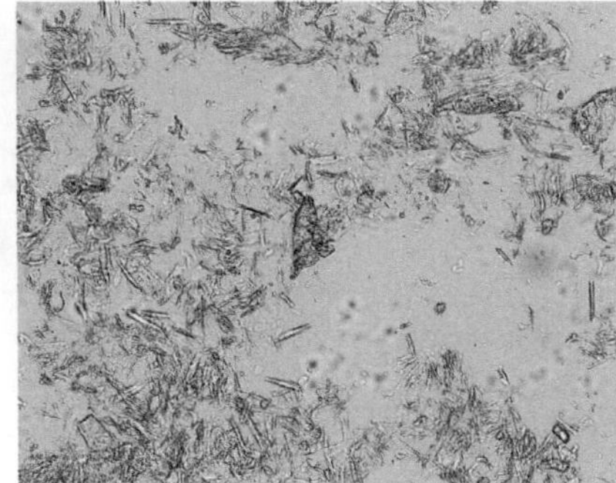

Figure 79b

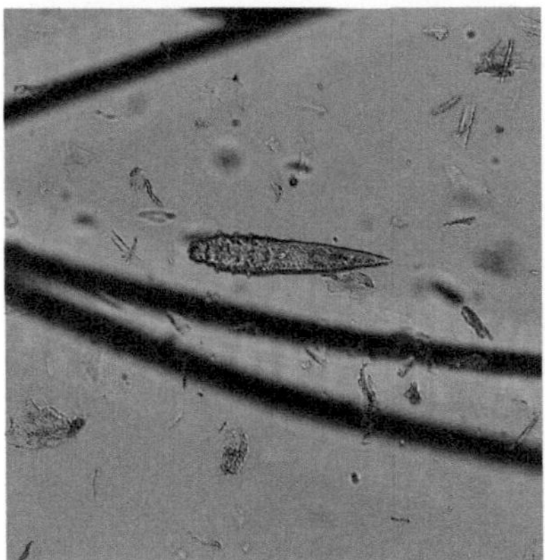

Figure 79c

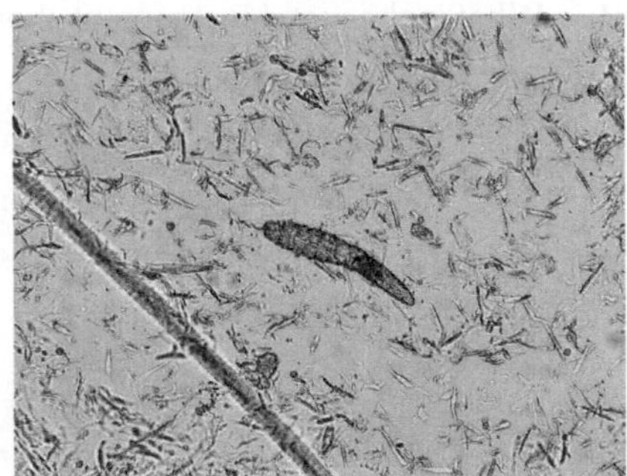

Figure 79d

80. **i.** Congenital X-linked alopecia or X-linked ectodermal dysplasia. It has been reported in many breeds of dogs and occasionally in cats. Affected animals may be born without hair or lose their hair coat over the first 4–6 weeks of their life. The hair loss is symmetrical and typically involves the frontotemporal, sacral, ventrum, and proximal extremity regions. There is no treatment for this disease.

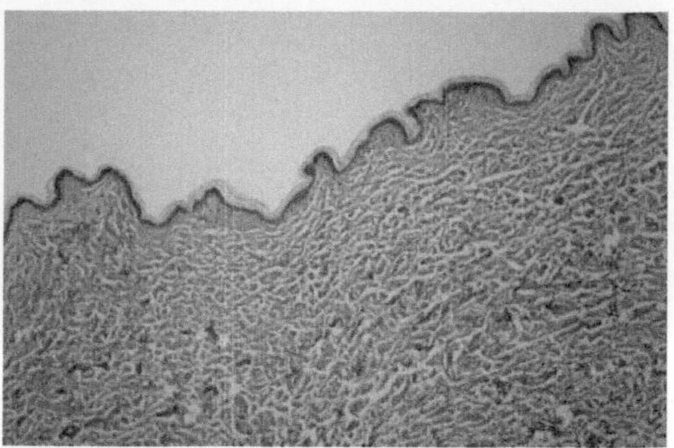
Figure 80b

ii. Skin biopsy results show a significantly reduced number, marked hypoplasia or complete absence of hair follicles, arrector pili muscles, sebaceous glands, and epitrichial sweat glands (**Figure 80b**).

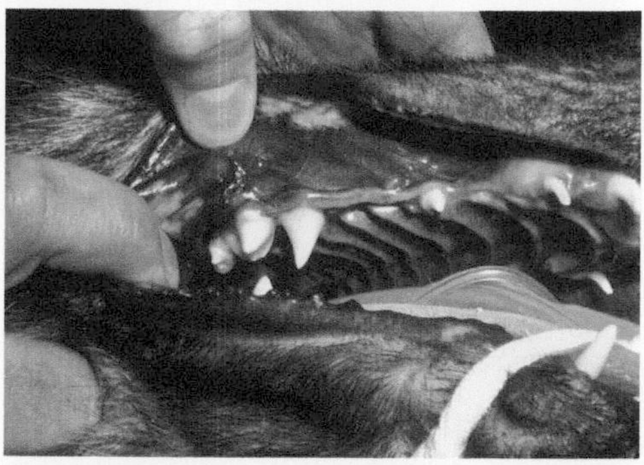
Figure 80c

iii. The other common ectodermal defect often present is abnormal dentition (**Figure 80c**). However, abnormal glandular (epitrichial and atrichial sweat glands, sebaceous, lacrimal, tracheal, and bronchial) development is also possible, which can lead to issues with thermoregulation, corneal disease, and respiratory infections.

81. The flat metal instrument is a skin-scraping spatula. This can be purchased from medical or chemical suppliers, and it is also used as a weighing spatula. This tool is used for obtaining superficial and deep skin scrapings. There are a number of advantages of the metal spatula over a traditional scalpel blade. First, the spatula is reusable and less expensive than using a new scalpel blade for every patient. Second, and more importantly, it is a safer method for collecting specimens for both the patient and the clinician. The edge of the blade is sharp enough for scraping the skin, but not sharp enough to cut either the patient or clinician. This tool is especially useful in small or struggling patients that may be easily injured and for scraping interdigital areas that may be difficult to adequately scrape with a scalpel blade. Another use of the tool is for the collection of cytological specimens from beneath claw beds, crevices in the skin, or for collection of surface material.

Figure 80b.

Figure 80c.

80. i. Congenital X-linked alopecia or X-linked ectodermal dysplasia. It has been reported in many breeds of dogs and occasionally in cats. Affected animals may be born without hair or lose their hair coat over the first 4–6 weeks of their life. The hair loss is symmetrical and typically involves the frontotemporal, sacral, ventrum, and proximal extremity regions. There is no treatment for this disease.

ii. Skin biopsy results show a significantly reduced number, marked hypoplasia or complete absence of hair follicles, arrector pili muscles, sebaceous glands, and epitrichial sweat glands (Figure 80b).

iii. The other common ectodermal defect often present is abnormal dentition (Figure 80c). However, abnormal glandular (epitrichial and atrichial sweat glands, sebaceous, lacrimal, tracheal and bronchial) development is also possible, which can lead to issues with thermoregulation, corneal disease, and respiratory infections.

81. The flat metal instrument is a skin-scraping spatula. This can be purchased from medical or chemical suppliers, and it is also used as a weighing spatula. This tool is used for obtaining superficial and deep skin scrapings. There are a number of advantages of the metal spatula over a traditional scalpel blade. [illegible] the spatula is reusable and less expensive than using a new scalpel blade for each patient. Second, and more importantly, it is a safer tool [illegible] the patient [illegible] the patient or clinician with tool [illegible] particularly useful in small or wriggling patients that may be easily injured and for scraping [illegible] which may be difficult to adequately scrape with a scalpel blade. Another use of the tool is for the collection of cytological specimens from lesions [illegible] the skin, or for collection of surface material.

82. Insect growth regulators are commonly used in available flea preventative products.

i. What are the two basic categories of insect growth regulators, and in general, how do they work?

ii. Give examples of each class of drugs.

iii. What are the advantages and disadvantages of each class of drugs?

83. A 5-year-old male Labrador retriever presented for a focal patch of hair loss over the tail. The owner notes that they first noticed the area about a month ago over which time the lesion has gotten slightly larger. The patient has no prior history of skin or ear issues, and the owner reports that the patient is not bothered by the lesion. Physical exam reveals an overall healthy patient with an unremarkable exam except for a 4 cm × 3 cm oval-shaped, raised alopecic plaque with mild scale formation over the dorsal tail (**Figure 83a**).

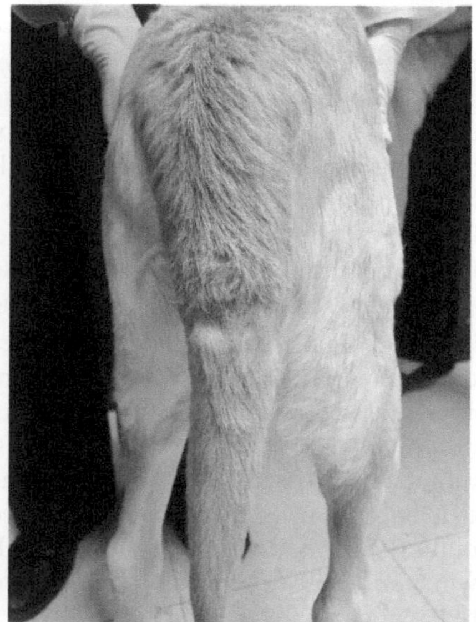

Figure 83a

i. What is your diagnosis, and what treatment options can you recommend to the owner?

ii. What is the condition known as in cats, and how does clinical presentation differ?

84. An 8 month-old spayed female Weimaraner presented for "warts" on her lips. The owner reported that over the last several weeks a single lesion had progressed to what is shown (**Figure 84a**). Lesions were present on both the inner and outer labial surfaces of both the left and right sides. The growths did not bother the patient, but lesions were noted to be easily traumatized and occasionally bleed.

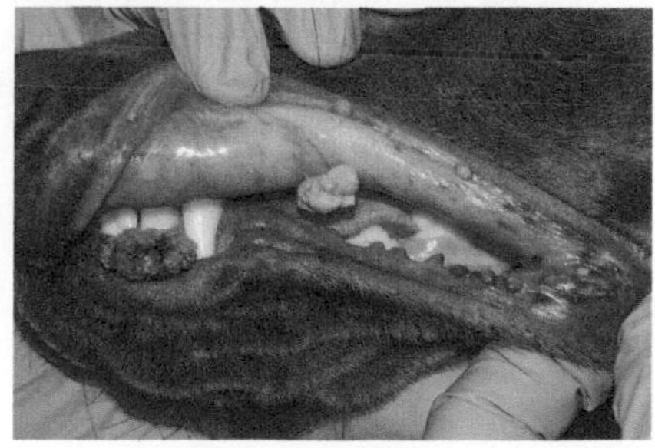

Figure 84a

i. What is the clinical diagnosis?

ii. What are possible treatment options?

82. i. Insect growth regulators are typically subdivided into juvenile hormone analogs or chitin synthesis inhibitors. Juvenile hormone analogs in essence mimic the effects of natural insect juvenile hormone. In the normal development of a flea, a fall in juvenile hormone concentrations triggers the development of the pupal stage. These drugs prevent pupation, and they are also ovicidal. Chitin synthesis inhibitors interfere with the development of the exoskeleton and affect nonadult stages of the life cycle. Although both can be used alone for flea control, both groups are much more effective as a preventative and when combined with other paraciticides.
ii. The most commonly used juvenile hormone analogs are fenoxycarb, methoprene, and pyriproxifen. Methoprene and pyriproxifen can be used on animals and are available in collars or topical products. Fenoxycarb is used in the environment. The most commonly known chitin synthesis inhibitors are lufenuron and cyromazine. Lufenuron is a benzylphenol that inhibits chitin, an important component of the flea exoskeleton. Cyromazine is an aminotriazine. It does not inhibit chitin but rather causes the exoskeleton to become stiff and results in lethal body wall defects. It is not widely used.
iii. Methoprene is directly and indirectly ovididal, embryocidal, and larvicidal. It does not readily wash off the animal or surfaces to which it has been applied. The product is safe for use on cats and can be used in combination with other products. The major disadvantages of the drug include sensitivity to UV radiation and that it can volatilize and move to other locations. Pyriproxyfen is ovicidal and larvicidal and is not sensitive to UV radiation. It is very stable even outdoors and is also safe for use on cats. It is not easily removed by bathing and will translocate to bedding. The major concern about this drug is its potential to harm nontarget species insects.

Chitin synthesis inhibitors are systemic drugs that have high margins of safety. They are an alternative to environmental insecticides although it can take greater than 3 months for fleas to be eliminated from a closed home environment. There is no residue problem on animals or people, and they are safe for use in cats. The major disadvantage of this drug is that it must be given with food to be absorbed, takes months to eliminate fleas from the environment, and has no adulticidal activity (Kunkle and Halliwell, 2002).

83. i. Tail gland hyperplasia. All dogs have an oval area along the dorsal surface of the tail near the proximal aspect that is composed of simple hair follicles and numerous sebaceous and circumanal glands. This normal cosmetic issue is not usually appreciated in geographic regions where routine spaying and neutering of canine patients is practiced. When glandular hyperplasia is present, the area may be alopecic, exudative, hyperpigmented, contain comedones or cysts, and may become infected, although this latter issue is uncommon. This is primarily a cosmetic defect that does not require treatment. However, neutering of this patient may improve the appearance but will unlikely complete resolve the issue. When this condition occurs in castrated individuals, their adrenal function should be evaluated.

ii. Feline tail gland hyperplasia or "stud tail." The difference in cats is that the glandular tissue is linear along the length of the dorsal tail rather than being found in a discrete single region. Presentation is similar to that of dogs, but cats tend to have more accumulation of debris and seborrheic material.

84. i. Canine oral papillomatosis. Canine oral papillomatosis is an infectious disease that is normally confined to the oral cavity or lips in young dogs. Lesions normally begin as flat white papules that progress over several weeks to cauliflower-like hyperplastic growths. Lesions typically spontaneously resolve, but in some cases they may persist or progress in severity (**Figure 84b**).

ii. Potential treatment options include surgical debulking (cold steel, cryosurgery, CO_2 laser), recombinant canine oral papillomavirus vaccination, oral azithromycin, injectable high-dose interferon or low-dose oral administration, oral cimetidine, and topical imiquimod.

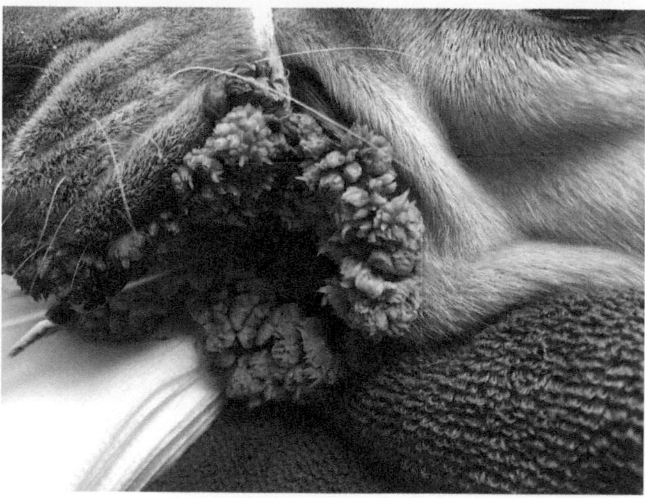

Figure 84b

85. A DSH cat presented for a lesion on its lip (**Figure 85a**). This type of lesion is very common in cats.

i. What is the name of this lesion?

ii. What are the treatment options for this patient?

iii. What is the most common cause for recurrence of these lesions in the cat?

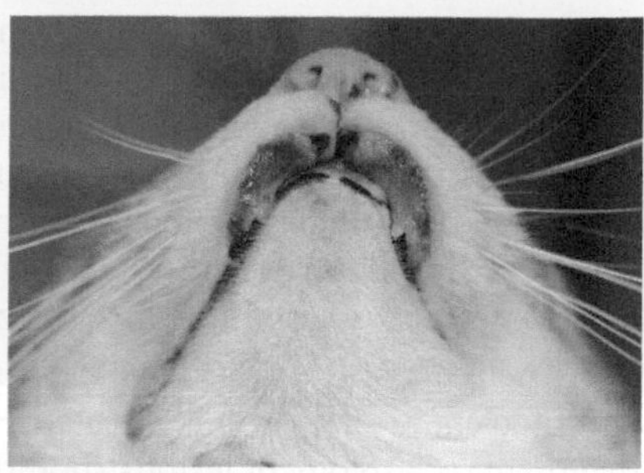

Figure 85a

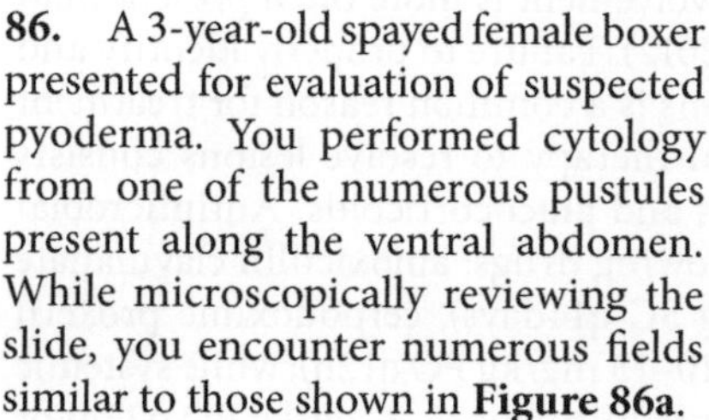

86. A 3-year-old spayed female boxer presented for evaluation of suspected pyoderma. You performed cytology from one of the numerous pustules present along the ventral abdomen. While microscopically reviewing the slide, you encounter numerous fields similar to those shown in **Figure 86a**.

What is being pointed out by the three green arrows?

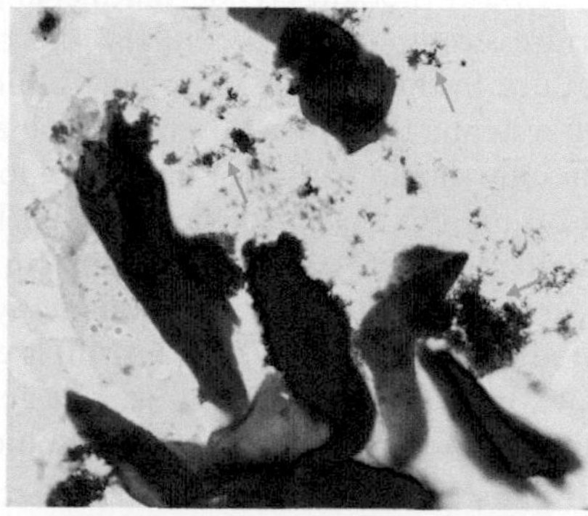

Figure 86a

87. A 4-year-old spayed female Labrador retriever presented for a complaint of head shaking, scratching, and severe ear pain with a malodorous discharge. The owner first appreciated clinical signs within the past week. Marked mucopurulent discharge was appreciated in both canals during examination. Cytologies of the exudate stained with a Romanowsky-type stain (**Figure 87a**) and Gram stain (**Figure 87b**) are shown.

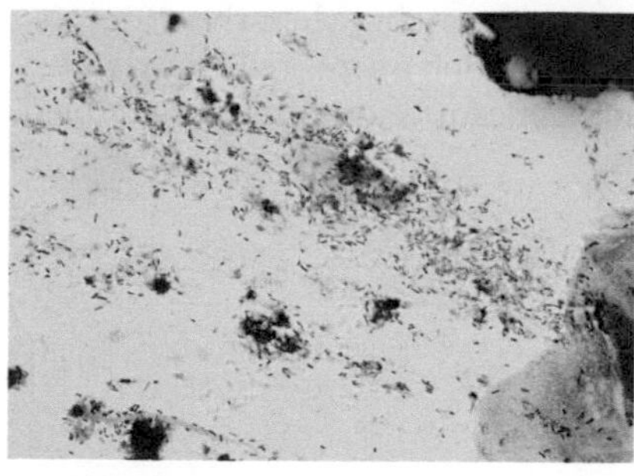

Figure 87a

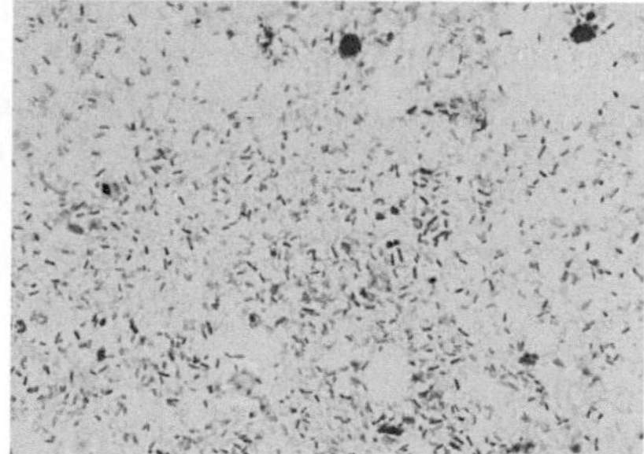

Figure 87b

i. What etiology is most likely causing the secondary infection in this patient?

ii. Empiric topical therapy with what antimicrobial agents are appropriate choices in this case?

iii. What are common reasons for treatment failure in canine otitis?

85. **i.** Indolent ulcer. This lesion along with the eosinophilic granuloma and plaque compose the group of feline eosinophilic skin lesions. This term is often used inappropriately as a final diagnosis, and the three lesions are actually a reaction pattern of the skin in cats to another primary condition. Indolent ulcers may be unilateral or bilateral and most commonly occur on the upper lip near the philtrum or canine teeth. Indolent ulcers may occur by themselves, or they may occur simultaneously with eosinophilic plaques and granulomas.
ii. Although small lesions have been reported to resolve spontaneously, cats with indolent ulcers should be treated as lesions can rapidly enlarge and become disfiguring. Cytology of lesions should be performed to identify if intracellular bacteria are observed, as bacterial involvement is more often present than previously thought (Wildermuth et al., 2012). Failure to properly identify and address complicating secondary infections is a common reason for treatment failure in the author's opinion. Clinical therapy to resolve lesions consists of systemic therapy with antimicrobials and glucocorticoids. Antimicrobial therapy should consist of one of the following drugs: amoxicillin clavulanate (62.5 mg PO q12h), cefovecin (8 mg/kg SC q14days), cefpodoxime proxetil (5–10 mg/kg PO q24h), or clindamycin (10–15 mg/kg PO q12h); while systemic glucocorticoid therapy with oral methylprednisolone (1–2 mg/kg PO q24h) or prednisolone (1–2 mg/kg PO q24h) is effective. In cats difficult to orally medicate, injectable methylprednisolone acetate (up to 20 mg/cat SC) is a possible alternative; however, this option should be used with caution.
iii. The most common reason for recurrent indolent ulcers in the cat is an underlying allergic hypersensitivity to parasites, fleas, food, or an environmental allergen. In rare instances, recurrent lesions have also been associated with viral or dermatophyte infections. Failure to properly identify and address the primary underlying cause will continue to lead recurrence in these patients.

86. This is stain precipitate. This is an artifact that in some instances is misidentified as bacteria by untrained veterinarians and staff. Stain precipitate formation occurs secondary to pH changes in the stain, when the stain gets excessively dirty, if stain solution is not changed or left uncovered for extended periods of time leading to evaporation and concentration of the agent, or if slides are not properly rinsed once stained.

87. i. Cytology reveals the presence of a Gram-negative rod-shaped bacterial population. Given the clinical symptoms and bacterial characteristics, *Pseudomonas aeruginosa* is the most likely etiologic agent. Other Gram-negative rod-shaped organisms that are associated with canine bacterial otitis include *Proteus* spp., *Escherichia coli*, and *Klebsiella*. Bacterial otitis externa associated with *Pseudomonas* frequently presents with acute, severe suppurative inflammation, canal ulcerations, discomfort, and pain that require immediate treatment.

ii. The majority of topical products approved for use in canine otitis contain a combination of an antibacterial, antifungal, and glucocorticoid. Several factors should be considered in product selection: (1) What is the target organism? (2) What is the probability that the chosen medication will completely kill the organism and decrease the chance for resistance development? (3) What product is least likely to result in a possible adverse event? and (4) How likely is it that the owner will adhere to the therapeutic protocol? Given the target organism, potential antimicrobial options commercially available would include fluoroquinolones (enrofloxacin, marbofloxacin, and orbifloxacin), aminoglycosides (neomycin and gentamycin), polymyxin B, or silver sulfadiazine. In a case such as this, where concerns may exist for tympanic membrane integrity due to poor visualization as a result of excessive exudate, a fluoroquinolone is likely the best option. Fluoroquinolones target the organism, can be delivered at high concentrations, are concentration dependent and facilitate once-daily dosing to help improve therapy compliance, and avoid potential ototoxicity concerns that exist with aminoglycosides and polymyxin B.

iii. The author has observed three common reasons for treatment failure of canine otitis externa. The first is a lack of appropriate treatment length. All cases of canine otitis externa should be medicated for a minimum of 2 weeks with follow-up examination and repeat cytology to determine if treatment should be extended. Although some of the newer commercial products entering the veterinary marketplace require less than 2 weeks of administration, most provide extended residual activity in the ear canal beyond the suggested 2-week time frame. The next reason for treatment failure is an inadequate volume of medication is instilled into the ear canal. Although the exact volume of medication to instill into a dog's ear to ensure appropriate contact is unknown, it is clear that the standard recommended amount of ear drops labeled on most commercial ear products is insufficient, especially in larger dogs. The last reason is actually perceived treatment failure due to recurrence of bacterial or fungal otitis externa. It is important to remember that in recurrent otitis externa, the bacterial or fungal component is a secondary infection due to a primary problem. Primary causes of canine otitis externa include parasites, allergic hypersensitivities, endocrine dysfunction, foreign bodies, keratinization disorders, or neoplasia. Failure to address and properly manage the primary cause of the secondary infection will continue to result in recurrence despite adequate therapy of the infectious component.

88. A 2-year-old neutered male DSH cat presented for evaluation following adoption from a local shelter. The owner did not have any concerns regarding the patient, and physical exam along with blood work were unremarkable. However, on fecal floatation the following was found (**Figure 88a**).

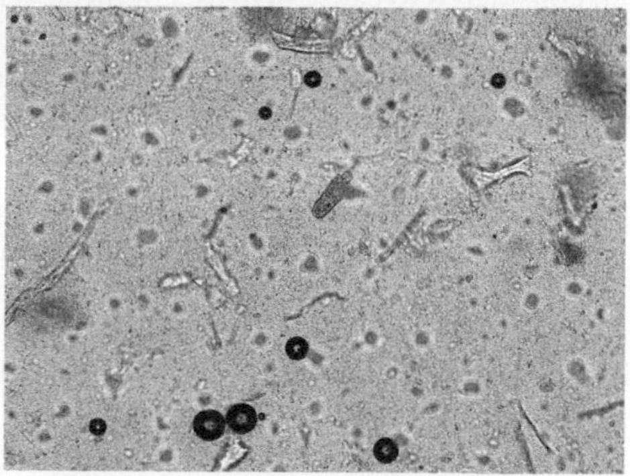

Figure 88a

i. What is the name of this parasite?

ii. What is unique about this species compared to other species of this mite family affect dogs and cats?

iii. What should be recommended at this time for this patient?

89. A *Cheyletiella* spp. egg is shown in **Figure 89a**.

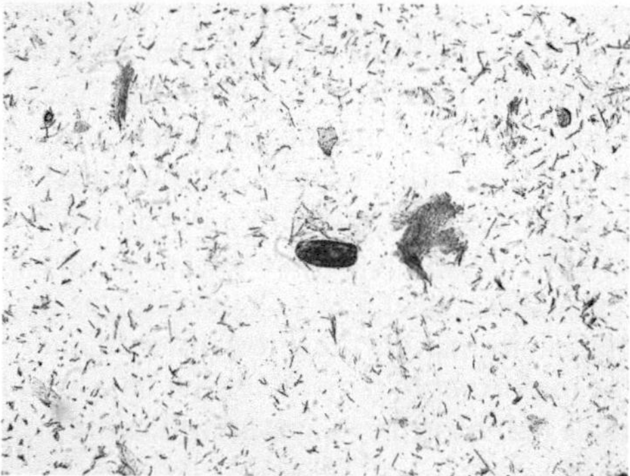

Figure 89a

What various diagnostic methods have been used to demonstrate this mite as a cause of disease in dogs or cats?

90. Pyriproxyfen and methoprene are both juvenile hormone analogs that are commonly utilized in flea treatment/preventative products.

What is the major difference between these two products that may need to be taken into account depending on the intended patient's lifestyle?

88. **i.** *Demodex gatoi.*

ii. The mite is unique with respect to other variants of *Demodex* spp. (1) It is the only contagious form of demodicosis known at this time and (2) is considered a primary cause of pruritus in cats. Other species of *Demodex* have historically not been considered to cause pruritus in the absence of secondary infections. (3) It resides on the surface of the skin. Other species of *Demodex* mites are considered follicular. (4) Lime sulfur is the most efficacious treatment option at this time, which is not the case with the other species known to cause disease in dogs and cats.

iii. Based on limited evidence-based reviews for feline demodicosis treatment protocols, there is evidence to support application of lime sulfur 2% as a topical dip once weekly (Mueller, 2004). To date, lime sulfur has been the most efficacious treatment for feline *D. gatoi* infestations. There is also evidence to support the recommendation of amitraz rinses (0.0125%–0.025% weekly). Cats may be more sensitive to the side effects of this treatment option compared with dogs; if considered, it is generally recommended to use a lower concentration. There are also case reports that describe the efficacy of a combination spot-on product containing imidacloprid 10% plus moxidectin 2.5% for treatment (Short and Gram, 2016). Anecdotally, a topical spot-on product containing a 28% solution of fluralaner has also been observed to be effective when applied at the labeled dose and frequency for flea prevention in cats. Well-designed clinical trials to evaluate these treatment options need to be performed prior to widespread acceptance as the standard of care. Additionally for the owner, all in-contact cats should be treated as this is a contagious parasite, and the shelter should be notified so that they are aware of possible exposure or endemic disease.

89. The diagnosis of cheyletiellosis is confirmed by demonstrating a mite or an ova. Many techniques have been suggested and include skin scraping, acetate tape impressions, and flea combing the patient and collecting the material into a Petri dish and then either examining the material with a dissecting microscope or dissolving the material in 10% potassium hydroxide and then fecal float the material to observe it similar to evaluating a patient for intestinal nematodes. In cats, a fecal float may be rewarding as this species can have meticulous grooming habits making the mites more difficult to identify readily on examination. It is important to remember that on a fecal float, *Cheyletiella* spp. eggs will resemble hookworm ova, just significantly larger.

90. The major difference with respect to these products is their stability in the presence of UV light. Methoprene is sensitive to UV light and therefore would be a questionable product selection for a dog or cat that predominantly lives outdoors.

91. The lateral aspect of a 5-year-old German shepherd is shown after the hair coat clipped (**Figure 91a**). The dog presented because of fever, depression, malodor, and pruritus. Upon examination, multiple hemorrhagic bullae and draining tracts with serosanguineous discharge were noted along the lateral rear legs and ventral abdominal region. The patient was also noted to have pain upon manipulation of these regions.

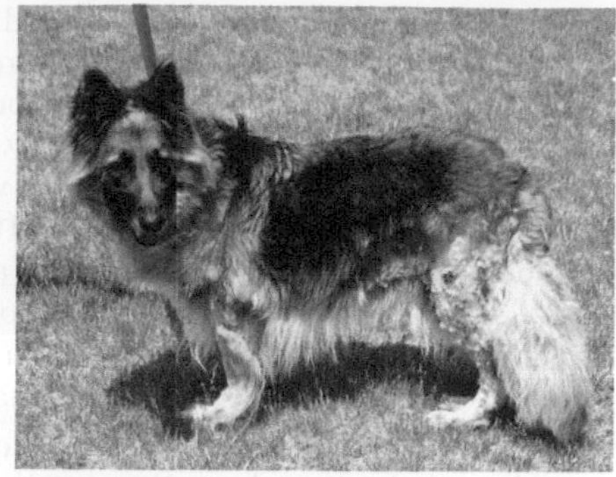

Figure 91a

i. What clinical entity is suspected based on presentation and exam findings?

ii. What diagnostics should be recommended?

iii. What is the recommended treatment for this patient?

92. A 4-month-old kitten presented for hair loss and crusting along both ears (**Figure 92a**). Further questioning of the owner revealed that the kitten was the only cat in the household and that it was adopted 2 weeks prior from a local shelter. The owner also noted the kitten frequently scratched at the area. A Wood's lamp examination of the kitten failed to reveal green fluorescence of hairs. Skin scrapings, flea combings, skin cytology, and ear swabs also failed to reveal any potential etiologic agents. A DTM plate was inoculated via a toothbrush culture technique. Given the presentation and signalment, dermatophytosis is still the top differential for this patient's clinical lesions despite the negative diagnostic findings.

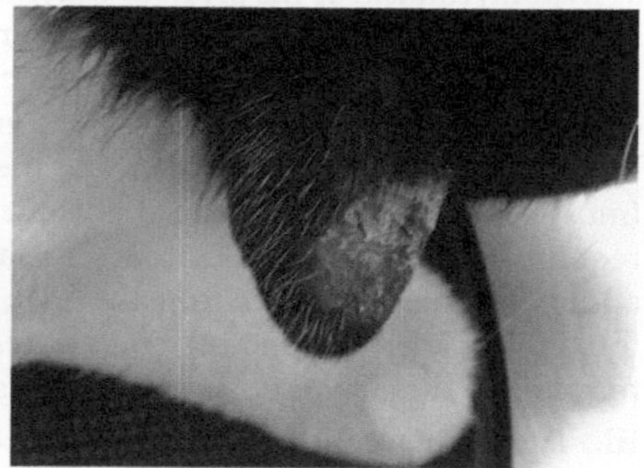

Figure 92a

i. What recommendations are important to make for the next 1–2 weeks until the final culture results are available?

ii. What is the most common error made when interpreting DTM cultures in-house?

91. i. The clinical presentation and findings in this case are consistent with German shepherd pyoderma. This syndrome is poorly understood, and the exact etiology at this time is unknown but thought to be multifactorial and the result of a possible immunodeficiency. This syndrome represents a unique presentation of recurrent deep pyoderma with lesions typically found over the lumbosacral region, ventral abdomen, and thighs. The condition is encountered in middle-aged German shepherds with a familial predisposition. Given the lack of complete understanding of this condition, it should be simply viewed as a classic clinical syndrome of German shepherds triggered by a variety of possible etiologies in susceptible individuals (Rosser, 2006).

ii. Initially, skin scrapings should be acquired to rule out demodicosis as a possible underlying etiology. Skin cytology samples should also be acquired to verify the presence of bacterial organisms from lesions. The consistent use of adulticidal flea prevention should be confirmed to rule out underlying flea allergy dermatitis as a triggering cause. Subsequently, routine blood work such as a CBC count, serum chemistries, urinalysis, and total thyroxine level should be obtained to screen the patient for a possible underlying endocrinopathy such as hypothyroidism as the primary cause for the secondary pyoderma. Finally, as this is a case of deep pyoderma, a bacterial culture should be acquired to aid in the appropriate selection of a systemic antibiotic. A culture is obtained in cases of deep pyoderma for several reasons: (1) many patients have previously been treated with prior antibiotics, and the incidence of resistance is increasing (most common bacteria isolated is *S. pseudintermedius*); (2) deep pyoderma requires extended therapeutic courses of antimicrobials, and an ideal systemic antibiotic should be chosen from the start; and (3) cultures should be submitted for aerobic, anerobic, and fungal cultures, as anerobic and fungal infections may mimic the clinical appearance of this syndrome.

iii. Treatment for this condition involves the use of a systemic antibiotic based on culture and sensitivity results. It is important that whatever antimicrobial agent is selected, that it be given at the appropriate dose and frequency. Additionally, it must be given for an appropriate length of time. The rule for treating deep pyoderma is to treat for 2 weeks past clinical resolution. This may result in some dogs being on antibiotics for up to 6–8 weeks, or even longer in severe cases. Some authors have also suggested the use of whirlpool soaks to hasten resolution of clinical lesions. The use of topical agents such as shampoos should be questioned in these patients as the pyoderma is deep not superficial, and many patients have pain during the initial phase of treatment. When possible, however, topical shampoo therapy should be brought into the treatment regimen. Rechecks should be scheduled every 2–4 weeks until clinical resolution is reached. It is also important to identify and treat the primary cause of the recurrent infection to prevent further episodes. Possible primary causes for this recurrent infection are flea allergy dermatitis, atopy, cutaneous adverse food reaction, and endocrinopathy (i.e., hypothyroidism, Cushing disease, etc.).

92. i. First, pending disease confirmation, the owner should restrict the kitten's access to areas of the home that are easily cleaned to prevent spreading spores around the environment. Second, the owners should clean the areas that the kitten has access to frequently to mechanically remove debris and wash laundry items to decontaminate them. Third, use disinfectants on items that cannot be thoroughly cleaned. Fourth, the owner should be encouraged to start topical therapy on the patient to minimize the spread of spores in the environment and begin treatment. Systemic antifungals should only be used in patients with confirmed disease via culture, dermatophyte PCR, or observation of fungal elements on cytology/trichogram. Fifth, any other health issues the kitten may have should be addressed. Finally, the owner should be instructed to use common sense and good hygiene after handling the kitten as dermatophytosis is a zoonotic disease.

ii. The most common problem encountered with in-house DTM fungal cultures is the high number of false-positive results when identification of a dermatophyte is made using only the color change as the sole diagnostic criteria. Although dermatophytes induce a color change, many nondermatophyte species will also induce a color change and may have similar colony morphology. Diagnostic confirmation requires microscopic identification. This is the step most often skipped due to the veterinarian's or the staff's lack of comfort with the appearance of fungal elements microscopically.

93. A 5-year-old DSH cat presented for a second opinion due to right-sided facial swelling and draining lesions that also affect the bridge of the nose (**Figure 93a**). The owner reports that the lesions initially began as a single bump and crust over the right side of the nose that has gradually enlarged and become more severe despite several courses of systemic antibiotics. The cat lives in the Midwest region of the United States and lives primarily indoors with occasional unsupervised time outdoors. Despite the rather shocking dermatologic lesions, the patient was otherwise healthy on examination with only a mildly elevated rectal temperature. To start, an impression smear was taken of the exudate from the open lesions, the results of which are shown in **Figure 93b**.

i. What is your diagnosis, and what is the likely source of this infection?

ii. What drugs have been used successfully to treat this disease in cats? What is the prognosis, and how can therapy be monitored?

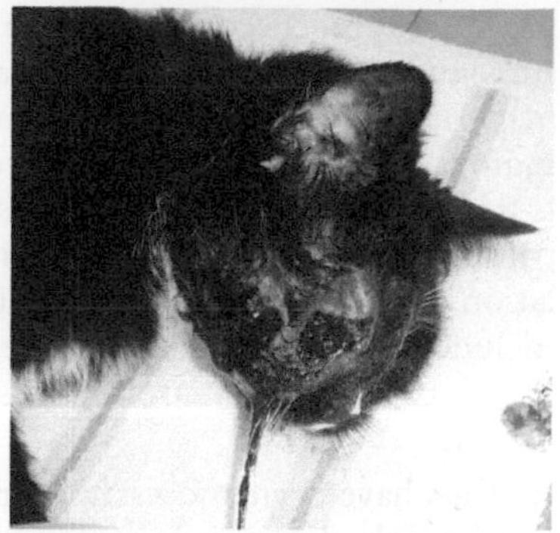

Figure 93a

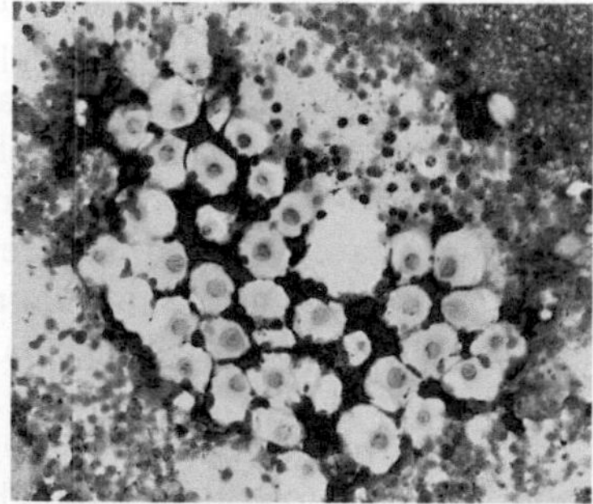

Figure 93b

94. **Figure 94a** shows a proprietary food that may be considered a novel protein diet for use during diet elimination trials.

i. What is meant by the term *novel*, and what are some examples of commercial novel protein sources?

ii. What are common documented food allergens of dogs and cats?

iii. What issues exists with finding appropriate novel protein diets for patients?

iv. While discussing recommendations with an owner for their nonseasonally pruritic dog, the owner says that they have done a lot of online research and want to know why you are recommending a diet elimination trial and not a blood test that they have read so much about. How should this owner's question be answered?

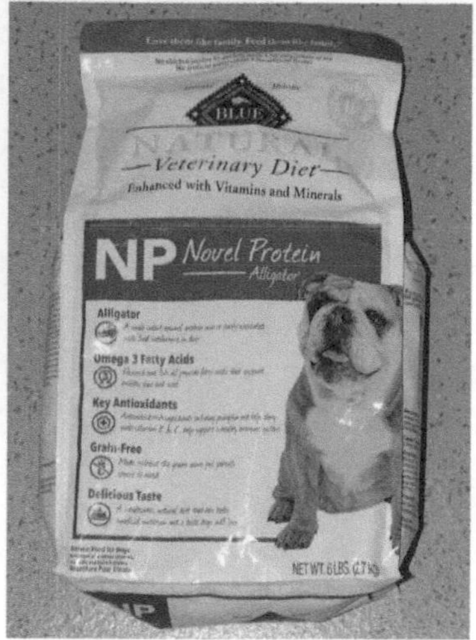

Figure 94a

93. i. Cryptococcosis. This organism is identified by the enormous capsule surrounding the yeast cells. This is a deep fungal disease caused by *Cryptococcus neoformans* or *C. gattii*. The fungus has a worldwide distribution and is commonly associated with decaying vegetation and pigeon feces. Cryptococcosis is the most common deep mycosis of cats. The agent is primarily an airborne pathogen with the nasal cavity being the primary site of infection, but inoculation and ingestion of the organism can also lead to disease. Clinical signs include upper respiratory disease, chronic nasal discharge, masses over the bridge of the nose, neurologic disturbances, cutaneous nodules, and ocular disease.

ii. Cats have been successfully treated with amphotericin B, ketoconazole, itraconazole, fluconazole, and terbinafine. However, amphotericin B and ketoconazole are not tolerated well by cats and should be avoided if possible. At this time, fluconazole is thought to be the treatment of choice as it is better tolerated by cats than the other options and also penetrates sites such as the CNS and eye better than itraconazole. Additionally, limited studies suggest that overall treatment duration is shorter with fluconazole (Pennisi et al., 2013). Overall, prognosis is favorable in most cases unless neurologic disease and dissemination have occurred. **Figure 93c** shows the patient after just 8 weeks of therapy with fluconazole and wound management. Therapy can be monitored by using the cryptococcal capsular antigen test, which can be run on serum, cerebrospinal fluid (CSF), or urine. Therapy is continued until the antigen test is negative. In cases where the owner does not wish to monitor this test or it is not available, treatment should be continued until at least 2–4 months after resolution of clinical signs.

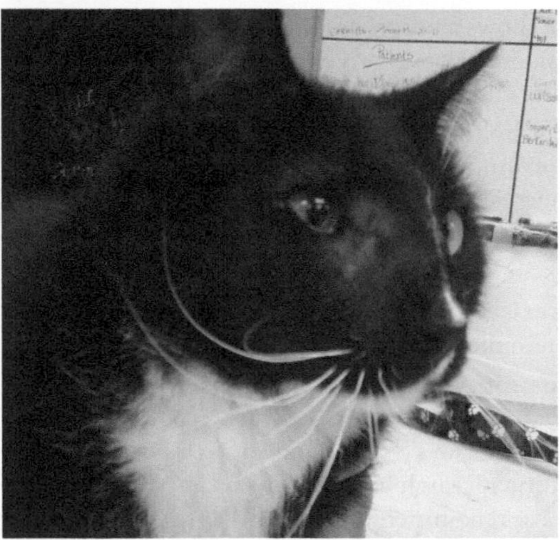

Figure 93c

94. i. The term *novel* is meant to refer to a new protein that the patient has never encountered. However many times, novel is interpreted as hypoallergenic, and this is simply not the case. There is nothing special about a novel protein other than the simple concept that the patient has not previously consumed the item, so therefore, the likelihood of having developed an allergic hypersensitivity to the food item is extremely low. Commercially available novel protein diets include items such as venison, rabbit, duck, kangaroo, lamb, alligator, bison, and horse.

ii. The most frequently reported food items in dogs associated with cutaneous adverse food reactions are beef, dairy products, chicken, wheat, lamb, soy, corn, egg, pork, and fish. In cats, the most commonly documented or reported food allergens are beef, fish, chicken, wheat, corn, dairy products, lamb, and egg (Mueller et al., 2016). It is important to remember that how common an offending food allergen is will vary geographically and mirror those ingredients commonly included in pet foods in that region.

iii. There are two main issues that exist with trying to find a commercially available novel protein diet for a small animal patient. The first is that it is often difficult to obtain an accurate diet history from many pet owners. Confounding this issue are studies showing identification of undeclared protein sources in over-the-counter diets via enzyme-linked immunosorbent assay (ELISA), PCR, and bone fragment sedimentation analysis (Ricci et al., 2013). What these studies showed is that even if you can obtain an accurate diet history, it is highly likely that the pet has been exposed to other proteins not included on the label. The second issue is the concern surrounding the potential for cross-reactivity. Theoretically speaking, the closer animals are taxonomically, the higher is the risk that an individual may be allergic to both species. Practically speaking, if a patient is allergic to beef, then it is possible that the patient may also be allergic to other ruminants such as lamb, venison, bison, and so on. Although this concept has not been well-documented in veterinary patients, it is indeed a consideration when trying to select the most appropriate diet for a patient during an elimination trial.

iv. The simple answer to this particular owner's question is that although companies offer blood testing for food allergens, these tests when evaluated independently fail to provide reliable differentiation between allergic and non-allergic pets, have low repeatability, and are inaccurate at identifying the offending food allergen in confirmed food allergic patients. Therefore, at this time, they are not reliable and cannot be recommended (Mueller and Olivry, 2017).

95. Recently, two similar long-acting otic medications Claro and Osurnia were introduced to the veterinary marketplace.

What are the major differences between these two products?

96. *Cuterebra* spp. infestations in the dog and cat typically manifest as large nodular swellings of the skin and subcutaneous tissues with a central opening.

i. Besides the cutaneous manifestations, what other symptoms have been reported as a result of *Cuterebra* infestation in dogs and cats?

ii. What nonsurgical method can be tried to remove a *Cuterebra* larva?

97. It is late spring, and the local television stations have been televising public service announcements about the dangers of sunbathing. The announcements included a list of various types of skin tumors that can develop in people as a result of excessive sun exposure (basal cell tumors, squamous cell carcinomas, and melanoma). They are stressing that people with any suspicious lesions are urged to seek a consultation with their physician. One day, a very distressed owner calls and requests a "skin cancer check" for her dog. During the examination, she points out a raised, solitary, pigmented lesion that has rapidly developed on the dorsum of her West Highland white terrier dog (**Figure 97a**).

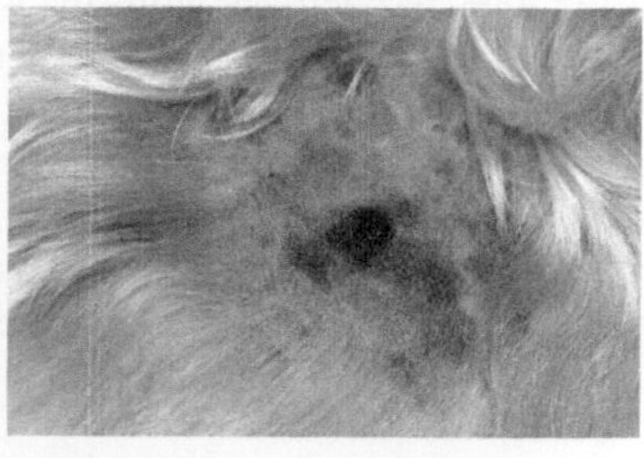
Figure 97a

i. What is the most likely diagnosis, and how should this lesion be managed?

ii. What role does breed play in predicting prognostic significance?

iii. What roles does lesion location have in predicting benign or malignant behavior?

98. A 5-year-old castrated male Rhodesian ridgeback dog presented for the recent appearance of firm, dark brown-black, "bumps" noticed within the last month. Physical exam reveals several, small, 5–6 mm diameter hyperpigmented papules that are firm on palpation and present over the lateral left rear leg and dorsal lumbar region (**Figure 98a**). The owner was recently diagnosed with melanoma and is concerned about the same possibility in their dog and asks you to biopsy a couple of the masses in order to determine their origin.

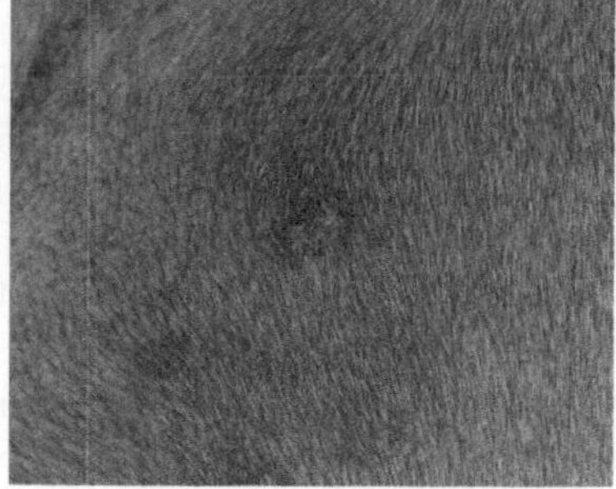
Figure 98a

Describe the basic steps for acquiring a punch biopsy sample.

95. Although these two products are similar in nature, there are several differences with respect to formulation and labeled administration that users should be aware of. The first difference between the two products has to do with the vehicle formulation, which in the case of Claro is a solution, while Osurnia is a gel. Second, the steroid that is found in both products also differs. In the case of Claro, it contains mometasone, while betamethasone is used in Osurnia. The next difference between the two is with respect to the concentration of antimicrobials each contains. In both instances, florfenicol and terbinafine are the active ingredients, but their content is slightly different in both products. In Claro, the concentrations of florfenicol and terbinafine are 1.66% and 1.48%, respectively, while in Osurnia they are both 1%. The final difference between the two products is how they are labeled to be administered. With Claro, the product is instilled into the affected ear once with duration of activity expected for 30 days, and during this time, the ear should not be cleaned as it may affect efficacy. In the case of Osurnia, the product is instilled into an affected ear once, with a second dose reapplied in 7 days, and the ear should not be cleaned for 45 days after the initial administration so as not to disrupt contact of the gel with the ear canal.

96. i. Other clinical symptoms that have been reported are commonly associated with aberrant migration of the larvae through tissues other than the skin. These include anaphylaxis, respiratory complications, ocular issues, and CNS symptoms. Neurologic symptoms are reported to include mental dullness and seizures. Helpful historical findings that may indicate a patient's neurologic symptoms are related to aberrant larval migration include time of year symptoms were first observed (July through September; northern hemisphere), outdoor exposure, or a recent upper respiratory infection (Glass et al., 1998). Additionally, a recent investigation suggests that small breed dogs may also have severe systemic manifestations such as protein-losing nephropathy, systemic inflammatory response syndrome, disseminated intravascular coagulation, or multiple organ dysfunction, which may result in death (Rutland et al., 2017).

ii. Encouraging the larva to "self-extrude" is a technique that can occasionally be successful when smaller larvae are present or when an owner is significantly limited financially. To perform this technique, an occlusive lotion, ointment, or substance (i.e., petroleum jelly) is placed over the breathing hole, which then triggers the parasite to back out of the hole.

97. i. The most likely cause is a melanocytic neoplasm or cutaneous melanoma. Cutaneous melanomas can be benign or malignant. Benign lesions (also called *melanocytoma*) are usually well-defined, deeply pigmented, less than 2 cm in diameter, and mobile. Areas of pigmentation that are congenital and are most likely part of a dog's normal skin coloration are called melanocytic nevi. The treatment of choice is radical surgical excision, and submission of the lesion for histological examination and determination of margins.

ii. Breed may have an important role in differential diagnosis development and likely biologic behavior. Cutaneous melanomas occur more commonly in dogs with heavy skin pigmentation such as the schnauzer (miniature and standard) and Scottish terrier. The prior breeds along with the Irish setter and golden retriever are at an increased risk of developing subungual melanoma. Chihuahuas, golden retrievers, and cocker spaniels develop melanoma of the lip more commonly, while German shepherds and boxers are prone to oral melanomas (Smith et al., 2002).

iii. Melanocytic tumors arising in the oral cavity are the most common oral malignant neoplasm and should always be considered aggressive. Cutaneous melanomas are common, but less than 5% of them end up classified as malignant. Subungual melanoma is the second most common tumor of the digit, and radiographic evidence of metastasis is present in greater than 50% of cases (Smith et al., 2002).

98. The first step is to either leave the site alone or gently clip the site and lightly soak the area with a solution of 70% alcohol if needed (**Figure 98b**). Care must be taken to ensure the skin is not traumatized or meaningful surface debris removed. If crusts are present or disorders of keratinization are suspected, clipping and light cleaning should be avoided. Biopsy sites for histopatology samples should never be scrubbed. These activities may remove important surface pathology or create iatrogenic inflammatory lesions. Next, the subcutaneous region under the lesion is infused with roughly up to 1 mL of local anesthetic (1%–2% lidocaine) per site (in smaller patients, the toxic dose of lidacaine should be calculated prior to this step as not to surpass the potential toxic threshold) with a 25-gauge or smaller needle (**Figure 98c**). Lidocaine can sting when injected and may cause some animals to object to the process. The use of sodium bicarbonate at a ratio of 10:1 (lidocaine:bicarb) can be done to buffer the lidocaine. Care should be taken to ensure lidocaine is not directly injected into the lesion or intradermally. The skin punch biopsy is then placed

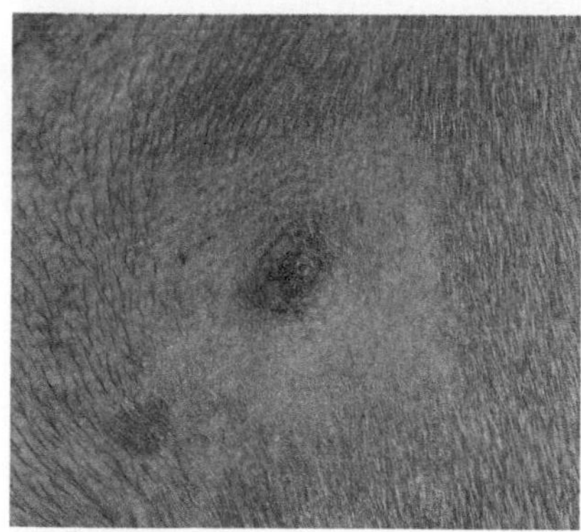

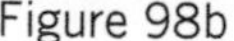

Figure 98b

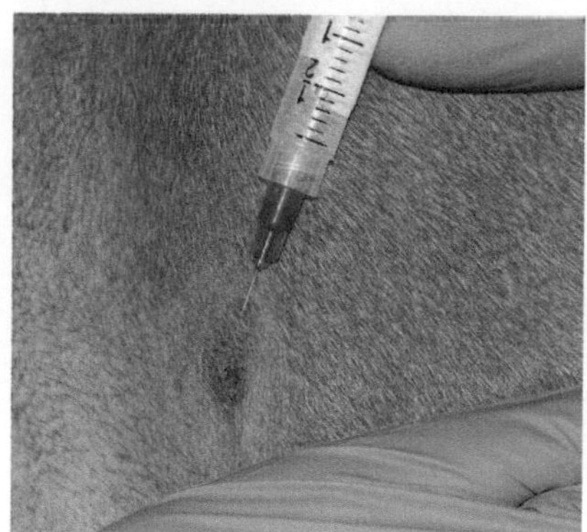

Figure 98c

directly over the lesion. A 6-mm punch biopsy sample normally provides a sufficient sample, but in this case an 8-mm punch biopsy was used to ensure complete removal of the lesion (**Figure 98d**). Next, the skin around the biopsy site should be tensed to prevent shearing the sample, and light but firm pressure is applied to the instrument while it is rotated in *one* direction until the sample is "free" from the surrounding tissue. It is not necessary when using a punch biopsy to bury it up to the hub when acquiring samples, especially in areas where the skin is thinner. The skin around the biopsy is then pinched to help "pop" the sample out and facilitate grasping the subcutaneous stalk of the sample, and it is then lifted up and excised with curved iris scissors or a scalpel blade (**Figure 98e**). Care needs to be taken during this step to prevent crushing artifact or removal of surface debris such as a crust. The sample is then placed on a tongue depressor and allowed to lightly dry and adhere prior to being placed in formalin (**Figure 98f**). This step helps prevent curling of the sample and allows the pathologist to better orient the specimen prior to trimming and sectioning. Finally, the defect is closed with a single cruciate or simple interrupted sutures (**Figure 98g**).

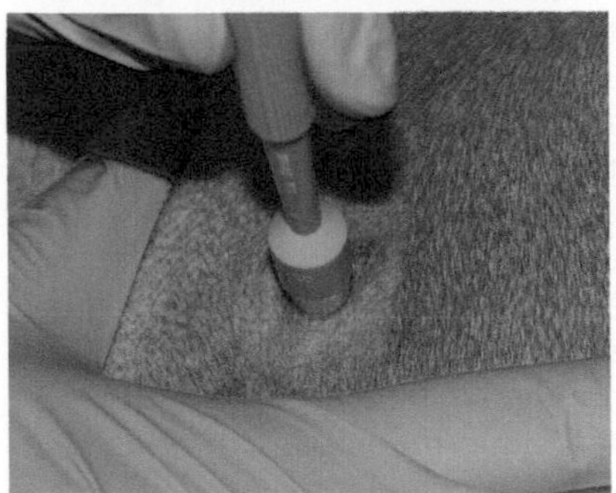

Figure 98d

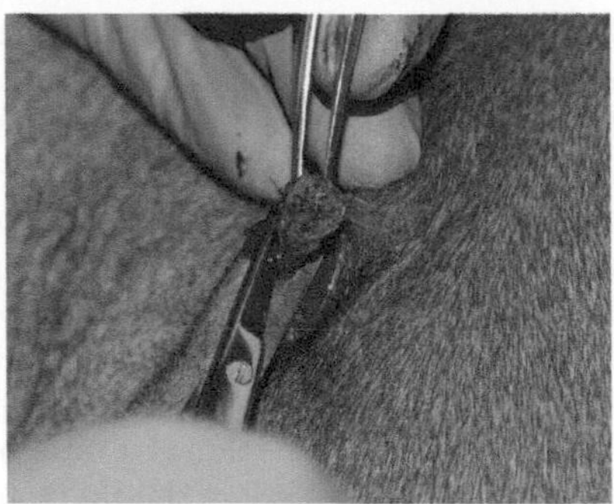

Figure 98e

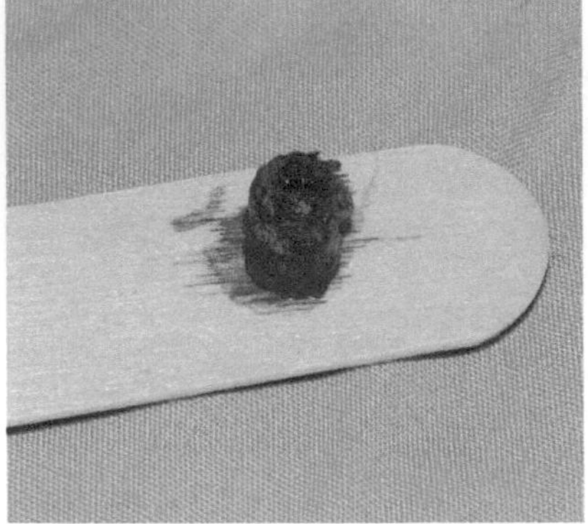

Figure 98f

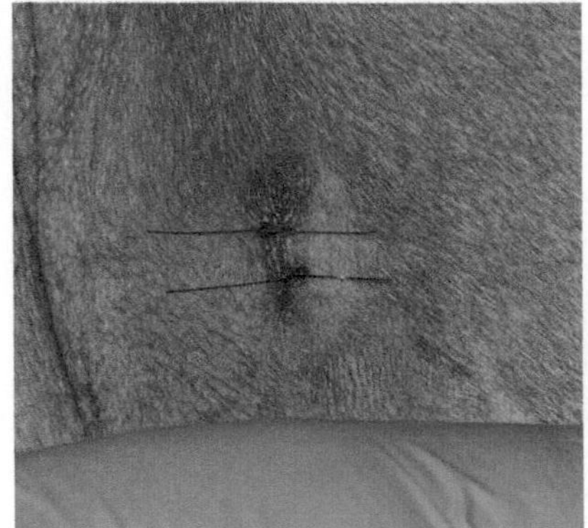

Figure 98g

99. Macrocyclic lactones are commonly utilized in therapeutic protocols for treating ecto- and endoparasitism in dogs and cats. Concern with the use of this class of medications arises in patients who have a multidrug resistant-1 (MDR-1) gene mutation affecting P-glycoprotein.

i. What exactly does the gene mutation do to P-glycoprotein?

ii. Where in the body is P-glycoprotein found?

iii. Besides macrocyclic lactones, what other drugs may create issues in patients with an MDR-1 gene mutation?

iv. What drugs when administered at clinically used doses in dogs can result in P-glycoprotein inhibition creating drug-drug interactions that can mimic adverse events observed in MDR-1 mutant dogs?

100. **Figure 100a** shows the three tablet strengths of oclacitinib (Apoquel) that are produced and currently available through Zoetis.

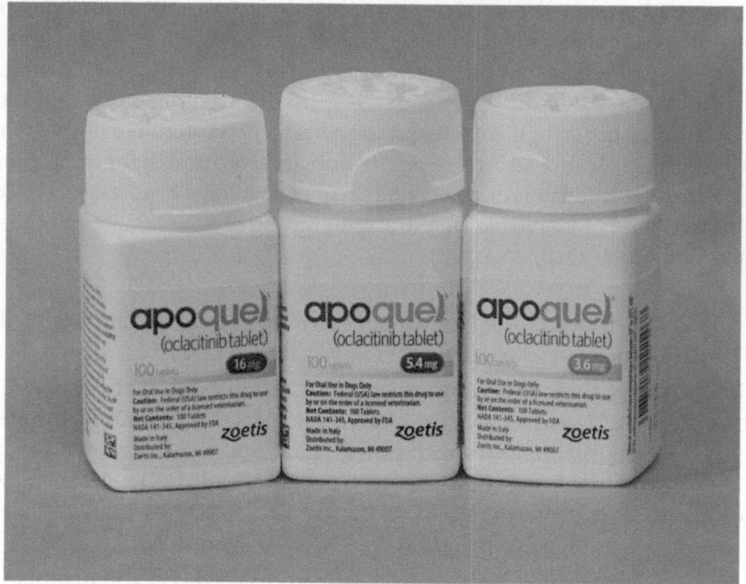

Figure 100a

i. What is the labeled indication for this drug?

ii. What is Oclacitinib's pharmacologic mechanism of action?

iii. What is the recommended dosing for this medication?

iv. What are possible adverse events associated with use of this medication?

101. Seborrheic dermatitis is a commonly used term in veterinary medicine. However, what does this term mean, what is the difference between primary and secondary seborrhea, and what are keratolytic and keratoplastic agents?

99. **i.** P-glycoprotein is a transmembrane efflux transporter. The MDR-1 gene mutation (also referred to as ABCB1-Δ1 gene) results in a 4-base pair gene deletion that generates several premature stop codons. This results in the production of a fragment of P-glycoprotein, which creates compromised transporter function.

ii. P-glycoprotein is present within the small intestine, colon, biliary ductules, renal tubules, CNS, blood-brain barrier, pancreas, placenta, blood-retinal barrier, and blood-testes barrier (Martinez et al., 2008).

iii. Other drugs where exaggerated side effects or toxicities have been observed in dogs with MDR-1 gene mutations include doxorubicin, vincristine, vinblastine, digoxin, butorphanol, loperamide, acepromazine, and ondansetron (Mealey, 2013).

iv. Many drugs based on data in humans or rodents can inhibit P-glycoprotein function and include fluoxetine, erythromycin, ketoconazole, itraconazole, diltiazem, quinidine, verapamil, cyclosporine, tacrolimus, and spinosad. However, evidence for these potentially clinically relevant drug-drug interactions in the dog exists only for ketoconazole and spinosad. Ketoconazole has been shown to increase brain penetration of ivermectin in dogs lacking an MDR-1 mutation when the drugs are coadministered, resulting in neurologic toxicity. Similar neurologic toxicity has also been encountered in dogs simultaneously receiving spinosad for flea prevention and ivermectin for management of demodicosis. Additionally, severe adverse events have been experienced in dogs prescribed ketoconazole that are undergoing concurrent chemotherapy (Mealey and Fidel, 2015).

100. **i.** Oclacitinib is labeled for the control of pruritus associated with allergic dermatitis and control of atopic dermatitis in dogs at least 12 months of age.

ii. Oclacitinib is a selective janus kinase (JAK) inhibitor that preferentially inhibits JAK-1, and to a lesser degree JAK-2 and JAK-3. Via inhibition of these pathways, oclacitinib interferes with pruritogenic and pro-inflammatory cytokine activity (interleukin-2 [IL-2], IL-4, IL-6, IL-13, and IL-31) associated with canine atopic dermatitis.

iii. The recommended initial dose of oclacitinib is 0.4–0.6 mg/kg of body weight administered orally twice a day for up to 14 days. The drug is then given at the same dose once daily for maintenance therapy. The requirement for long-term therapy should be based on an individual patient assessment. Oclacitinib can be given with or without food.

iv. Potential adverse events attributed to the administration of oclacitinib at this time are relatively low but include vomiting, diarrhea, anorexia, lethargy, development of nonspecific dermal lumps, development of pyoderma or otitis, weight loss/gain, behavior changes, lymphadenopathy, development or reactivation of demodicosis, potential increased susceptibility to papilloma viral infections, and neoplasia. Although several dogs did develop neoplastic disease during various phases of clinical trials, there is currently no definitive evidence that the use of oclacitinb is associated with the development of cancer in dogs.

101. The general term for scaling is *seborrhea.* This is not a clinical diagnosis but rather a clinical description of a type of skin lesion. Seborrhea has two basic etiologies: primary seborrhea and secondary seborrhea. Primary seborrhea is caused by an inherited disorder of keratinization of the epidermis. Examples of primary seborrheic conditions are primary seborrhea of the American cocker spaniel and ichthyosis of golden retrievers. Secondary seborrhea occurs when any external or internal disease alters the normal development of the skin. It is simply the skin's response to insult. It may occur as a result of secondary infections, parasites, allergic dermatitis, endocrine disorders, nutritional disturbances, immune-mediated conditions, and owner factors (excessive bathing). A keratolytic agent creates decreased cohesion between keratinocytes increasing desquamation. This results in a softening of the stratum corneum and removal of scales. Examples of keratolytic agents are benzoyl peroxide and salicyclic acid at high concentrations (3%–6%). A keratoplastic agent attempts to normalize the process of keratinization and includes active ingredients such as salicyclic acid at low concentrations (0.1%–2%), sulfur, and coal tar.

102. A 4-year-old spayed female Siamese cat presented for examination of progressive skin lesions that have failed to respond to prior treatment with antimicrobials. Lesions began acutely developing on the cat's skin 2 months ago, and since that time she is reported to be lethargic with a decreased appetite. There is one other cat in the household with no reported skin issues, and the two have been housemates for the past 3 years. Dermatologic examination revealed the presence of adherent crust symmetrically affecting the periocular, perioral, auricular, and dorsal muzzle regions along with numerous paw pads and claw bed regions (**Figure 102a–d**). Small crusts could be palpated in the hair coat, and careful examination of the cat revealed crusts around the nipples. Additionally, the physical exam revealed a slightly elevated rectal temperature.

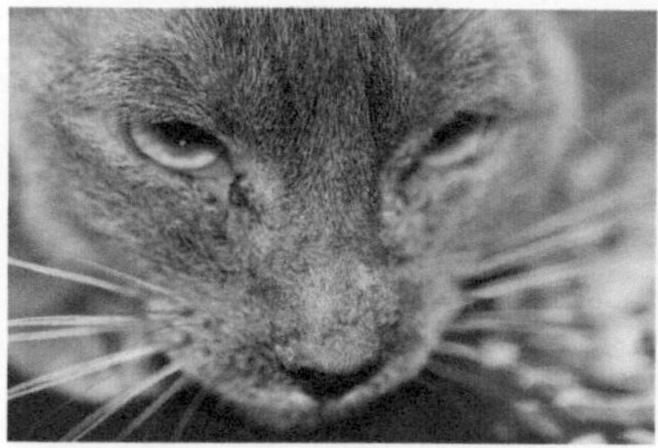

Figure 102a

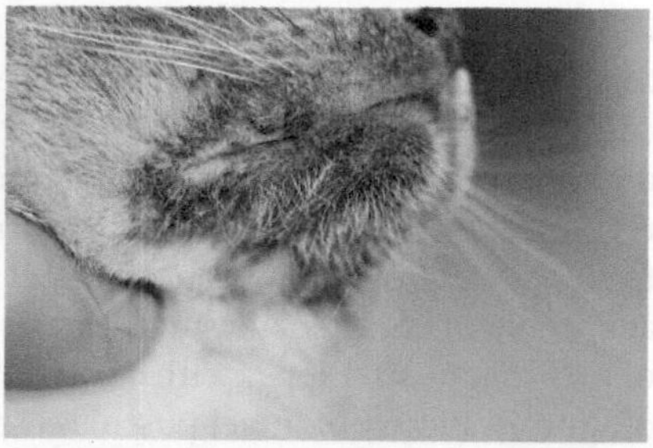

Figure 102b

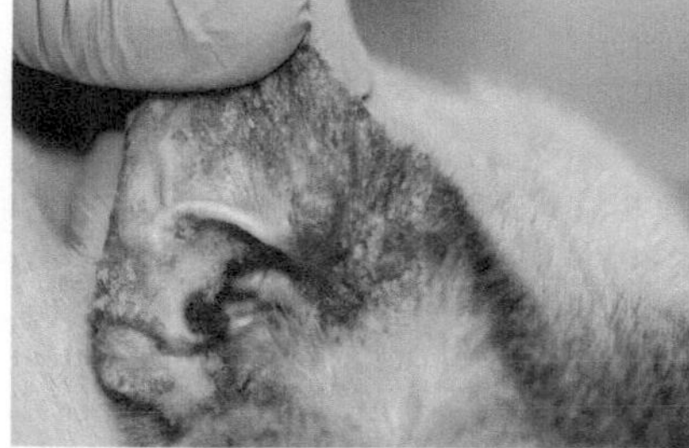

Figure 102c

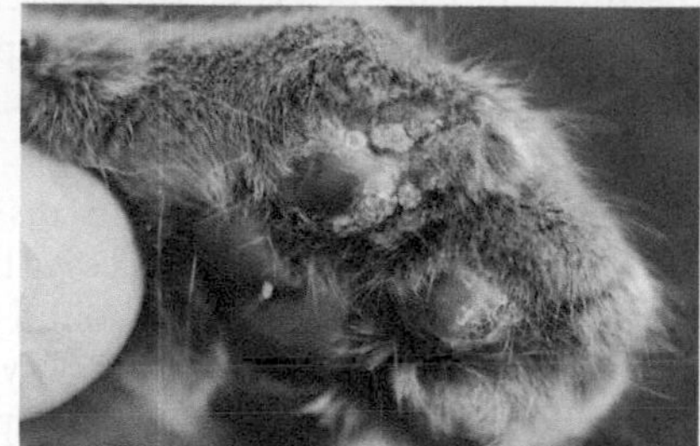

Figure 102d

i. Given this patient's history and physical examination findings, what is the most likely diagnosis?

ii. What diagnostic tests should be performed?

iii. How is this disease treated, and what is the prognosis?

102. i. Although dermatophytosis should be considered in any case of generalized scaling and crusting seen in a cat, the symmetrical facial, auricular, perinipple, and footpad crusting, in combination with systemic signs observed in this case, are most suspicious for pemphigus foliaceus (PF). PF is an uncommon immune-mediated skin disease of cats (probably the most common autoimmune skin disease) that in many cases is idiopathic but may be drug related. Pruritus is common in cats with PF. There are no breed or sex predilections seen with the disease in cats. The hallmark lesion is a superficial pustule; however, intact pustules are often difficult to find as they easily rupture resulting in crust formation as seen in this case. PF tends to have symmetrical lesion formation at characteristic locations such as the ear pinnae, rostral muzzle, nasal planum, and footpads along with the unique locations of the perinipple region and claw beds in cats.

ii. Skin scrapings should be obtained to rule out mites. Even though dermatophytosis is unlikely, a fungal culture should be performed to eliminate this cause as early cases of PF in cats can look surprisingly similar. Cytology from an intact pustule or exudate should be examined to rule out a secondary bacterial infection. When intact pustules are present, they should ideally be saved for biopsy, but in cases where an intact pustule can be sampled, the presence of acantholytic keratinocytes in the absence of bacteria can be highly supportive of a PF diagnosis. Biopsy with dermatohistopathology is required for definitive diagnosis. Biopsy of intact pustules is preferred, but if no pustules are present, samples obtained from crusted areas should then be pursued. When performing a biopsy in cases of suspected PF, it is important to take care and preserve the intact pustule or crust. In these cases, an elliptical skin biopsy using a scalpel blade may be preferred, as inappropriate skin punch biopsy selection may rupture the fragile pustules or dislodge the crust. Ideally, several samples should be submitted for examination.

iii. The overall prognosis for PF in cats is generally good. PF is an autoimmune disease that normally requires lifelong therapy with remission occurring rarely unless an inciting cause can be found and removed. Initially, treatment normally involves the administration of systemic glucocorticoids at immunosuppressive doses. Prednisolone or methylprednisolone (2–6 mg/kg PO q24h) and triamcinolone (0.4–2 mg/kg PO q24h) are the most commonly used steroids for this condition in cats. Daily administration should continue until clinical signs resolve (normally 2–4 weeks), at which time slow (e.g., every 10–14 days), steady tapering of the dose should begin until the lowest alternate day dose (q48–72h in the case of triamcinolone) that maintains control of clinical symptoms is obtained. In the author's opinion, changes of more than 25% to any given dose are more likely to result in relapse of clinical signs when performing a dose taper. In cases that are slow to improve, glucocorticoids' side effects are excessive, or combination therapy is preferred, the addition of chlorambucil (0.1–0.2 mg/kg PO q24–48h) or cyclosporine (5–10 mg/kg PO q24h) may be pursued (Irwin et al., 2012). When chlorambucil is used, routine CBC monitoring should be performed.

103. A 4-year-old Cavalier King Charles spaniel presented for the problem of nonseasonal paw licking of 3 years' duration. According to the owner, the dog's activity was diagnosed as an anxiety-related behavioral issue. Over the last 3 years, the owner tried various activity-related interventions, including hiring a dog walker and sending the dog to kennel to play every day. The dog walker and the kennel operator reported the dog chewed its feet regardless of the activities they offered the dog. The owner is seeking a second opinion because the problem seems to be worsening. The patient is current on vaccinations, and the owners administer monthly heartworm (ivermectin) and flea preventatives (afoxolaner) year-round. Physical exam revealed barbering alopecia and salivary staining most notably on the rear paws along with perianal alopecia, erythema, and hyperpigmentation (**Figure 103a, b**).

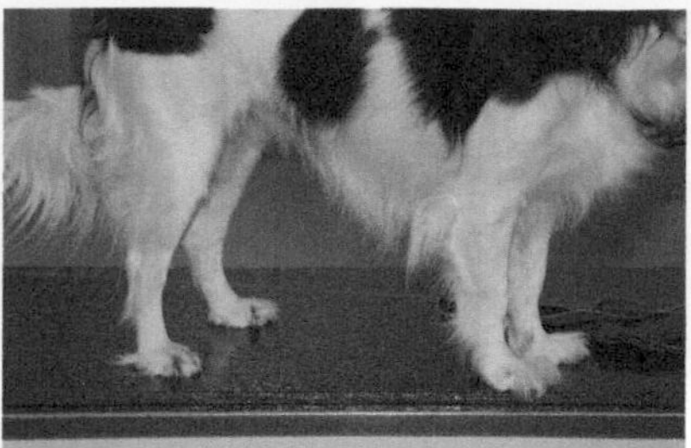
Figure 103a

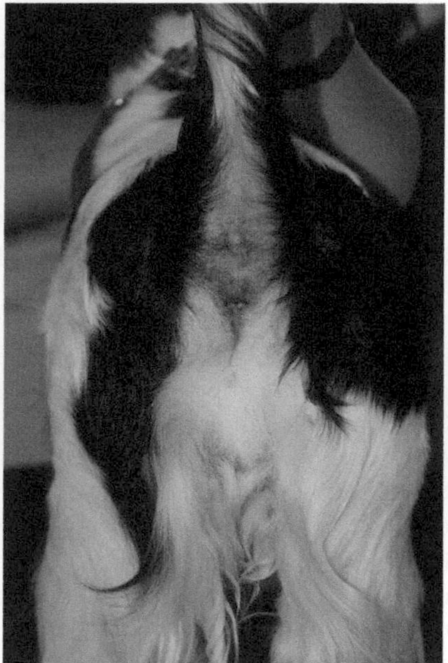
Figure 103b

i. What are the most common causes of excessive paw licking/chewing in dogs?

ii. What diagnostic tests are indicated for this patient, and how should the workup proceed to determine the underlying cause of the patient's pedal pruritus?

iii. What antipruritic options exist that may provide immediate relief for this patient?

iv. If this patient's pruritus is determined to be the result of atopy, what long-term disease-targeted treatment options are available that should be discussed with the owner?

103. **i.** The most common causes of pedal pruritus include demodicosis, atopy, cutaneous adverse food reactions, contact allergy, and secondary bacterial or yeast infections.

ii. Material for a cytological examination should be collected before doing a skin scraping using mineral oil. Debris from around the claw or between the interdigital webbing should be scraped off with a skin-scraping spatula or scalpel blade and smeared onto a glass slide, stained, and examined microscopically. Additionally, impression cytology should be acquired via acetate tape from the interdigital and perianal regions and examined. If secondary infections are present, they should be treated topically with medicated bathing, wipes, or mousse given the focal lesion distribution. If symptoms resolve with treatment of secondary infections, then preventative topical therapy may be all that is needed. However, if pruritus persists or recurs despite resolution of secondary infections, then the patient should continue to be worked-up for the likely underlying allergic hypersensitivity. As the patient is on monthly flea prevention that is also effective for other contagious parasites, flea allergy dermatitis or parasite hypersensitivity are unlikely. Given the nonseasonal distribution of symptoms and young age of onset, a diet elimination trial would be warranted. If the patient failed to respond to an appropriate diet elimination trial, atopy would be the most logical diagnosis for this patient's pruritus, and appropriate disease-specific therapy should be pursued.

iii. Glucocorticoids, oclacitinib maleate (Apoquel), and lokivetmab (Cytopoint) are the current antipruritic therapies that exist with a quick onset of action. Glucocorticoids and oclacitinib should provide relief within 24 hours at appropriate dosing, while lokivetmab is effective in most patients who respond to the therapy within 72 hours. Cyclosporine has a much slower onset of action and may take 2–6 weeks to appreciate therapeutic benefit.

iv. Long-term therapy options for patients with atopy are allergen-specific immunotherapy (injectable and sublingual), lokivetmab, oclacitinib, cyclosporine, and glucocorticoids. All of these options have varying degrees of efficacy along with pros and cons of their use. It is important when discussing options with owners that they understand there is no right option, and no option is 100% effective and safe. The most appropriate therapy for an atopic patient should be made on an individual basis taking all patient- and owner-related factors into account.

104. A 3-year-old mixed breed dog presented for swollen paws. On physical examination, marked interdigital erythema, mild swelling, and alopecia are observed to affect all four paws. You elect to perform an impression smear from the feet. A microscopic image (100×; oil immersion) from that sample is indicated in **Figure 104a**.

What is present in the center of the image indicated by the green arrow?

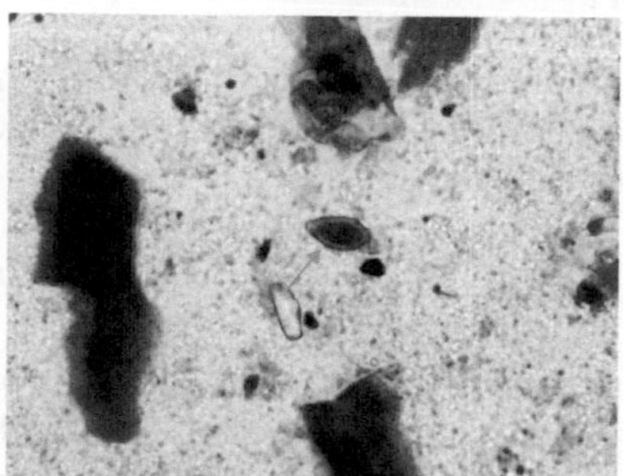

Figure 104a

105. An 8-year-old spayed female golden retriever who is the only dog in the household and predominately lives indoors presented for annual examination and vaccinations. The owner reports that over the last several months the dog has been observed to be itchy, especially along her dorsum. The patient has no prior skin or ear issues, and the owner has never previously thought their dog was pruritic. Physical examination revealed mild generalized erythema of the skin, mild to moderate thinning of the hair coat along the dorsal lumbar and flank regions likely secondary to self-trauma, and the presence of mild scale formation. There were no obvious signs of ectoparasites, and flea combing along with skin scrape samples were negative. Annual blood work consisting of a CBC and serum biochemistries was fairly unremarkable, with the exception of a mild eosinophilia. The following was found on the patient's fecal flotation (**Figure 105a**).

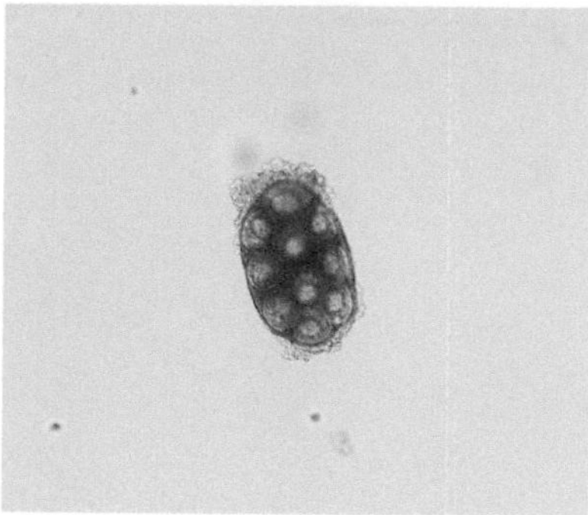

Figure 105a

Given the physical and diagnostic findings, what is the most likely cause of this patient's recent onset of pruritus?

104. This is a *Cladosporium* spp. spore. The shape of the spores can vary from spherical, to barrel like, or lemon shaped, which is the variant shape present in the image. *Cladosporium* is one of the more common molds to which an individual may develop an allergic sensitization. The mold is found in wet, damp areas, carpets, or plants. In this particular instance, this is an insignificant finding, but the contaminant can be misinterpreted as an infectious fungal spore (*Cryptococcus* spp., dermatophyte ectothrix spore) or a parasite egg (due to shape and appearance of "operculum") by the untrained observer. The size and shape relative to the anucleated keratinocytes in the image make either of the infectious fungal agents unlikely, while the stain uptake and coloration are not typical for parasitic organisms.

105. Flea allergy dermatitis. **Figure 105a** shows a *Dipylidium caninum* (the "flea" tapeworm) egg packet. *D. caninum* requires the flea for completion of its life cycle. The flea acts as the intermediate host for the parasite when its larval stages ingest a *D. caninum* egg that then goes through its life cycle before becoming an infective cysticercoid in the adult flea. The definitive host, the dog or cat, becomes infected upon ingesting an adult flea during grooming, licking, or chewing as a result of pruritus. The prepatent period for *D. caninum* has been reported to be roughly 4 weeks. *Trichodectes canis* may also serve as an intermediate host but is unlikely the cause of pruritus in this case due to the patient's lifestyle, pruritus and lesion location over the caudal dorsum, and lack of finding adult lice or nits on examination.

106. You are presented with a 1.5-year-old intact male border collie with a 3-month history of progressive alopecia and increasing pruritus. Prior therapy with glucocorticoids has provided some symptomatic relief, but the owner reports it is becoming less and less beneficial. On examination, marked generalized erythema was present along with patchy alopecia, crusting, comedone formation, and occasional draining tracts affecting the face, trunk, and distal extremities (**Figure 106a–c**). Trichography revealed numerous *D. canis* mites of all life stages, while cytology from draining tracts demonstrated neutrophilic inflammation with numerous intra- and extracellular coccoid-shaped bacteria. A clinical diagnosis of generalized, juvenile-onset demodicosis with a secondary deep pyoderma was made.

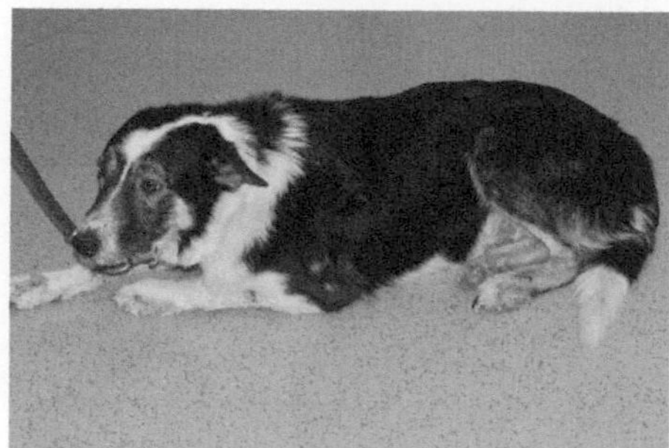
Figure 106a

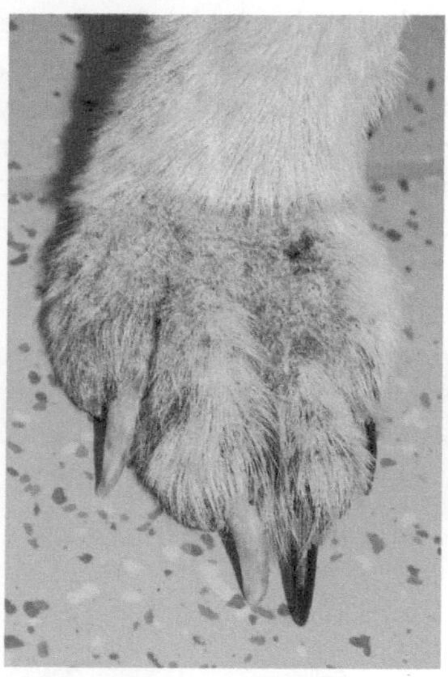
Figure 106b

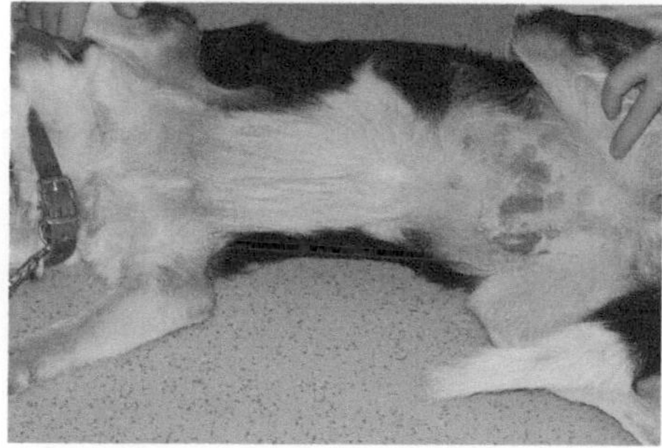
Figure 106c

i. Given your diagnosis, what is concerning about this patient?

ii. How can you determine whether your concerns are justified with this particular patient?

iii. What other breeds are known to require this same consideration?

106. i. The patient is a border collie. Border collies are part of the herding breed family, which are known to possess the ABCB1-Δ1 (formerly MDR-1) genetic mutation. This mutation alters P-glycoprotein function increasing the likelihood of severe or fatal adverse events when patients are treated with macrocyclic lactones (i.e., ivermectin).

ii. A commercial test is now available through Washington State University (WSU). The test allows screening of dogs for the mutation genotype prior to therapy rather than just adhering to the old adage of "white feet, don't treat." Blood or cheek swab samples can be used to evaluate patients for the presence of the mutation. This test is available through WSU's diagnostic laboratory for approximately \$60–\$70. Information on sample collection and test kits can be obtained from the WSU Veterinary Clinical Pharmacology Laboratory (https://vcpl.vetmed.wsu.edu). Results are available within approximately 2 weeks.

iii. Other breeds known to possess this mutation are shown in **Figure 106d** along with the reported frequency of mutant allele occurrence. Although these breeds have a well-documented increased occurrence of the genetic mutation, any dog could possess the mutation, and macrocyclic lactone toxicity has been observed in dogs that did not possess the genetic alteration.

Breed	Mutant Allele Frequency	Breed	Mutant Allele Frequency
Australian Shepherd	50%	Long-Haired Whippet	65%
Australian Shepherd, Mini	50%	McNab	30%
Border Collie	<5%	Mixed Breed	5%
Collie	70%	Old English Sheepdog	5%
English Shepherd	15%	Shetland Sheepdog	15%
German Shepherd	10%	Silken Windhound	30%
Herding Breed Crosses	10%		

Information taken from: Washington State University's Veterinary Clinical Pharmacology Website 2017

Figure 106d

107. A 3-year-old neutered male mastiff presented for a second opinion of a previous diagnosis of generalized demodicosis with a secondary pyoderma. The patient had previously been prescribed sarolaner, cephalexin, and a benzoyl peroxide shampoo 3 weeks ago. The owner has given all medications as directed but notes that the patient is getting worse and now has bloody discharge from multiple sites along his back and legs. Physical exam reveals marked alopecia, generalized erythema, and truncal papules, pustules, hemorrhagic bullae, along with multiple draining tracts and serosanguineous discharge (**Figure 107a**). A skin scraping reveals numerous, dead, adult *D. canis* mites, while a cytology sample from one of the draining lesions shows large numbers of intracellular and extracellular coccoid-shaped bacteria. Based on your findings, you suspect a possible resistant secondary infection and recommend a bacterial culture.

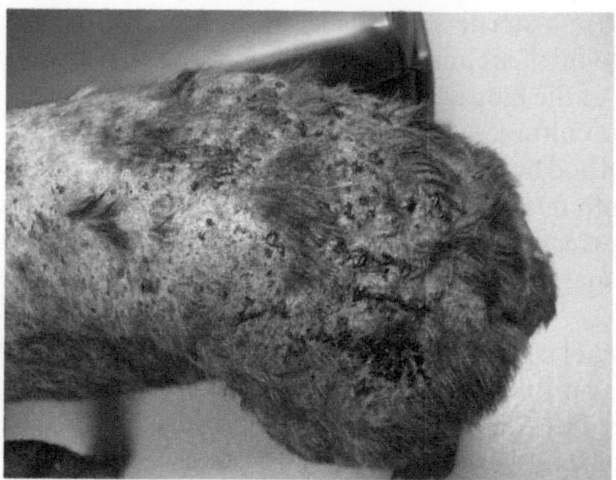

Figure 107a

How should this sample be acquired?

108. What is mycophenolate mofetil, what dermatologic conditions has it been used for, and what are the major adverse events encountered with use of the drug?

107. This is an example of deep pyoderma, and culturing technique varies a little from that associated with superficial disease. There are three possible methods for obtaining a sample for bacteriologic culture from this patient.

The first is to sample one of the unruptured hemorrhagic bullae. This can be accomplished by either aspirating the lesion and transferring the aspirated material to a culture swab or simply rupturing one with a sterile needle and inserting a culture swab.

The second method is to obtain the sample via biopsy. This method is indicated when severe exudation is present, the surface is heavily contaminated, and/or a mixed population of bacteria are observed on cytology. To obtain a sample via this method, the surface is prepped as it would be for a surgical procedure and then rinsed with sterile saline to remove any residual antiseptic solution that could potentially inhibit growth of bacteria. A sample via punch biopsy is then aseptically collected. The author prefers that once the biopsy is collected to use a sterile scalpel blade and remove the surface from the deeper dermis to further eliminate the chance for surface contamination. The dermal portion of the biopsy is then placed in sterile saline and submitted for macerated tissue culture.

The third method by which a sample can be collected is to insert the culture swab directly into one of the active draining tracts. This method is less ideal as the draining tract is likely to be contaminated with additional secondary pathogens that may make interpretation of culture results more difficult.

108. Mycophenolate mofetil (CellCept) is a prodrug whose metabolite mycophenolic acid is an immunomodulatory agent. The drug exerts its effect via inhibition of inosine-5′-monophosphate dehydrogenase, which is an enzyme involved with purine synthesis and leads to arrest of T- and B-cell activation and expansion. The drug is rarely used as a primary or sole therapeutic agent but is instead used as an adjunctive or alternative immunosuppressive agent when standard therapies fail. It has been primarily used for pemphigus foliaceus and supepidermal blistering dermatoses. A wide range of dosing regimens have been proposed with twice-daily dosing being the most common. Severe adverse events reported include bone marrow suppression and GI symptoms (possible intestinal hemorrhage). The medication should not be used in conjunction with azathioprine as both drugs have a similar mechanism of action, which may lead to an increased risk of bone marrow suppression.

109. A 1.5-year-old spayed female pit bull terrier presented for a second opinion for a 3-month history of the progressive lesions shown in **Figure 109a–d**. The owner reports that the patient is pruritic and prior therapy with Apoquel and two different 10-day courses of systemic antibiotics (cephalexin and amoxicillin-clavulanate) have failed to provide any perceivable benefit. The patient is the only dog in the household, has supervised access to a rural farm, and neither owner has a rash affecting their own skin. The owner also notes that there has been no change in the patient's appetite, energy level, or urination/defecation habits. Other than the skin lesions, physical exam findings were fairly unremarkable.

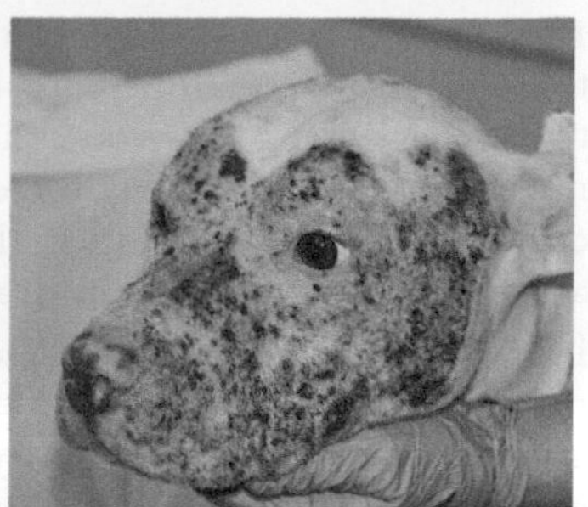

Figure 109a

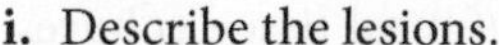

i. Describe the lesions.

ii. What are your primary differentials for this patient, and what initial diagnostic tests should be performed?

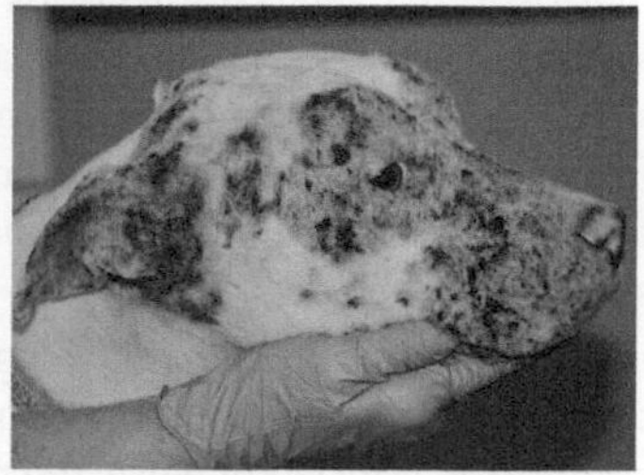

Figure 109b

iii. **Figure 109e** shows a microscopic image (100×; oil immersion) that is representative of multiple fields from a cytology sample acquired from draining tracts on the face. What is your diagnosis, and what further diagnostic tests should be recommended at this time?

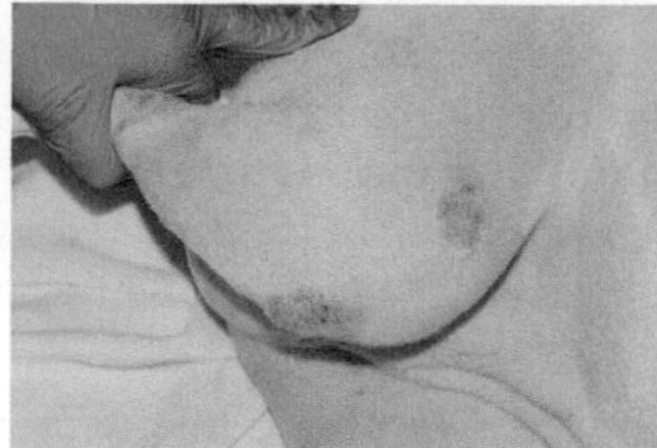

Figure 109c

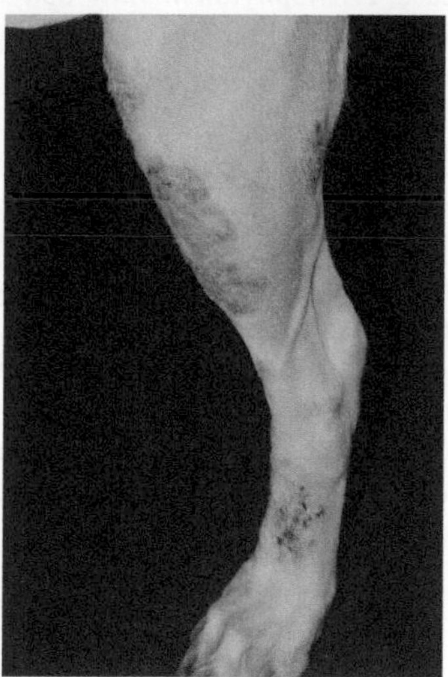

Figure 109d

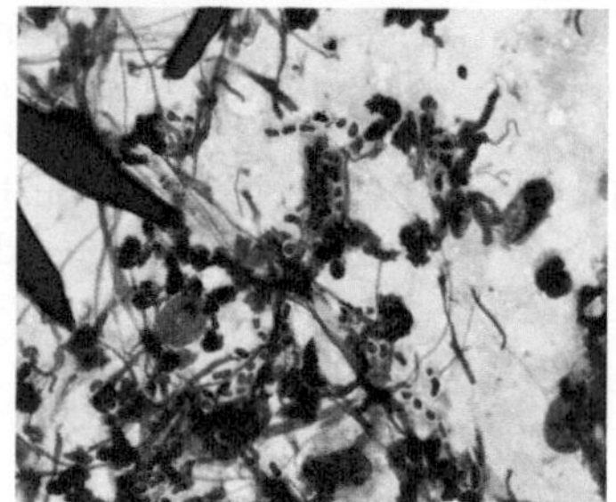

Figure 109e

110. What is a hygroma, and how is it managed?

109. i. There is well-demarcated alopecia of the face and muzzle with erythema, multiple small hemorrhagic bullae, crusting, and punctate draining tracts that extend to involve the pinnae and dorsal head while sparing the nasal planum. Additionally, there are circular, erythemic, alopecic patches with crusting and scaling over the right cranial and lateral stifle with similar lesions and the presence of punctate draining lesions along the left rear leg.

ii. Given the patient's age, clinical presentation, and lesions present, the primary differentials for this patient should include causes of furunculosis in a young dog. The three primary differentials for this patient are demodicosis, dermatophytosis, and deep pyoderma. Other less likely differentials that should be considered pending results of initial diagnostics include juvenile cellulitis, dimorphic mycotic infections (i.e., blastomycosis), severe solar dermatitis, rare bacterial infections (actinomyces, nocardia, or mycobacteria), or an adverse drug eruption. Initial diagnostics for this patient should include skin scraping and cytology samples from under crusts and the draining tracts. If these initial diagnostics fail to yield a definitive diagnosis, then additional tests such as biopsy with histopathology and bacterial/fungal tissue cultures should be pursued.

iii. Dermatophytosis. The image shows nuclear streaming from inflammatory cells along with multiple small, circular to oval, encapsulated basophilic structures consistent with dermatophyte arthroconidia (ectothrix spores). Dermatophytes never form macroconidia in tissue but rather form hyphae and these structures on keratinized tissues. At this time, a fungal culture or dermatophyte PCR with reflex culture should be pursued to definitively identify the causative fungal species so that the owners can be informed about how the infection was acquired, the likelihood of recurrence, and for treatment monitoring purposes. In this particular case, *Trichophyton mentagrophytes* was determined to be the causative agent, which was likely acquired from exposure to rodents or their dens while playing on the farm.

110. A hygroma is a false or acquired bursa that occurs over bony prominences and pressure points, especially the olecranon in large breed dogs. They develop as the result of a repeated trauma-induced inflammatory response. They manifest initially as soft, fluctuant (fluid-filled), painless swellings that contain a clear, yellow to red-tinged fluid. Over time, they may develop into abscesses or granulomas, with or without draining tracts. Early on, hygromas can be managed medically via bandaging, protective covering (such as DogLeggs), and corrective housing. In chronic cases with significant inflammation or resistant infections, drainage, flushing, drain placement, surgical correction, or skin grafting may be required.

111. A 3-year-old castrated male Pomeranian presented for the problem of progressive hair loss and skin color changes over the past 6 months. Physical examination revealed noninflammatory alopecia on the dog's trunk, tail, and proximal extremities with marked hyperpigmentation of the skin in the affected regions (**Figure 111a**). The dog was nonpruritic and was otherwise healthy with no other abnormalities noted. All diagnostics were normal or negative including a CBC, serum chemistries, and urinalysis. Skin biopsies were compatible with an endocrine alopecia. The results of the thyroid and adrenal function screening are presented.

i. What is the interpretation of the endocrine function tests?

ii. What is the likely diagnosis in this case?

iii. What is the prognosis for this patient, and what treatment options exist?

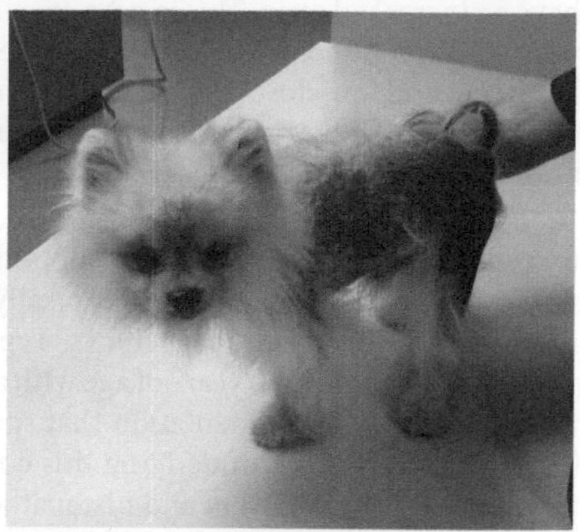

Figure 111a

Michigan State University—Thyroid Panel	Results	Normal
Total thyroxine (TT4)	30	15–67
Total triiodothyronine (TT3)	1.1	1–2.5
Free T4 by ED	15	8–26
T4 autoantibody	5	0–20
T3 autoantibody	0	0–10
Thyroid-stimulating hormone	21	0–37
Thyroglobulin autoantibody %	7	<10

Low-Dose Dexamethasone Suppression Test (ng/mL)	Results	Normal
Pre-	2.57	1.0–5.0
4 h	0.64	
8 h	0.85	

Note: Interpretation: Cortisol level less than 1.4 at 8 is normal; Cortisol level greater than 1.4 at 8 hours post-dexamethasone supports hyperadrenocorticism.

Urine Cortisol/Creatinine Ratio	Results
Urine cortisol	26.1 μg/dL
Urine creatinine	180.0 mg/dL
Urine cortisol/creat ratio	45

Note: Interpretation: <34 hyperadrenocorticism is highly unlikely; ≥34 hyperadrenocorticism is a possibility.

ACTH Stimulation Test (ng/mL)	Results	Normal
Pre-	2.47	1.0–5.0
Post-	7.18	5.5–20.0

111. **i.** When interpreted as a whole, the thyroid hormone screening panel indicates normal function. The UCCR is high, however urine samples collected from stressed dogs, dogs in the hospital, or dogs with nonadrenal illness can have an increased ratio. This is not a specific test for hyperadrenocorticism, but when the ratio is normal, Cushing disease is highly unlikely. The ACTH stimulation test and low-dose dexamethasone suppression test revealed normal basal cortisol levels and normal suppression results. At this point, hypothyroidism and hyperadrenocorticism are unlikely.

ii. Based on the breed, age of onset, and lack of other symptoms or laboratory abnormalities, a diagnosis of alopecia X should be made. Alopecia X is a noninflammatory condition that typically affects Pomeranians, Alaskan malamutes, keeshonds, and chow chows. Typical age of onset for alopecia is anywhere between 1 and 10 years of age with affected dogs developing symmetrical alopecia and hyperpigmentation that spares the head and distal extremities. The exact mechanism underlying this condition is not fully understood. This is a diagnosis of exclusion, and histopathology is not helpful in differentiating this condition from other noninflammatory endocrine causes of alopecia.

iii. The overall prognosis for this condition is good as it is primarily a cosmetic disorder. The ability to establish new hair regrowth is highly variable, with no treatment being consistently successful. Also, any new hair growth may not be permanent. Numerous treatment regimens have been proposed that include neutering intact animals, melatonin administration, deslorelin implant, medroxyprogesterone acetate injections, trilostane and lysodren administration, and causing micro skin trauma with either a pumice stone or cosmetic microneedling device. No treatment is guaranteed to be successful, and the severe potential adverse events of some of these options need to be considered given this is a cosmetic condition.

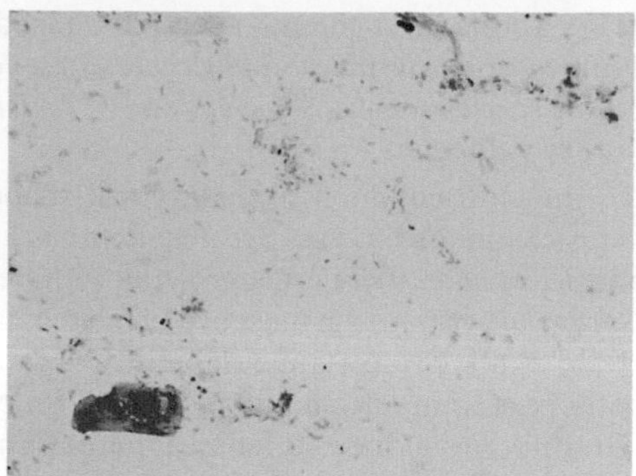
Figure 112a

112. Otitis externa is a common disease of the canine external ear that is the result of an underlying primary disease. Diagnosis is based on physical examination findings and compatible cytological findings. In cases of otitis externa, cytological smears from the ears may show the presence of coccoid-shaped bacteria, rod-shaped bacteria, peanut-shaped organisms, or some combination of these various organisms (**Figure 112a**—Gram stain).

i. What coccoid-shaped bacteria are most commonly isolated from the ears of dogs with otitis externa?

ii. What rod-shaped bacteria are most commonly isolated from the ears of dogs with otitis externa?

iii. What is the most likely identity of the peanut-shaped organisms?

113. A 2-year-old spayed female Scottish terrier that weighed 12.5 kg presented for multiple sores on her belly. The owner reported that the lesions were first observed 2 weeks ago and have progressively worsened since that time. The patient has no prior history of dermatologic issues and was reported to be non-pruritic. Physical examination revealed multiple papules, pustules, and epidermal collarettes along the ventral abdomen and medial rear legs. The patient was diagnosed with a superficial pyoderma based on negative skin scraping results and the presence of paired coccoid-shaped bacteria on cytology. The owners inform you that they are unable and unwilling to treat the patient topically, and that they struggle giving her oral medications. Based on this, you elect to treat the patient with cefovecin (Convenia).

i. What generation of cephalosporin is cefovecin classified as, and what other commonly used drug in dogs falls within this same classification?

ii. What side effects have been observed with this class of medications?

iii. Calculate the dosage of cefovecin for this patient.

iv. What is the concern/controversy with using either one of these drugs as first-line antimicrobials in dogs with pyoderma?

112. i. The most common coccoid-shaped bacterial species associated with canine otitis externa is *Staphylococcus pseudintermedius*, but other staphylococcal species such as *S. aureus* and *S. schleiferi* along with *Streptococcus* spp. may be pathogens.

ii. The most common secondary rod-shaped bacterial pathogens recovered from canine otitis cases are *Pseudomonas aeruginosa, E. coli, Proteus* spp., and *Klebsiella*. There are a growing number of cases in the literature where *Corynebacterium* spp. have been isolated as the primary pathogen (Aalbaek et al., 2010). Gram stain can be utilized to help quickly sort these possible pathogens from one another and is useful clinically as *Corynebacterium* spp. (Gram-positive) have different inherent antimicrobial susceptibilities compared to Gram-negative pathogens (Henneveld et al., 2012).

iii. Peanut-shaped organisms found on otic cytology specimens are *Malassezia* spp.

113. i. Third-generation; cefpodoxime proxetil (Simplicef).

ii. The most common adverse events seen with either one of these medications are anorexia, diarrhea, vomiting, and lethargy. Other reactions with a very low frequency of occurrence observed with any cephalosporin included hypersensitivity reactions, anaphylaxis, myelotoxicity, immune-mediated thrombocytopenia/hemolytic anemia, prolongation of clotting times, transient increases in serum aminotransferases, and cutaneous adverse drug eruptions (pemphigus-like, erythema multiforme, vasculitis, and toxic epidermal necrolysis).

iii. The recommended dose for cefovecin is 8 mg/kg:

Patient weight—12.5 kg

Dosing—8 mg/kg

Dosage—12.5 kg × 8 mg/kg = 100 mg

Cefovecin when reconstituted is provided as an 80 mg/mL solution:

Administered dosage—100 mg ÷ 80 mg/mL = 1.25 mL SC injection

In this scenario, the patient should be rechecked at 2 weeks to ensure complete resolution of the infection has occurred and to readminister cefovecin if needed.

iv. The two major concerns regarding the use of either of these agents as first-line antimicrobials are (1) the potential selective effect they may exert on the bystander Gram-negative microbiota given their broader spectrum of activity compared to first-generation drugs (specifically, highly resistant extended-spectrum β-lactamase-producing *E. coli*) and (2) the selection of methicillin-resistant *S. pseudintermedius* (Hillier et al., 2014). As a result, consensus for their tier status has not been agreed upon, and they fall within a "gray zone" between first- and second-tier antimicrobials. At this time, it is best to reserve their use as a first-tier option only where medicating may be difficult to impossible and/or compliance is expected to be poor.

114. A litter of 10-week-old kittens presented for evaluation of scratching at their ears. Upon examination, there was black-brown waxy debris in the ears. A swab of the debris was taken for a mineral oil prep sample to evaluate microscopically. The following was observed from that sample (**Figure 114a**).

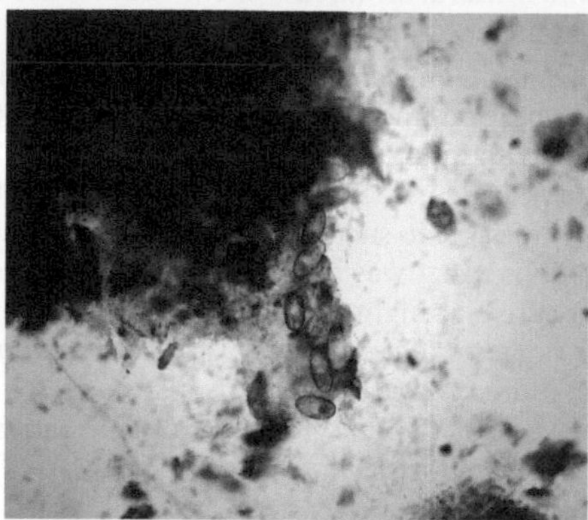

Figure 114a

i. What is the diagnosis?

ii. List three other pediatric diseases that can present with a similar history and physical exam in a kitten.

iii. What is the zoonotic implication of this infestation?

115. The dorsal back of a 5-year-old male schnauzer dog is shown in **Figure 115a**. The dog has just been diagnosed with atopy. The owner reports that the dog has had "bumps" over its back almost its entire life. Palpation of the dorsum reveals diffuse crusted papules from the neck to the lumbosacral area. When the hair coat is clipped, numerous comedones are seen.

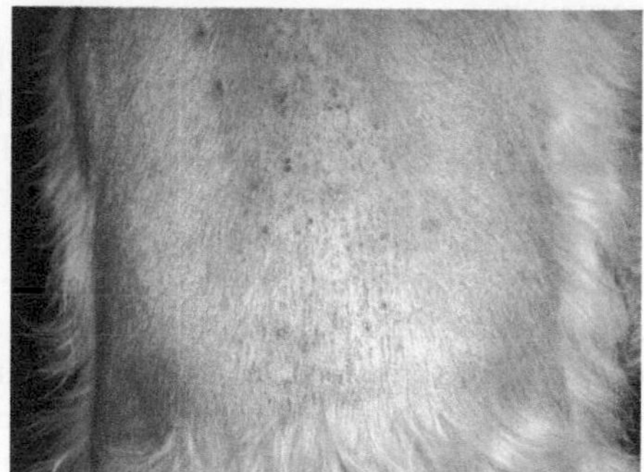

Figure 115a

i. What is the name of this dog's condition?

ii. What other differentials should be considered for the lesion formation in this case?

iii. How does it relate to the dog's atopy?

iv. How should this patient be treated?

116. There are two major categories of adverse drug reactions. What are they? Give an example of each type.

114. **i.** *Otodectes cynotis* (ear mites). Multiple eggs are present in the photomicrograph taken at 4× power.

ii. *Microsporum canis* and *Malassezia* spp. yeast can cause otic disease in kittens. *Demodex cati* can also be found in the ears of kittens. Otic examinations, ear swab cytology, and mineral oil smears of ear exudate are the minimal diagnostics for cats or kittens presented with pruritic ears.

iii. Although rare, *Otodectes cynotis* is considered a zoonotic disease. Lesions in people have been reported and consist of a papular eruption on the hands and arms (Harwick, 1978). In one anecdotal report (Lopez, 1993), a veterinarian took mite-infested ear debris from a cat and placed it into his own ear, on several occasions. He was able to successfully infest himself with ear mites and reported intense itching. What was most interesting was his observation that the mites were most active at night and could be heard chewing and moving around his ear. This suggests that ear mite preparations would be best applied in the evening. On a more practical level, this also suggests that veterinarians and owners cleaning the ears of pets with ear mite infestations should practice good handwashing hygiene post-treatment.

115. **i.** Schnauzer comedone syndrome.

ii. When comedone formation is encountered, the most common differentials are demodicosis and hyperadenocorticism (iatrogenic or naturally occurring), which would be differentials in this case, along with pyoderma and dermatophytosis.

iii. This condition is unrelated to the dog's atopy. The syndrome is a disorder of keratinization characterized by dilated cystic hair follicles that develop into comedones.

iv. This is a genetic skin disease that can be controlled but not cured. Owners should be educated not to manipulate the comedones or to scrub the area aggressively, as these dilated hair follicles rupture easily and may become infected. These dogs may have secondary bacterial and yeast infections that are often overlooked. Impression smears of the contents of the comedones should be cytologically examined and concurrent infections treated. The hair coat should be kept short to facilitate bathing one to two times a week. Shampoos containing benzoyl peroxide, ethyl lactate, salicylic acid, or sulfur are most beneficial in helping manage the condition. The most important aspect of treatment is to clean the skin without being unduly harsh.

116. Adverse drug reactions can be divided into predictable and unpredictable/idiosyncratic reactions. Predictable adverse drug reactions are usually dose related and are often related to the pharmacology of the drug. An example would be the vomiting associated with cyclosporine administration. Unpredictable or idiosyncratic drug reactions are dose-independent and are related to the host's immune response and/or the breed of the dog. An example would be acute renal toxicity with sulfonamides in Doberman pinschers.

117. A 2-year-old dog presented for evaluation of a mass on its forepaw (**Figure 117a**). The lesion was raised, alopecic, firm, erythematous, and moist with extensive salivary staining. Closer examination revealed an erosive area with peripheral crusting and a raised border that was slightly "crater-like." The owner reported the lesion had developed over the last several weeks, and this was the first occurrence of the lesion.

i. What is the clinical diagnosis?

ii. What are the two major causes of this syndrome, and what core diagnostic test needs to be done at this time?

iii. What is considered appropriate first-line therapy in this case?

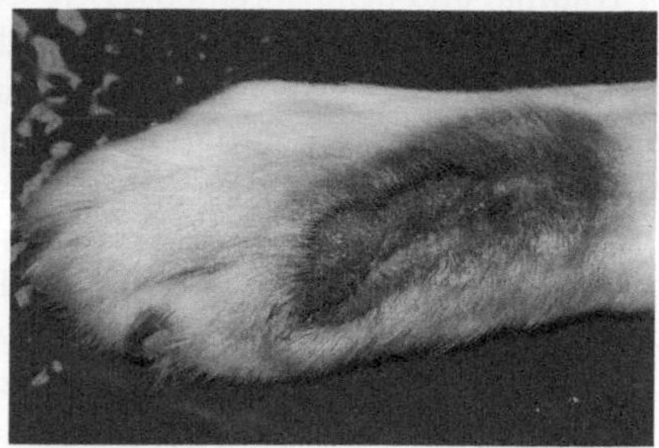

Figure 117a

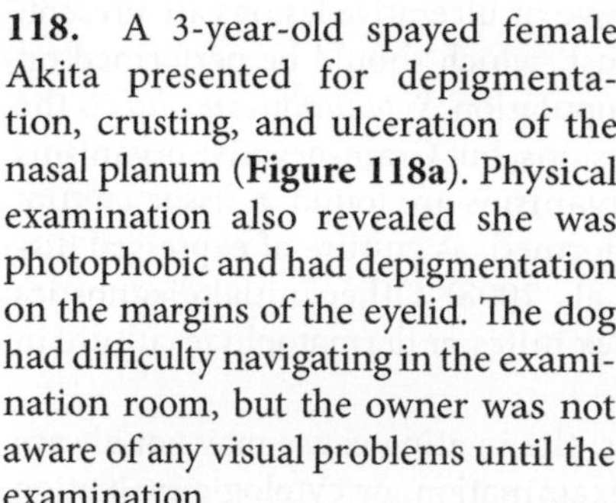

118. A 3-year-old spayed female Akita presented for depigmentation, crusting, and ulceration of the nasal planum (**Figure 118a**). Physical examination also revealed she was photophobic and had depigmentation on the margins of the eyelid. The dog had difficulty navigating in the examination room, but the owner was not aware of any visual problems until the examination.

i. What is the most likely diagnosis?

ii. What will the dermatologic and ophthalmic examinations be looking for?

iii. How should this disease be managed?

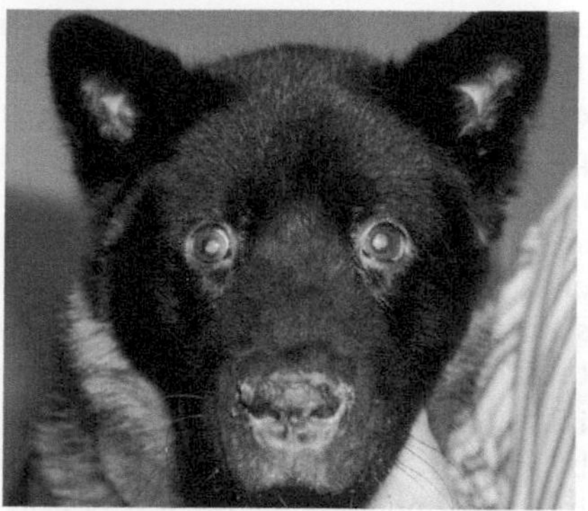

Figure 118a

119. A microscopic image (100×; oil immersion) from a skin impression of the interdigital space of the front right paw of a dog is shown in **Figure 119a**. What does the green arrow indicate present on the slide?

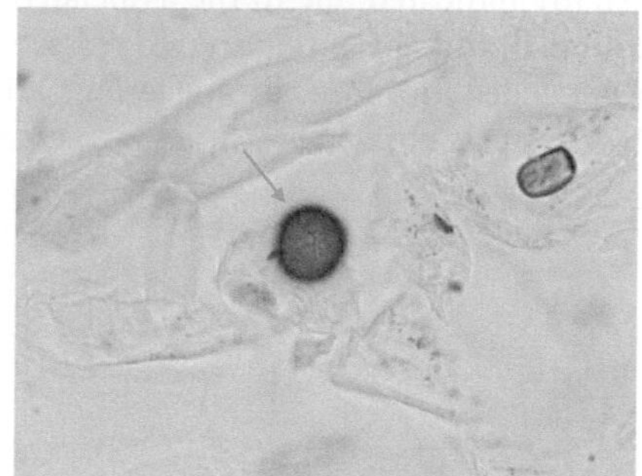

Figure 119a

120. Enrofloxacin is a commonly used fluoroquinolone antibiotic in veterinary medicine. However, its use in cats, specifically at higher doses, is contraindicated due to an unusual and species-specific adverse drug reaction.

What unique adverse event is seen in cats treated with doses greater than 5 mg/kg/day, and what is the proposed mechanism for this side effect?

117. i. Acral lick granuloma or dermatitis.

ii. The two major causes of this lesion are organic diseases (allergic hypersensitivity, foreign body, endocrine dysfunction, arthritis/osteopathy, neuropathy, or trauma) and behavioral (obsessive-compulsive disorder). Although the latter may be a contributing factor, it is a diagnosis of exclusion, and it cannot be emphasized enough that other causes are usually much more important and likely to be the precipitating cause. Pruritus in dogs is manifested by licking, and in many dogs, this may be the only clue that the dog is pruritic. Sometimes the differentiation between the two major causes is obvious (the dog has other compelling clinical signs of an underlying skin disease, there is a clear history of separation anxiety, or recent trauma/disruption in the dog's life). Clinical clues of an underlying pruritic skin disease may include signs of salivary staining on other limbs, a history of lesions developing on other legs in random fashion, and/or multiple lick granulomas occurring at the same time, or a history of trauma. A secondary infection should be suspected in all cases of acral lick dermatitis, especially when erosive or ulcerative lesions are present. Therefore, cytologic examination is a must, which should be performed on exudate expressed from the lesion on manipulation. *S. pseudintermedius* is the primary organism recovered from these lesions, but Gram-negative organisms may also contribute. If Gram-negative organisms are found, a tissue culture acquired via sterile biopsy should be performed, as culture of expressed discharge may be misleading (Shumaker et al., 2008). Other initial diagnostics such as skin scrapings to rule out *Demodex* mites or dermatophyte culture in the case of acute lesions may be indicated.

iii. With initial first-time solitary lesions, the inciting cause may not always be evident. Unless the history, physical examination, or cytologic evaluation indicate a potential cause, it is best to first focus on resolving the secondary infection with first-time lesions. Prolonged systemic antimicrobial therapy is usually indicated due to the associated scar tissue formation. A 4- to 8-week course of therapy is required to resolve lesions, with longer courses occasionally needed for more chronic lesions. Ideally, therapy should be continued for 2 weeks past clinical resolution as gauged by the clinician, not the owner.

118. **i.** Canine uveodermatologic syndrome (Vogt-Koyanagi-Harada [VKH]-like syndrome). This is a rare autoimmune disease involving the skin and eyes. It is believed to be a T-lymphocyte-mediated autoimmune process where lymphocytes attack melanocytes. However, the exact antigen(s) associated with the melanocyte that triggers the disease is still unknown. There is no age or sex predilection. Although many breeds have been described as being affected by uveodermatologic syndrome, the Akita, chow chow, Siberian husky, and Samoyed are seen most commonly.

ii. The disease is characterized by depigmentation of the skin and acute concurrent uveitis. Depigmentation may occur on the nose, lips, eyelids, footpads, scrotum, prepuce, anus, and hard palate. The disease causes uveitis, photophobia, blepharospasm, lacrimation, injected conjunctiva, corneal edema, retinal detachment, cataracts, and secondary glaucoma. If left untreated, these dogs may develop permanent blindness.

iii. The skin lesions usually develop within 7–10 days of the ocular lesions; however, the owner is more likely to notice the depigmentation first. Because this disease can cause secondary glaucoma and blindness, aggressive treatment to control the ocular disease is indicated. Skin biopsies should be taken of the depigmented areas, and a thorough ocular examination for symptoms of uveitis should be performed. Lifelong systemic glucocorticoids and azathioprine are usually needed to control the disease. Skin lesions may respond to therapy but should not be used as an indicator of remission as dogs may have active ocular lesions even though the skin lesions are static or have repigmented. As a result, periodic ocular examinations should be performed to monitor uveitis.

119. This is a pollen spore. Recovery of pollen spores from the skin of dogs and cats is a common finding on impression cytology samples, especially during times of the year when plant pollen counts are high.

120. Acute retinal degeneration that results in permanent blindness. Although the exact pathogenesis is unknown, this adverse event is thought to be subsequent to ABCG2 dysfunction. ABCG2 is a transmembrane efflux pump (similar to P-glycoprotein) that is located at the blood-retinal barrier, which normally restricts fluoroquinolone access to retinal tissue. When exposed to light, fluoroquinolones generate reactive oxygen species (ROS) that can cause tissue damage. Outside of the skin, the eye is the organ most susceptible to phototoxicity. Therefore, in cats, a dysfunctional blood-retinal barrier results in the accumulation of a photoreactive drug within the retina that, upon exposure to light, generates ROS that create tissue damage and retinal degeneration (Mealey, 2013). Retinal damage has also been observed in cats exposed to higher doses of orbifloxacin.

121. Two DTM plates are shown (**Figure 121a, b**). Both have been inoculated with a fungal culture from a dog.

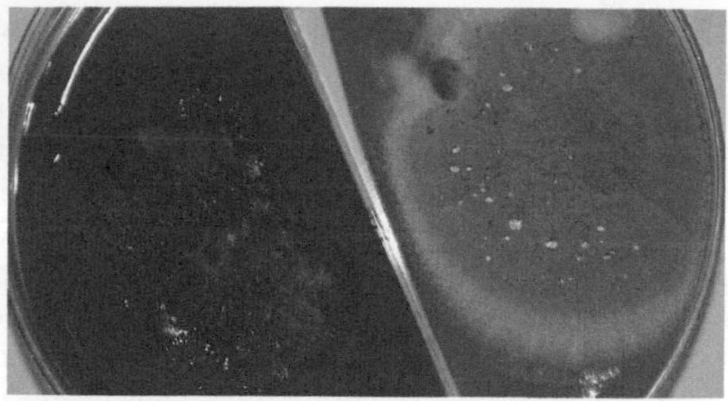

Figure 121a

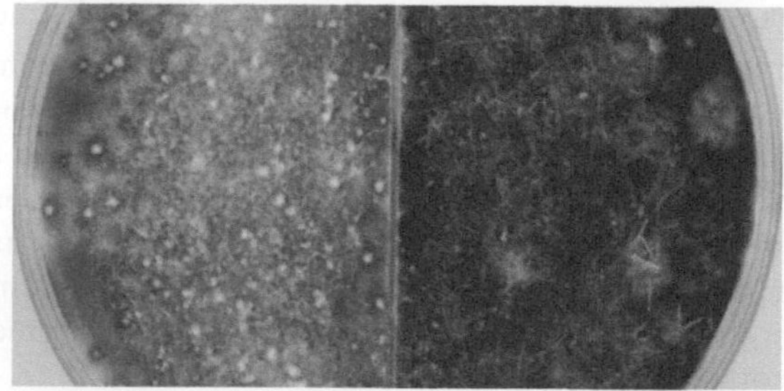

Figure 121b

i. What is DTM, and what is the principle of its use?

ii. How can the gross characteristics of fungal colony growth be used to aid in the differentiation of possible pathogens and contaminants? Which culture plate has colony growth compatible with a suspect pathogen and why?

iii. What factors may be most important in the development of false-negative fungal cultures when incubated in private practice?

122. A continually evolving and growing concern in veterinary medicine is the increasing frequency with which resistant infections are encountered in patients. As a result, terminology for the classification of these infections is becoming commonplace in everyday veterinary practice.

i. What do methicillin resistant, multidrug resistant, and extensively drug resistant mean?

ii. What drugs are classified as β-lactams?

121. **i.** DTM consists of plain Sabouraud's dextrose agar, phenol red as a pH indicator, and antimicrobials to inhibit the growth of bacterial and fungal contaminants. Although there are a variety of commercially available plates, the author prefers the use of agar plates that are easy to inoculate and contain adequate media to prevent desiccation. The illustration shows a dual-compartment plate, which allows for inoculation of more than one media type to aid in colony growth and promote macroconidia formation for species identification. The dual-compartment plate normally combines DTM with either plain Sabouraud's dextrose agar or rapid sporulation medium. DTM is popular because it contains a color indicator that signals the growth of a possible pathogen. Pathogens use the protein in the media first, producing the color change. In general, contaminants use the carbohydrate source first and do not produce a color change until the entire carbohydrate source has been exhausted. The color indicator (phenol red) may alter the gross and microscopic appearance of fungal colonies and/or depress macroconidia growth. In addition, some common contaminants will grossly mimic pathogens and turn the media red.

ii. The plate with the pale white, fluffy colonies is the one most compatible with a possible dermatophyte pathogen as seen in **Figure 121b**. Dermatophyte pathogens are pale in color and are never heavily pigmented as seen in **Figure 121a**. The red color change in the medium indicates the organism is consuming the protein in the media; both pathogens and some contaminants can turn DTM red. Contaminants tend to use the carbohydrates in the medium first before using proteins. Old fungal culture plates growing contaminants may eventually turn red as the organisms utilize the protein in the DTM.

iii. Two published studies have indicated that incubation at room temperature or use of an inadequate commercial fungal culture media might account for false-negative culture results in practice. In the first study (Guillot et al., 2001), increased incubation temperature (24°C–27°C [75.5°F–80.6°F]) resulted in a more rapid color change and improved sporulation of fungi. The second investigation (Moriello et al., 2010) evaluated multiple commercially available media inoculated with control strains of dermatophytes under different conditions. What the investigators of this second study concluded was that the majority of commercially available media preparations were comparable with respect to first growth, first color change, and first sporulation. The exception to these findings was one commonly used self-sealing culture plate, which was significantly less reliable and prone to desiccation.

122. **i.** Methicillin resistance is probably the most important resistance mechanism of staphylococci and is acquired via the expression of the *mecA* gene. *mecA* is a mobile genetic element carried on the staphylococcal chromosome cassette *mec* (SCCmec) that encodes for an altered penicillin binding protein (PBP2a) with a low affinity for β-lactam antibiotics that confers resistance to all derivatives of this antimicrobial class (Morris et al., 2017). *Multidrug resistant* (MDR) has several definitions that are in the veterinary literature, but the most widely accepted is that of a bacterial isolate that is resistant to three of more classes of antibiotics. Those classes would include β-lactams, macrolides, lincosamides, fluoroquinolones, aminoglycosides, tetracyclines, potentiated sulfonamides, chloramphenicol, and rifampin. Given this, a staphylococcal isolate can be methicillin resistant but not multidrug resistant or methicillin and multidrug resistant. The author has found this latter point to be a source of confusion for practitioners from time to time. Finally, the term *extensively drug resistant* (XDR) has entered the veterinary literature and is used to describe a bacterial isolates that are susceptible to two or fewer antimicrobial classes.

ii. The β-lactam antimicrobial class includes the following:

a. *Penicillins*: penicillin G and penicillin V

b. *β-lactamase resistant penicillins*: methicillin and oxacillin

c. *Aminopenicillins*: ampicillin, amoxicillin, and their combinations with β-lactamase inhibitors

d. *Carboxypenicillins and Ureidopenicillins*: ticarcillin and piperacillin

e. *Cephalosporins*: cephalexin, cefadroxil, cefazolin, cefpodoxime, and cefovecin

f. *Monobactams*: Aztreonam

g. *Carbapenems*: imipenem and meropenem

123. An 8-year-old castrated male West Highland white terrier presented with a chief complaint of excessive oily skin along his back. On examination, the hair coat along the dorsum was noted to have a pronounced "greasy" feel with a noticeable texture difference from the surrounding hair (**Figure 123a**). When the hair coat was parted along the dorsum, mild erythema and scaling were also appreciated (**Figure 123b**). Based on physical exam findings, skin scraping samples were acquired (**Figure 123c**).

i. What is the diagnosis?

ii. Where does this mite reside in relation to the skin?

iii. How do treatment recommendations for this mite compare with the other species affecting dogs?

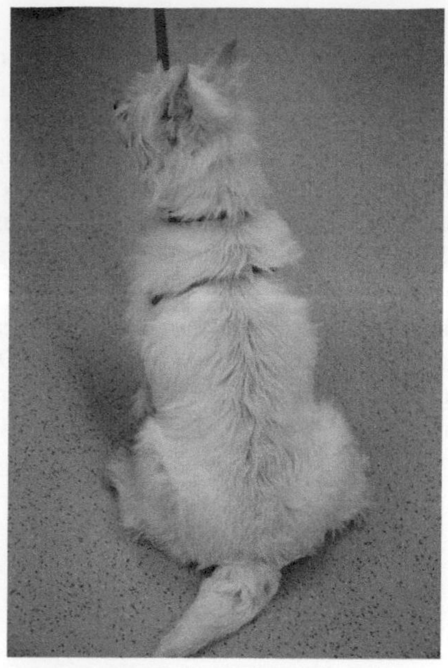
Figure 123a

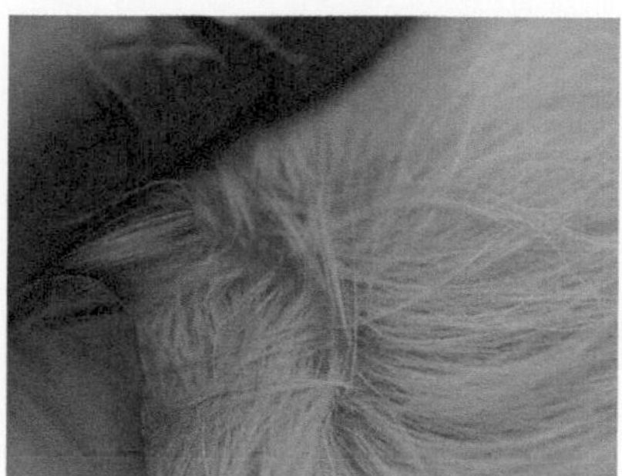
Figure 123b

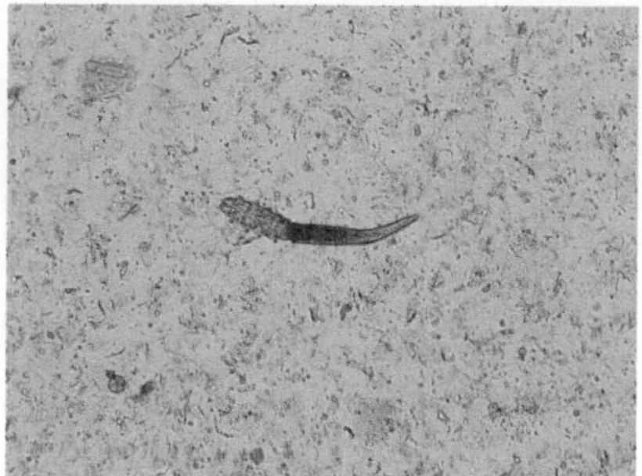
Figure 123c

123. i. *Demodex injai.*

ii. This mite lives in the hair follicle similar to *D. canis* and has been observed occupying the space from the follicular opening to the level of the sebaceous glands. It has also been observed within the sebaceous ducts and entering the sebaceous glands, which may explain the difference in presentation from *D. canis* with excessive seborrhea oleosa being a predominant complaint by owners in cases of demodicosis associated with *D. injai* (Hillier and Desch, 2002). Overall, this form of demodicosis is uncommon with terriers and shih tzus potentially being predisposed.

iii. Treatment recommendations, treatment length, and response rates are similar to that for disease caused by *D. canis*. Drug options utilized in therapeutic protocols include topical amitraz, topical moxidectin, oral/injectable macrocyclic lactones, and isoxazolines.

124. An intensely pruritic dog presented for examination. The dog's pruritus developed acutely approximately 3 weeks ago. The dog had no history of skin disease prior to this episode. The dog was normal on physical examination except for being intensely pruritic and having alopecic, erythemic, and excoriated elbows (**Figure 124a**). The organism shown in **Figure 124b** was found on a skin scraping from the elbow of the patient.

i. What is the organism?

ii. What is the life cycle of the mite, how long can it live off the host, and what body sites are reported to be favored by the mite?

iii. What are the identifying structures of this mite that aid in its identification?

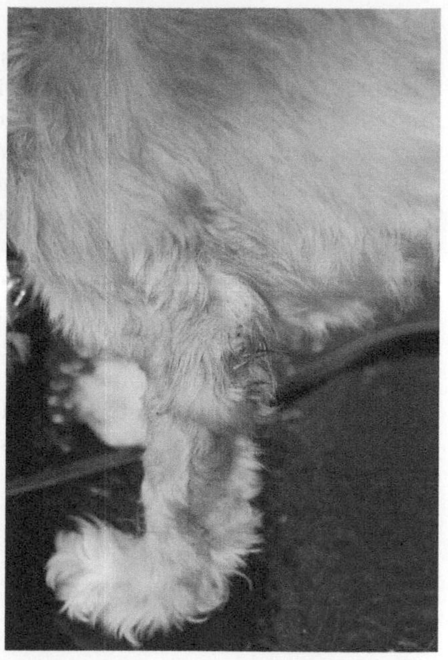

Figure 124a

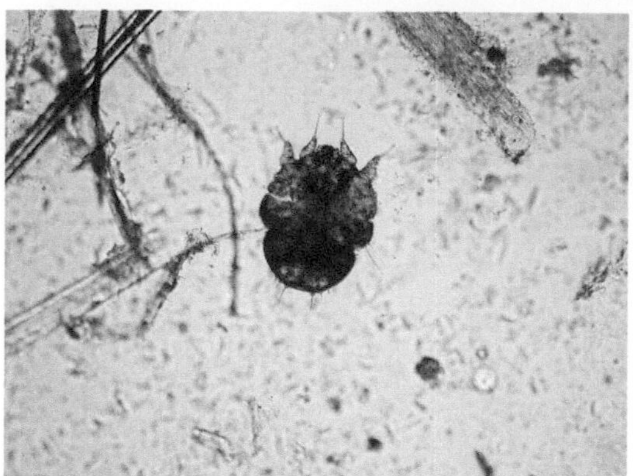

Figure 124b

124. **i.** *Sarcoptes scabiei* mite.

ii. The general life cycle of *Sarcoptes* spp. mites is that the female lays eggs in "tunnels" within the keratinized epidermis, the eggs hatch to larvae that migrate and feed on the skin surface prior to resting in a molting pocket where they molt to nymphs and eventually into adults. This cycle is completed in roughly 17–21 days. Mites can potentially live off the host for 4–21 days with the length of time dependent on relative humidity and temperature. At room temperature (20°C–25°C), all life stages can survive 2–6 days. The mites prefer thinly haired areas such as the ventrum, elbows, hocks, and ear margins of the dog.

iii. The structures used on routine light microscopy to identify scabies are their oval shape, long unjoined stalks with suckers off the anterior pair of legs, short/rudimentary posterior legs that do not usually extend beyond the boarder of the body that have long bristles without suckers and the presence of a terminal anus.

125. A 2-year-old mixed breed dog presented for progressive licking and itching that had been ongoing since the time of his adoption from a local shelter 3 months ago. The owners report that he was neutered, vaccinated, and treated with a flea product prior to his adoption but no further preventative medications had been administered since that time as no fleas have been seen on him. His owners have been bathing and giving him an over-the-counter antihistamine, but neither has provided relief. Physical exam revealed mild generalized erythema with thinning of the hair coat along the caudal dorsal lumbar region, flanks, and rear legs. A small amount of brownish dirt-like material was noted in the hair coat near the base of the tail. In addition, marked salivary staining of the caudal half of the body along with the paws was appreciated (**Figure 125a, b**). The remainder of the physical exam was unremarkable, including a normal otoscopic exam.

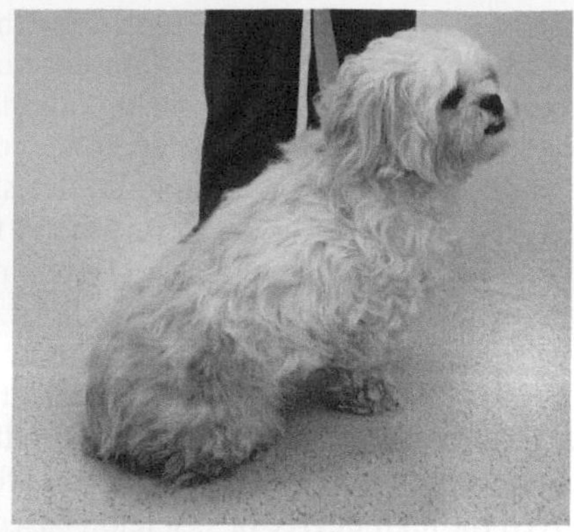

Figure 125a

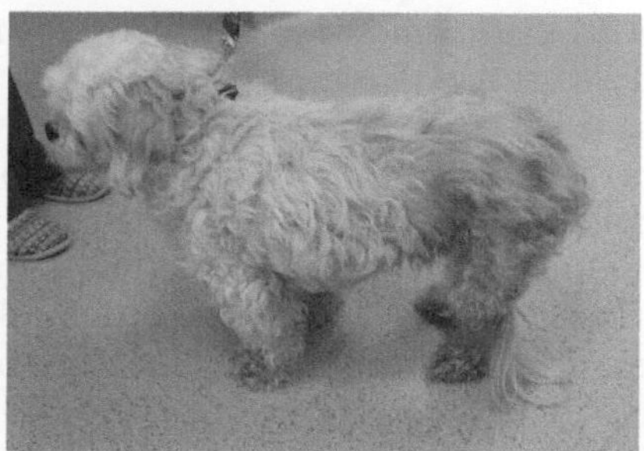

Figure 125b

i. At this time, based on the history and physical findings, what is your primary differential diagnosis, and what initial diagnostics should be performed?

ii. Addressing environmental issues is a major feature of any successful therapeutic plan for treatment of a diagnosed flea infestation. What aspects of environmental control measures should be considered in any treatment protocol?

125. i. The primary differential for this case is flea allergy dermatitis given the distribution of pruritus, presence of debris near the tail base, history of recent acquisition from a shelter, and lack of regular flea prevention. Initial diagnostics for this case included flea combing, skin scraping, and skin cytology via impressions with an adhesive slide. No live fleas were found, but the dirt-like material was determined to be flea dirt after rubbing some on a damp white paper towel. Skin scrapings were negative, and cytology samples did not reveal any secondary etiologic agents (i.e., bacteria or yeast), thereby confirming the clinical suspicion of flea allergy dermatitis. Had the flea dirt not been found, initial treatment for this patient should still have been aggressive flea control for 2–3 months prior to proceeding with a diagnostic workup for other causes of pruritus (cutaneous adverse food reaction or atopy) in a young dog given the high degree of suspicion based on clinical presentation.

ii. Environmental control involves addressing the inside of the home and the pet's outdoor space. To address the inside of the home, there are three basic steps that should be outlined to a client. The first is thorough vacuuming to dislodge eggs, larvae, and pupae from the carpet. This also stimulates emergence of fleas and therefore increases the frequency with which vacuuming needs to be performed. Vacuuming should address all areas visited by the pet, paying particular attention to furniture (needs to be moved to ensure area around and under is cleaned), and along baseboards/corners. A vacuum with a beater bar is preferred, and when finished the canister should be emptied into the trash and removed from the home immediately. The second step is to wash or replace the pet's bedding. This also includes washing all human bedding if the pet shares this space. The final step is to apply pesticides to the premises. A professional or the homeowner can do this task. The author recommends professional services as these individuals are trained, possess experience, have access to superior products, and in many cases include retreatment in initial prices. Although many homeowners wish to address this problem themselves, many are unaware of the thorough treatment that is required along with the time and effort this process takes. Also, most are uneducated with regard to proper product selection, which leads to incorrect application, and many fail to retreat in an adequate time frame. For outdoor spaces, five strategies should be considered: (1) decrease organic debris within the yard, (2) cut the grass short to increase sun exposure, (3) restrict access to crawl spaces and uncultivated areas, (4) apply a registered pesticide, and (5) decrease access to wildlife and stray animals. The efficacy of environmental management, however, should be realistically discussed with the clients in terms of expectations. For example, a single-family home with a fenced backyard will be much more effectively managed than a client living in an apartment complex or one living on a large piece of land where the pet (and other animals) has free roaming access.

126. A 6-month-old Newfoundland female dog presented for a recurrent infection. The owner says that this is the third time this has happened since they got her as a 6-week-old puppy. The patient's record indicates that she is current with all recommended vaccines, is on an appropriate-size oral monthly flea preventative (afoxolaner), and has previously been treated with two, 2-week courses of oral cephalexin at a proper dosage. Physical exam reveals scattered ventral thoracic, abdominal, axillary, and inguinal pustules and epidermal collarettes. No other skin or hair coat abnormalities are present. Skin scrapings were negative, and cytology of a ruptured pustule revealed intracellular coccoid bacteria. You diagnose the patient with a superficial pyoderma, and the owner asks if the infection could possibly be resistant. You inquire about the previous episodes to which the owner reports all prior occurrences had completely resolved while on antibiotics with lesions recurring 2–3 weeks after discontinuation of therapy. Although there is no indication from the history that this infection could be resistant, a bacterial culture was acquired to appease the owner, and the identification and sensitivity report are as follows:

Culture Summary

Animal ID	Specimen	Growth	Organism
001	Skin swab	Heavy, pure	*Staphylococcus pseudintermedius*

i. Which of these drugs is likely to be effective in the treatment of the current infection but should be avoided in this patient?

ii. If this patient were a Doberman pinscher instead of a Newfoundland, what drug, although effective, should be avoided?

iii. What are potential adverse events associated with the use of rifampin and trimethoprim/sulfamethoxazole?

iv. What are plausible primary causes for this patient's recurrent pyoderma?

Antimicrobial	*S. pseudintermedius*
Amikacin	S
Ampicillin	R
Amoxi/Clav acid	R
Cefazolin	R
Cefpodoxime	R
Cephalexin	R
Chloramphenicol	S
Clindamycin	S
Doxycycline	S
Enrofloxacin	S
Erythromycin	S
Minocycline	S
Oxacillin	R
Tetracycline	S
Rifampin	R
Trimethoprim/Sulfa	S

Abbreviations: S, susceptible; I, intermediate; R, resistant; NI, no interpretation.

126. i. Enrofloxacin. This antibiotic is a fluoroquinolone and should be avoided for several reasons in this patient. The first is that the patient is a young, rapidly growing, large breed dog, and the use of fluoroquiolones has been associated with cartilage defects in young, growing animals. As a result, use of enrofloxacin is not recommended for dogs under 1 year of age or in large to giant breed dogs under 18 months of age. The second is that fluoroquinolones are classified as second-tier antimicrobials and given the current isolate is still susceptible to first-tier drugs, they should be utilized in any therapeutic protocol before enrofloxacin. Finally, the use of fluoroquinolones, specifically first-generation drugs, is a known risk factor for selection of methicillin resistance in *Staphylococcus aureus* and for selection of extended spectrum β-lactamase-producing *E. coli.* Although a direct link with the development of MRSP has not been shown, given the similarities between MRSA and MRSP, enough evidence exists that this class of antimicrobials should not be used for treatment of superficial pyoderma when first-tier drugs or safe, reasonable second-tier alternatives still demonstrate susceptibility (Morris et al., 2017).

ii. Sulfadiazine/sulfamethoxazole + trimethoprim. Doberman pinschers, Samoyeds, and miniature schnauzers have been reported to have a higher risk than other breeds to develop reactions to sulfonamides, and these drugs should only be used in these breeds when the potential therapeutic benefit outweighs the significant potential of the known adverse events (Trepanier et al., 2003). Specifically, studies in Doberman pinschers have suggested this sensitivity may be genetic and due to a limited capacity to detoxify metabolites of sulfas (Campbell, 1999).

iii. Known adverse events associated with the use of rifampin in small animals include hepatoxicity, pancreatitis, red/orange discoloration of body secretions (urine, saliva, tears, etc.), thrombocytopenia, hemolytic anemia, GI symptoms, and pruritus with erythema (cats). Adverse events associated with the use of potentiated sulfas include fever, thrombocytopenia, hepatopathy, keratoconjunctivitis sicca (dry eye, small dogs potentially at greater risk), neutropenia, hemolytic anemia, cystitis, arthropathy, uveitis, cutaneous adverse drug eruptions, facial swelling, proteinuria, facial neuropathy, drug-induced hypothyroidism, GI symptoms, and seizures.

iv. Primary causes of recurrent pyoderma in dogs include an allergic hypersensitivity, endocrinopathy, follicular dysplasia, keratinization disorder, ectoparasites, iatrogenic immune suppression, an autoimmune disorder, or neoplasia. Given the dog's young age, absence of prescribed immunosuppressant medications, and lack of other symptoms (growth and developmental abnormalities), differentials such as neoplasia, iatrogenic immune suppression, or an endocrinopathy are highly unlikely. Negative skin scrapings, a lack of evidence of fleas, and the monthly use of an isoxazoline antiparasitic agent eliminates *Demodex* or flea allergy dermatitis as potential differentials. The finding of a normal hair coat on physical along with a lack of excessive scaling and thickening of the skin renders a keratinization disorder or follicular dysplasia unlikely. That leaves cutaneous adverse food reaction, atopy, or idiopathic bacterial folliculitis as the plausible culprits in this case. The next step in prevention and management of this case would be to start a diet elimination trial with a balanced home-cooked, novel protein, or hydrolyzed diet given the patient's young age and potential nonseasonality prior to considering allergy testing, allergen-specific immunotherapy, or pharmaceutical management for atopic dermatitis.

127. The rear paw of an adult cat is shown (**Figure 127a**).

i. What is this condition called?

ii. What treatment, if any, is required?

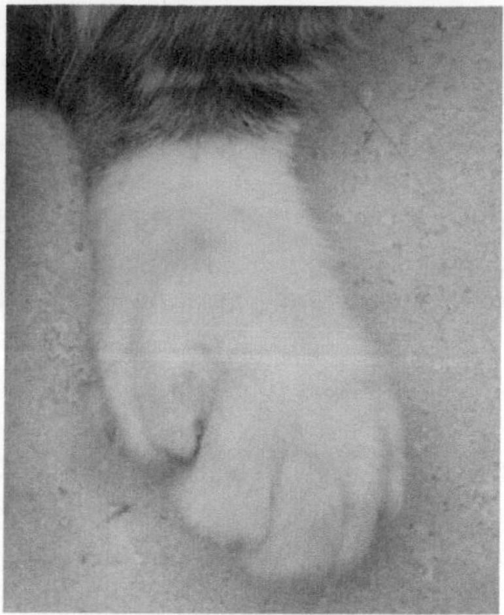
Figure 127a

128. A 3-year-old female, black Labrador retriever presented for a recent onset of a rash over the past 1–2 weeks. Physical exam reveals multiple papules and pustules along the ventral abdomen and medial aspect of the rear legs. As a result, you elect to acquire cytology and a skin scraping from the affected region. The skin scraping had no significant findings, and a microscopic field (100×; oil immersion) from the cytology stained with Diff-Quik is shown in **Figure 128a**.

What is present at the end of the green arrow?

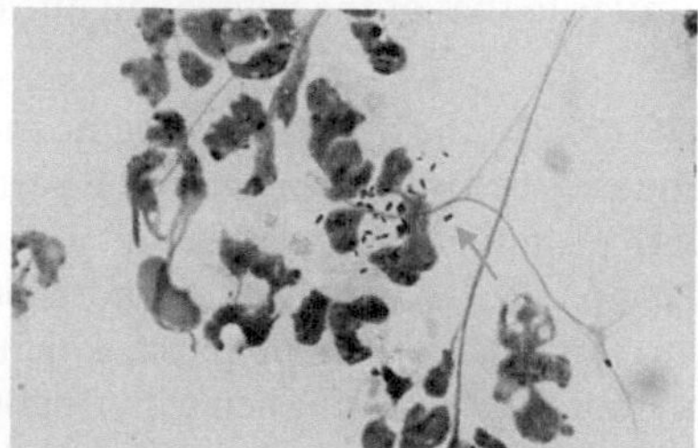
Figure 128a

129. **Figure 129a** is a video otoscopic image of the tympanic membrane of a 1-year-old spayed female mixed breed dog.

i. What structures are letters A, B, and C highlighting, and the dark area marked by the green * corresponds to what middle ear structure?

ii. How does structure C differ in appearance between dogs and cats?

iii. What is meant by the term *epithelial migration*?

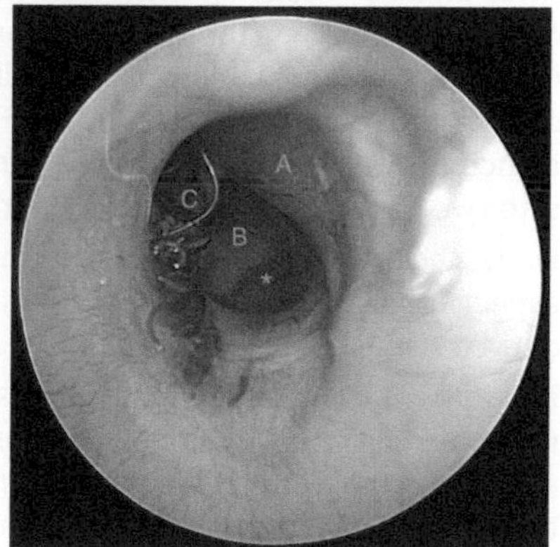

Figure 129a

127. i. Polydactyly. This is a hereditary disorder seen in cats in which there is an extra digit. Affected cats appear to have "thumbs." A common lay term for this condition is "mittened."

ii. This condition is cosmetic and causes the cat no discomfort provided that the claws of the extra toes do not grow into the associated pad or extra digits affect mobility. Owners should be educated that they need to look at the cat's claws and trim the claws, as needed. If the claw does grow into the pad, the cat will become lame. Most owners are very fond of the appearance of these cats, and although surgical removal of the extra digit will prevent ingrown claws, owners often prefer not to have this done.

128. This is a melanin granule. Melanin granules can be misinterpreted as bacteria by inexperienced veterinarians and technicians. Notice the dark brown-black coloration of this structure along with the variable shape of the other pigmented structures in the area. It is this coloration and variation in shape that help distinguish these structures from bacteria. Bacteria when present and stained with Diff-Quik will appear pale to dark purple/violet in color, similar to that of the neutrophil nuclei shown.

129. i. In the dog, the tympanic membrane is divided into two distinct sections. Structure A represents the pars flaccida, which is located caudodorsally with prominent vasculature and may appear flat or distended. A distended pars flaccida can be mistaken for a possible mass, foreign body, or parasite. Letter B corresponds to the pars tensa, which comprises the majority of the tympanic membrane surface. When a myringotomy is performed, it is done through the caudal ventral portion of this structure. Letter C corresponds to the manubrium of the malleus. The malleus along the incus and stapes comprise the three auditory ossicles, which transmit tympanic membrane vibrations to the oval or vestibular window. The * corresponds to the tympanic bulla, which is separated from the tympanic cavity proper by the septum bulla, which is seen as the prominent white ridge in the image. In the dog, the septum bulla is incomplete, while in the cat it is complete and separates the tympanic cavity into two distinct portions (dorsolateral and ventromedial).

ii. In the dog, the manubrium of the malleus is C-shaped with the concave aspect oriented rostrally. In the cat, this structure is straight and lacks the curved shape (Njaa et al., 2012).

iii. *Epithelial migration* is the process of the normal lateral and outward movement of keratinocytes and debris from the tympanic membrane and external auditory canal. In essence, it is the normal "self-cleaning" mechanism by which the ear prevents accumulation of cerumen.

130. A 1.5-year-old, intact, female Shetland sheepdog presented for a second opinion concerning recurrent crusting and hair loss on the face (**Figure 130a**, **b**) and ear tips. The affected regions are not pruritic. These lesions first developed when she was 20 weeks of age and have gradually progressed. Skin scrapings have been consistently negative for *Demodex* mites, and repeated fungal cultures were negative. Several other littermates had similar lesions, and a contagion was suspected but none were found. Finally, the lesions did not respond to oral antibiotic therapy. The owners also report that she is a "sloppy eater" and has not had a heat cycle yet.

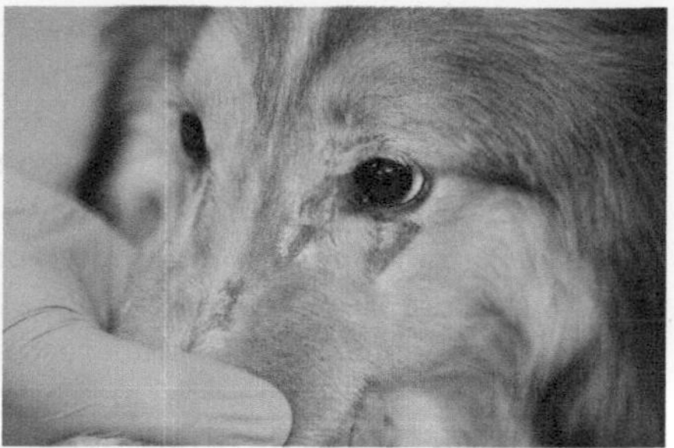
Figure 130a

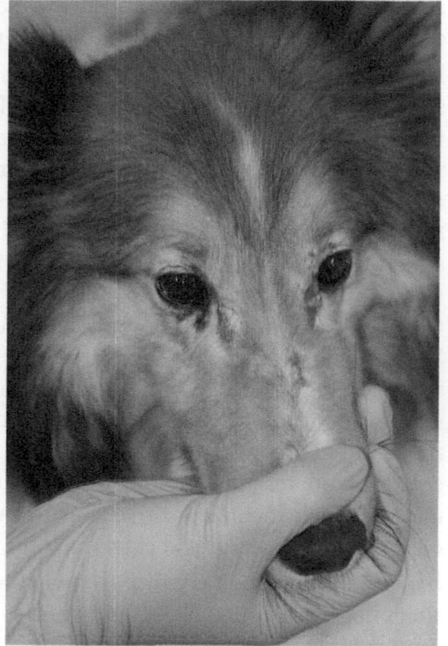
Figure 130b

i. Based on the information provided, what is the most likely diagnosis, and what other clinical signs are commonly associated with this disease?

ii. How is this disease diagnosed?

iii. This is a heritable disease. What is the mode of transmission, and how is this disease treated?

130. i. Dermatomyositis. This is an uncommon condition that predominantly affects the skin and to a lesser extent muscles. The exact cause is unknown, but an immune-mediated pathogenesis is suspected that results in an ischemic dermatopathy. Dermatomyositis is predominantly seen in Shetland sheepdogs and collies (canine familial dermatomyositis). Clinical signs are variable, may wax and wane, and range from mild to severe and debilitating. Cutaneous lesions usually appear before 6 months of age and may consist of cicatricial (scarring) alopecia, erythema, scaling, and crusting around the eyes, on the ear tips, in the metatarsal and metacarpal areas, on the digits, and on the tip of the tail. Myositis is a feature of this disease and, when present, correlates with the severity of the skin disease. Dogs with more severe signs may present with a history of difficulty chewing and/or swallowing, a high stepping gait, megaesophagus, and/or aspiration pneumonia. The most common signs of myositis are atrophy of the muscles of mastication and hindlimbs.

ii. A clinical diagnosis can be made based on the history, breed, and clinical signs, and ruling out other differentials. Differential diagnoses include dermatophytosis, bacterial pyoderma, and demodicosis. These are easily ruled out via skin scrapings, dermatophyte culture, and response to treatment. Other differential diagnoses include cutaneous lupus variants and vasculitis. With the latter being a possibility, a thorough history of vaccination and medication administration should be documented; particularly, timing of the last rabies vaccination prior to the development of clinical signs should be investigated. Canine dermatomyositis is confirmed via biopsy and dermatohistopathology. Skin biopsy findings show hydropic degeneration of basal cells, intrabasalar or subepidermal clefting, pigmentary incontinence, follicular atrophy, and possibly vasculitis. Muscle biopsy and electromyography aid in the diagnosis of myositis but are not routinely performed. Muscle biopsy findings show inflammatory exudates, muscle fiber necrosis, and muscle atrophy. Electromyography abnormalities include positive sharp waves and fibrillation potentials in muscles of the head and distal extremities.

iii. This is a hereditary disease, with a familial predisposition in Shetland sheepdogs and collies. Breeding studies have shown an autosomal dominant mode of inheritance in collies (Morris, 2013). The goal of treatment is to minimize the worsening of clinical signs and maintain a good quality of life for the dogs. General recommendations include minimizing UV exposure and restricting activities that traumatize the skin, as both may exacerbate lesions. Daily supplementation with fatty acids and vitamin E may be beneficial in mild cases. In recurrent moderate-to-severe disease, pentoxifylline is commonly implemented therapeutically and has historically been the drug of choice for this condition. In cases where these recommendations do not control clinical signs, combination therapy with additional immunomodulatory agents (e.g., tetracycline derivatives and niacinamide, glucocorticoids, cyclosporine, topical tacrolimus) should be pursued. Prognosis is highly variable and depends on disease severity as well as the ability to control signs while minimizing adverse events associated with pharmaceutical intervention. Regardless of disease severity, affected dogs should not be bred.

131. How much blood can an actively feeding female cat flea (*Ctenocephalides felis*) consume?

132. A 3-year-old mixed breed spayed female dog presented for a "rash" on the ventral abdomen (**Figure 132a**). This is the first occurrence of this issue in the patient who has a history of no prior skin problems. Physical examination revealed lesions on the ventral abdomen and thorax along with the medial rear legs. Close examination of the patient revealed intact papules, pustules, crusts, and epidermal collarettes. Skin scrapings were acquired and revealed no parasites.

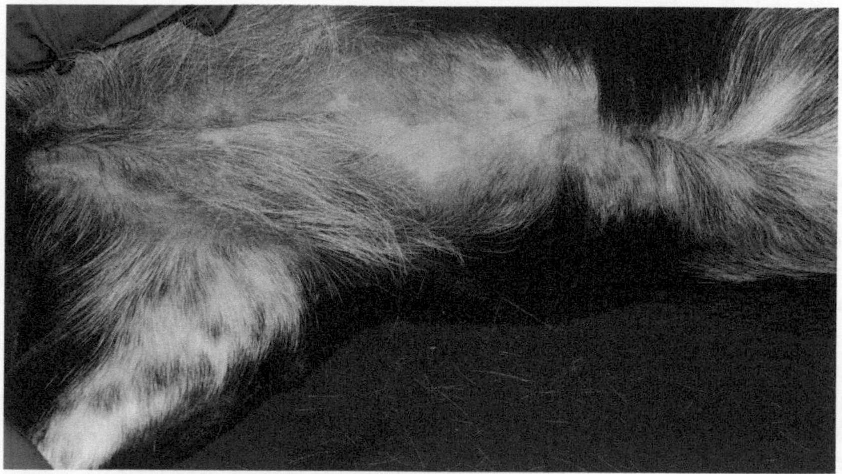

Figure 132a

i. What is the most likely clinical diagnosis, and how is it be confirmed?
ii. If a bacterial culture is acquired from these lesions, what bacteria are most likely to be isolated?
iii. The owners in this case are unable to treat the patient topically. What systemic antibiotics are considered first-tier antimicrobials? Which is considered appropriate for use in this patient, and how long should they be administered?

131. An adult cat flea has been shown to be able to consume an average of 13.6 μL of blood per day. This volume corresponds to approximately 15.15 times the flea's body weight (Dryden and Gaafar, 1991). As a result, a heavy flea infestation can easily cause anemia in a puppy or kitten. To put this in a practical example, a 0.5 kg kitten has approximately a 30 mL blood volume. If the kitten is in a heavily infested environment, 110 female fleas could potentially consume 5% (1.5 mL) of the kitten's blood per day.

132. i. Superficial bacterial folliculitis. The clinical signs are consistent for bacterial pyoderma. In this patient, all of the classic lesions of pyoderma are present: papule, pustule, crusted papule/pustule, and epidermal collarette. Skin cytology from an unruptured pustule, under a crust, or along the margin of an epidermal collarette should be acquired, and if intra- or extracellular bacteria are observed from lesional skin, the diagnosis is made.

ii. The most common pathogen associated with superficial bacterial folliculitis in dogs is *Staphylococcus pseudintermedius.* Other potential *Staphylococcus* spp. associated with infection but seen much less frequently are *S. aureus*, *S. schleiferi* (coagulase-variable bacterial species), and other coagulase-negative staphylococci. Other bacteria encountered on rare occasions include *Streptococcus canis, Pseudomonas aeruginosa*, and other Gram-negative bacteria, usually in association with *S. pseudintermedius* (Hillier et al., 2014).

iii. Several recent papers and working groups have provided treatment guidelines for superficial bacterial folliculitis that tier systemic antimicrobials into those that are appropriate for empiric therapy and those that should be reserved for cases with sensitivity reports justifying their use (Beco et al., 2013; Hillier et al., 2014). Those antimicrobials that are considered first tier and appropriate for the empiric therapy of a first occurrence pyoderma include: clindamycin (10 mg/kg q12h), cephalexin or cefadroxil (15–30 mg/kg q12h), amoxicillin-clavulanate (12.5–25 mg/kg q12h), and potentiated sulfonamides (dose and frequency are formulation dependent). Due to possible adverse events encountered with potentiated sulfonamides during therapy, the author does not use this class for empiric therapy and reserves them for methicillin-resistant cases when safer alternatives are not an option. There is considerable debate surrounding the third-generation cephalosporins cefovecin and cepodoxime as to whether or not they should be classified as first or second tier. The author prefers not to use these as first-line drugs for empiric therapy but will use them as a first-tier option when patient medicating is difficult to impossible or owner compliance is poor. Superficial bacterial folliculitis should be treated for 1 week past clinical resolution. Given this guideline, 14 days is the absolute minimum any superficial pyoderma should be treated for, and in most cases, this means that 3 weeks of therapy are likely required to resolve the infection when systemic antimicrobials are utilized.

133. A 1-year-old spayed female Chinese pug presented for acute onset of hair loss and rash. The owner reports that the patient has no history of ear or skin disease prior to 2 weeks ago. Review of the patient's medical record reveals that she is current with recommended vaccinations and routinely purchases topical imidacloprid and oral milbemycin oxime products for monthly flea and heartworm prevention. Physical exam reveals the presence of diffuse truncal, patchy "moth-eaten" alopecia with papules, pustules, crusts, and epidermal collarettes. Due to owner financial concerns, you elect to start with a simple cytology from an intact pustule. Shown are 4× (**Figure 133a**) and 100× (**Figure 133b**) microscopic images from this patient's cytology.

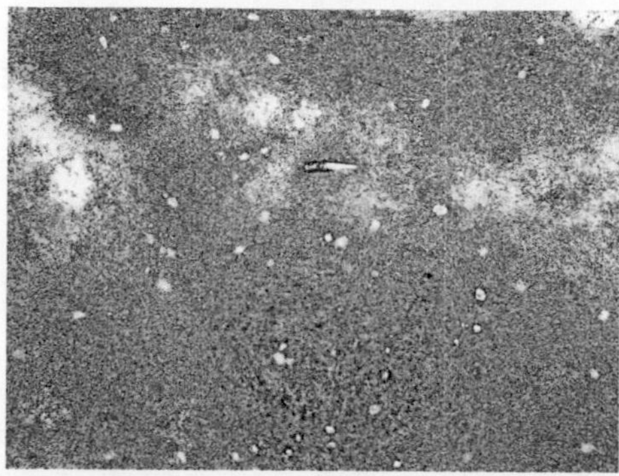

Figure 133a

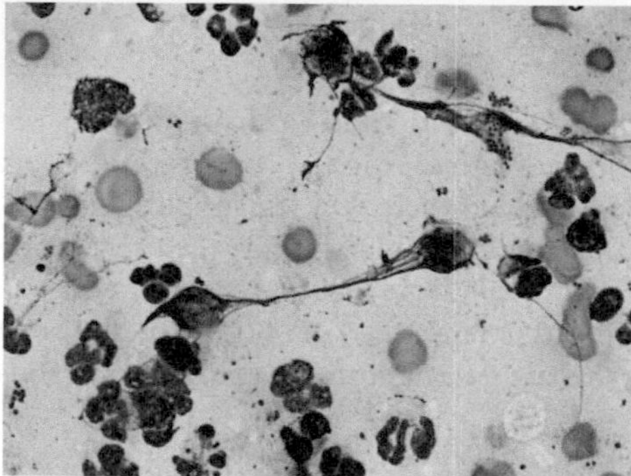

Figure 133b

What is your diagnosis?

134. House dust mites are a common environmental allergen implicated in atopic dermatitis that are thought to play a vital role in the development and propagation of disease.

What are the two most common species of house dust mites associated with atopic dermatitis, and what are their respective environmental niches?

133. Juvenile-onset generalized demodicosis with a secondary pyoderma. This case illustrates the importance of scanning acquired cytology specimens on lower microscopic power prior to proceeding with observation under high magnification. Scanning under low microscopic power is important to do for a couple of reasons. First, it prevents the observer from missing larger objects such as mites or foreign material, and second, it aids in identifying fields of interest to be observed under higher magnification as it is not practical or an efficient use of time to review all slides, or all fields on a single slide, under oil immersion. **Figure 133c** is a microscopic image at 10× power from the same field as **Figure 133a**. The adult *Demodex canis* mite is highlighted by the green arrow.

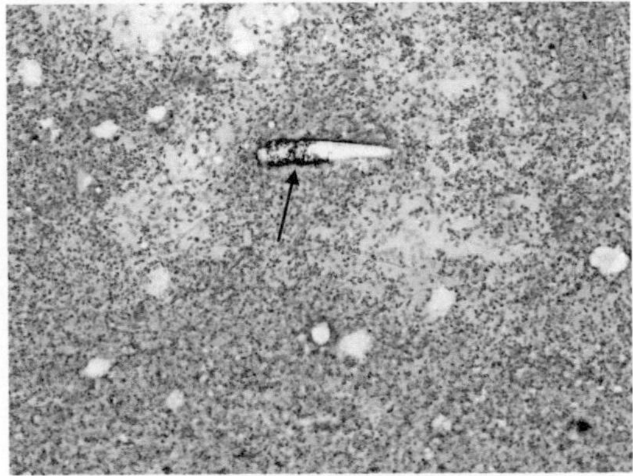

Figure 133c

134. *Dermatophagoides farinae* and *Dermatophagoides pteronyssinus*. Both mites are found in homes, with the highest concentrations located in furniture, carpeted floors, and bedding, where they feed on fungal spores and skin scales. For the most part, they require moderate temperatures (20°C–30°C) with high relative humidity (70%–90%). *D. farinae* prefers drier continental climates and is the most common species identified in the United States. *D. pteronyssinus* is more vulnerable to fluctuations in humidity and favors costal climates (Nuttall et al., 2006).

135. A 1.5-year-old castrated male orange cat presented for examination of black spots on his nose. The owner is concerned due to a family member's recent diagnosis of melanoma and is worried the cat is developing cancer as well. Physical examination reveals several macular hyperpigmented spots on the nasal planum (**Figure 135a**) that were first noted by the owner several months prior to presentation. The spots do not bother the cat, and the patient is otherwise healthy with no history of prior skin issues.

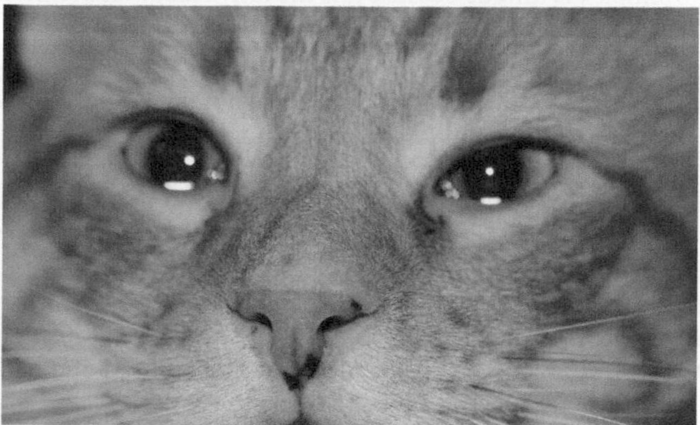

Figure 135a

i. What is this condition called?
ii. How should this condition be treated?
iii. What is unique about this syndrome?

136. What is the difference between a pyrethrin and a pyrethroid?

137. Recently, organisms previously identified as *Staphylococcus intermedius* underwent reclassification into the *Staphylococcus intermedius* group (SIG) of bacterial pathogens.

What organisms comprise this group, and what is the practical significance of this reclassification?

135. **i.** Lentigo simplex of orange cats. This is a very common hereditary pigmentary condition found in orange cats, in which well-demarcated, asymptomatic macular melanosis is observed on the lips, nose, gingiva, and eyelids. Lesions begin as very small black spots in cats, typically at less than 1 year of age, and with time become more numerous and enlarge.

ii. This condition is a cosmetic defect, which does not warrant therapy. Lesions do not progress over time to melanoma or any other neoplastic condition.

iii. Lentigo simplex is unique because it is the only recognized inherited form of hypermelanosis in small animals.

136. Pyrethrins are extracted from chrysanthemum plants and have immediate flea-killing activity (fast knockdown). They have little residual activity and are very sensitive to UV light. They are relatively nontoxic and are safe to use on young animals, including cats. Pyrethroids are synthetic drugs that are very stable in UV light. They work on sodium channels of insect nerve axons and cause nerve excitement and paralysis. They are rapidly adulticidal and have some repellant (prevent the parasite from coming near) activity. Examples of pyrethroids include D-*trans*-allethrin, resmethrin, fenvalerate, and permethrin. Cats are especially sensitive to these drugs, causing potentially lethal, toxic side effects; they are best avoided in this species.

137. The *Staphylococcus intermedius* group (SIG) is composed of *S. pseudintermedius*, *S. delphini*, and *S. intermedius* based on multilocus sequence analysis (Fitzgerald, 2009). Historically, *S. intermedius* had been considered the primary pathogen of canine pyoderma since its description in the 1970s. Under this new classification scheme, the primary pathogen of canine pyoderma is *S. pseudintermedius*. From a practical perspective, this means isolates historically identified as *Staphylococcus intermedius* from dogs are now believed to all have been *S. pseudintermedius* and are commonly found designated in the literature as *[pseud]intermedius.*

138. An indoor/outdoor cat presented after it had gone missing for several days. The owners note the patient is not using its left leg and has pain and is vocal when touched over the lumbar region. The hair coat was matted with exudate present and foul odor emanating from the tail-head region. Following light sedating and clipping, the following was revealed (**Figure 138a, b**).

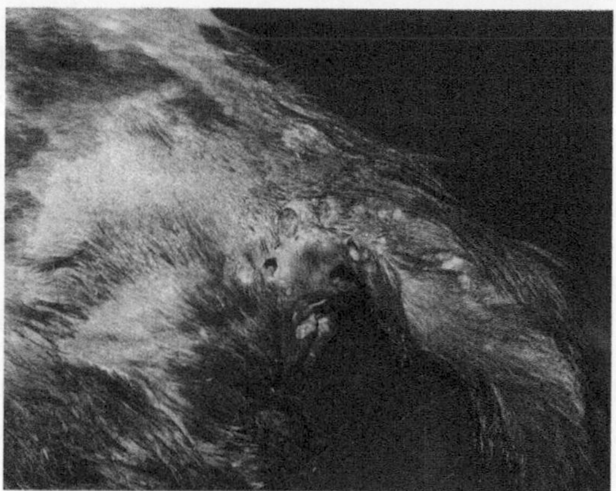

Figure 138a

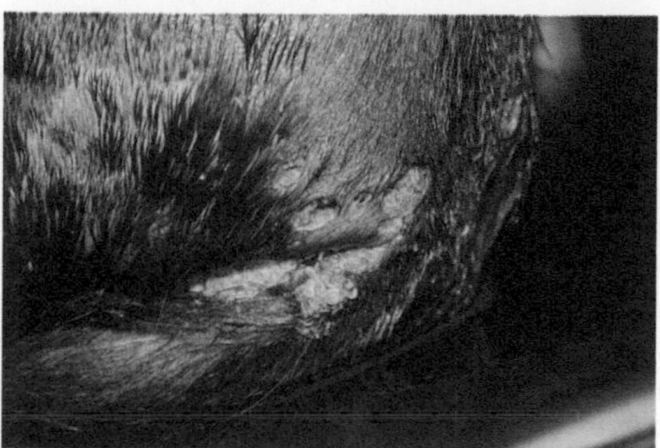

Figure 138b

i. What is your diagnosis, and what is the etiology of this condition?

ii. A classification scheme to describe the host-parasite relationship that is divided into obligatory, facultative, or accidental is commonly utilized for this condition. What does each mean, and what are examples of each?

iii. What are the possible ways that the causative species can be identified?

iv. How should this patient be managed?

138. **i.** Myiasis. This is an infestation of tissues by larvae of *Dipterous* flies. The condition is a disease of inattention to the pet. Adult flies lay eggs in wounds, on moist skin, or on soiled/unkempt hair coats, particularly in debilitated or recumbent patients. Larvae then hatch and secrete enzymes that liquefy tissue and facilitate tissue damage and destruction that can occur quickly.

ii. Obligatory myiasis is caused by flies whose larvae require living tissue to complete their life cycle. Fly species that cause obligatory myiasis can lay eggs in uninfected wounds or penetrate through the skin of their host to invade deeper tissues. Examples of flies that fall under this classification are primary screwworm flies (*Chrysomya bezziana* or *Cochliomyia hominivorax*) and bot flies (*Cuterebra* spp.). Facultative myiasis happens when a nonparasitic fly's larvae infest a patient. Normally these flies lay their eggs in decomposing organic debris, but they can also lay their eggs on animals with infected open wounds or soiled, unkempt hair coats. Flies that fall under this category are *Calliphora* spp., *Lucilia* spp., *Musca* spp., *Phormia* spp., and *Sarcophaga* spp. Accidental myiasis occurs when dogs or cats consume fly eggs or larvae, but the larvae do not cause clinical disease or proceed through further life stage development.

iii. If necessary, it is possible to identify the causative fly species. This can be done one of two ways. The first is that larvae can be collected and submitted for examination of characteristic structures, specifically the larval mouthparts, posterior spiracles, or stigma plates. The second is keeping larvae until they become adult flies at which time they can also be easily identified.

iv. First assess the patient to ensure they are stable, as a patient suffering from myiasis can progress to shock, intoxication, or sepsis. The wounds should then be clipped, cleaned, and flushed with providone-iodine or dilute chlorhexidine. It is important to shave beyond the immediate lesion borders as distant pockets of larvae commonly occur as a result of larval migration along the deeper tissue planes. If a few larvae are present, simple mechanical removal may be easiest, but in most cases, systemic drugs to quickly kill larvae are utilized. Drugs used for this purpose have included pyrethrin-based products, ivermectin, nitenpyram, and spinosad/milbemycin (Correia et al., 2010; Han et al., 2017). Nitenpyram is a neonicontinoid that is rapidly absorbed and excreted. Administration of nitenpyram as soon as myiasis is detected allows for quick larval kill to start before mechanical removal in patients where sedation may need to be delayed due to stabilization efforts. Administration of nitenpyram can also be performed rectally (off-label use) in severely debilitated patients. Finally, secondary infection of the wounds is common, and patients should be prescribed an appropriate broad-spectrum antibiotic (i.e., amoxicillin-clavulanic acid).

139. A 5-year-old spayed female Labrador retriever presented for head shaking and scratching at the ears (**Figure 139a**). The patient is the only dog in the household, spends a large amount of time outdoors, and lives on a small hobby farm with numerous other animals. The owner reported intermittent use of flea and tick preventatives. On physical exam, alopecia, erythema, and mild crusting were noted on both ears along with an accumulation of tightly adherent brownish-colored insects on the convex portion of the right pinna (**Figure 139b**). One of the insects was removed from the patient and examined under low microscopic power (**Figure 139c**).

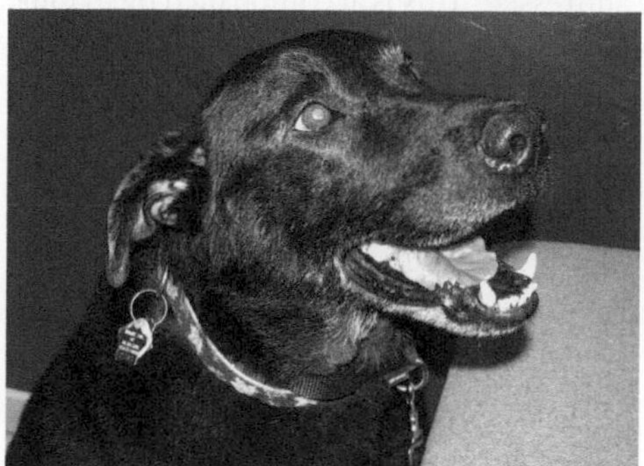

Figure 139a

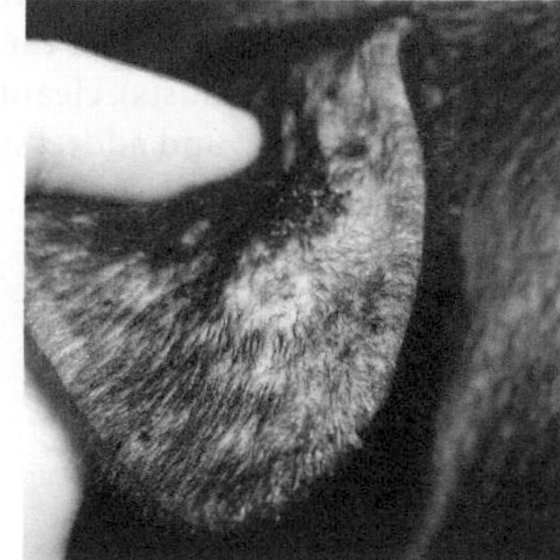

Figure 139b

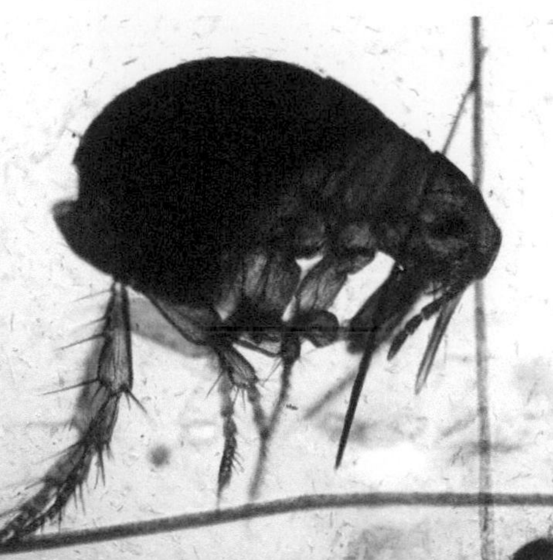

Figure 139c

i. What is your diagnosis, and what is the natural host for this organism?

ii. How is this condition treated/prevented?

139. **i.** Flea dermatitis due to *Echidnophaga gallinacea* (sticktight poultry flea). This flea is a major pest of domestic chickens and was likely acquired from those on the farm as a result of inconsistent use of flea preventatives. The parasite is known to cause issues with dogs and cats that have contact with infested fowl. When problematic in small animals, it is usually found along the ear margins or interdigitally around pads. The parasite is identifiable due to its small size, lack of genal and pronotal combs, and the shape of the flea's head.

ii. Treatment of this patient requires manual removal followed by consistent use of any of the number of insecticides registered for the treatment and prevention of flea infestations. To prevent further occurrence of this condition, the poultry and premises will need to be addressed. This is accomplished by manually removing the fleas from the chickens, treating them with an appropriate product (sprays and dusts), cleaning the environment (removal of bedding litter and treat nest box), and addressing the outdoor area for fleas.

140. A 4 mg tablet of methylprednisolone is shown in **Figure 140a**.

What do the score lines on this tablet indicate, what are the pros and cons of splitting tablets, and what advice should be given to owners when they are instructed to fraction tablets?

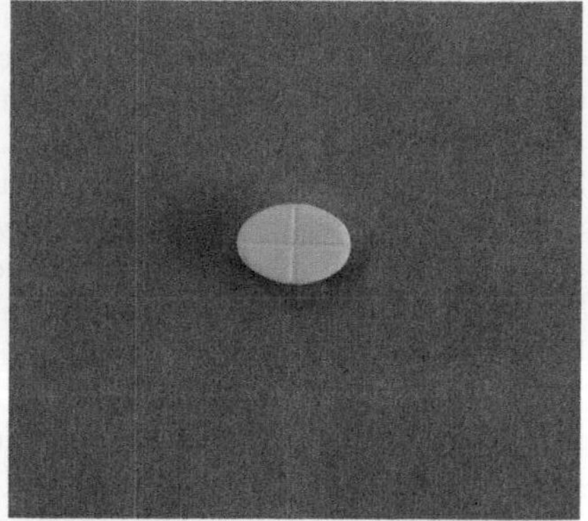

Figure 140a

141. The dorsal nasal planum of a 4-year-old spayed female boxer dog is shown in **Figure 141a**. This lesion started to develop when the dog was 1–2 years of age and has slowly progressed. The area is not reported to bother the dog but is considered unsightly by the owner. The rest of the physical examination was considered unremarkable.

i. What is the clinical name for the most likely condition this dog has, and how is it clinically managed?

ii. If this lesion occurred suddenly in an older dog, what is considered reasonable differential diagnoses?

iii. What skin disease has been described in Labrador retriever dogs that appears similar to this one?

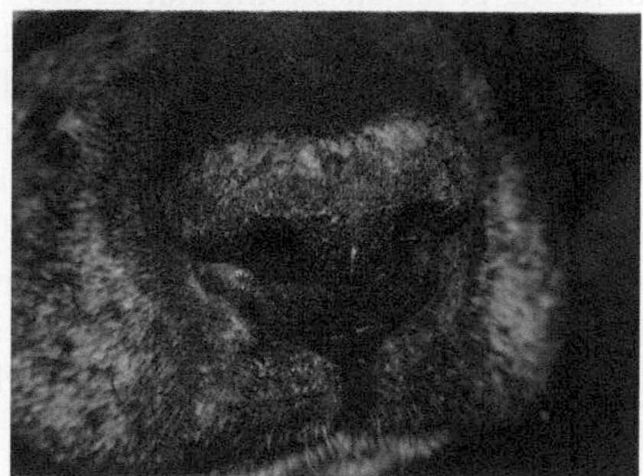

Figure 141a

142. A clinical condition similar to that observed in Labrador retrievers discussed in **Question 141** is seen in a particular breed of cat.

What is the name of the condition, and what breed of cat is affected?

143. What is the name of the medical/cosmetic device shown in **Figure 143a**, and what dermatologic condition in dogs is it been used for?

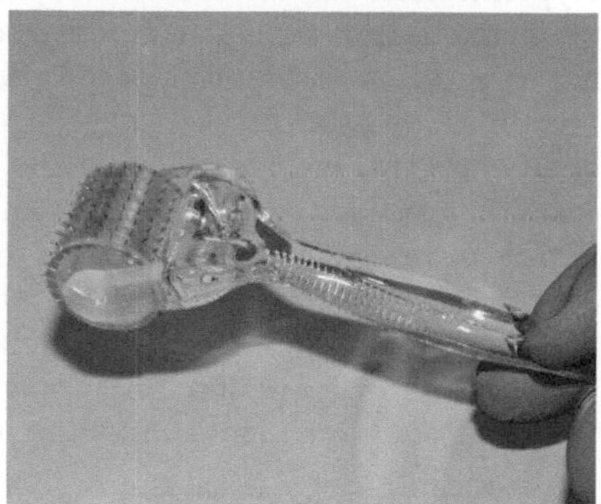

Figure 143a

140. The score lines on this tablet indicate that it could potentially be divided or split into fourths, and that when done properly, the content uniformity of the tablet would result in four 1 mg-containing portions. The pros of being able to split a tablet are that it allows dose flexibility in patients with a wide range of body sizes routinely encountered in veterinary medicine; it may aid in ease of administration in patients who may have difficulties swallowing; and the more common reason is it potentially may decrease the cost of therapeutic regimens. The disadvantages of tablet splitting are that they may be difficult for owners to break, it may create unequal portions resulting in significant dose fluctuations, there may be drug content loss due to crushing/powdering at the break site, or it may potentially expose owners to drugs with hazardous pharmacological effects. Overall, tablet splitting should have minimal clinical significance for drugs with long half-lives, wide therapeutic ranges, or where dose fluctuations are not a major concern. The same is not true for drugs with narrow therapeutic windows such as chemotherapeutics and immunosuppressive medications. Splitting of tablets should not be advised for medications that are extended release, enteric coated, or with formulations that lack score lines imprinted on the unaltered tablet. Owners should be instructed to break tablets by hand when possible as studies in human medicine have shown hand-splitting to be more reproducible than when tablet-splitters or kitchen knives are utilized (van Riet-Nales DA, 2014; Somogyi et al., 2017). When splitters or a kitchen knife are required, a demonstration should be performed for the owner to highlight proper technique. Pre-breaking tablets prior to dispensing should be reserved for cases where owners are unable to split the tablets, as this may subject the medication to stability issues.

141. **i.** Idiopathic nasodigital hyperkeratosis. The young age at onset, slow progression, and lack of other clinical findings support this clinical suspicion. Hyperkeratosis may affect the nose, pads, or both and can occur as a congenital, hereditary, or senile change. This condition is primarily a cosmetic one, but in severe cases, fissuring of the affected region may become painful. This keratinization issue can be managed and requires lifelong treatment. The main goals of therapy involve softening and removal of excessive keratin. In severe cases, this may require trimming with scissors or claw trimmers. Otherwise, in mild to moderate cases such as this one, the use of humectant or keratolytic agents is usually successful. Daily application (7–14 days) of products such as petroleum jelly, ichthammol, salicyclic acid, or propolyene gycol should be done until the nasal region is near normal and then their use decreased to one to two times a week in an effort to maintain the condition.

ii. The acute onset of nasal and/or footpad crusting should make the clinician suspicious of pemphigus foliaceus, cutaneous lupus variants, and hepatocutaneous syndrome. Other differential diagnoses for nasodigital hyperkeratosis include zinc-responsive dermatosis, leishmaniasis, canine distemper, or cutaneous horns. Biopsy is useful in differentiating these causes when they are suspected.

iii. Hereditary nasal parakeratosis of Labrador retriever dogs (Peters et al., 2003). This is an uncommon condition of Labrador retrievers or their crosses that is believed to have an autosomal recessive mode of inheritance. Lesions are often first seen between 6 and 12 months of age and start as mounds of hyperkeratosis on the dorsal aspect of the nasal planum. The severity varies, with some dogs having only small amounts of brownish dry adherent keratin on their nose, while others develop severe fissures and erosions. Histologically, this syndrome is characterized by parakeratotic hyperkeratosis and the presence of serous lakes within the epidermis. Dogs with this condition are treated primarily via application of moisturizers.

142. Ulcerative nasal dermatitis of Bengal cats. This condition is characterized by early onset (4–12 months of age) of mild nasal planum hyperkeratosis that may gradually progress to severe crusting, fissuring, erosions, and depigmentation. Histopathology reveals marked parakeratotic hyperkeratosis with pleocellular dermatitis. Limited details on treatment of the condition suggest that similar interventions used for nasal hyperkeratosis in dogs are effective. However, anecdotal reports of rapid lesion resolution with topical tacrolimus question the exact etiology of the condition (Bergvall, 2004).

143. This is a microneedler. This device varies by the material it is composed of along with the number and length of microneedles on the roller. The device has been used by the cosmetic dermatology industry as a method of skin tightening to improve the skin's surface appearance or minimize scars in people. The device is used by rolling it across the skin's surface and the needles create pinpoint punctures inducing superficial trauma to the skin. The minor trauma produced is enough to induce local wound repair substances TGF-β3, fibroblast growth factor 7, and collagen I. As a result of these functions, a recent investigation looked at the application of this device in Alopecia X, a condition where previous reports had documented induced hair growth at the site of skin trauma. The device was used on two spayed female Pomeranian dogs with a diagnosis of Alopecia X that had previously failed other forms of medical therapy. The authors reported that hair growth was observed in both by 5 weeks, with significant regrowth appreciated at 12 weeks post-procedure. The hair condition at 12 months was considered stable in both dogs with no loss of the regrown hair coat (Stoll et al., 2015). Whether or not this procedure produces permanent hair regrowth is unknown at this time, but it may provide a safe cosmetic option for a condition that is predominantly a cosmetic issue.

144. Cyclosporine is a commonly used medication in veterinary dermatology.
i. What is this drug derived from?
ii. What is the mechanism of action for this medication?
iii. What are the label indications of the drug?
iv. What conditions is this medication used for in veterinary medicine?
v. What are the most prevalent adverse events associated with use of this drug?

145. A 2-year-old cocker spaniel presented with the complaint of bilateral epiphora and periocular pruritus (**Figure 145a**). On physical examination, mild signs of primary seborrhea were noted (nasal digital hyperkeratosis and scaling). The discharge in the periocular area was thick and malodorous, and impression smears of this area revealed bacterial and yeast organisms. The initial working diagnosis was primary seborrhea with mild facial fold pyoderma. The epiphora and periocular pruritus did not resolve after a 21-day course of oral antibiotics and ketoconazole; however, impression smears of the skin revealed that the microbial infection had resolved. Closer examination of the patient revealed there was no evidence of face rubbing, chewing, or whole-body pruritus. The dog's conjunctivae were reddened, and the sclera injected. Excessive tearing was noted.

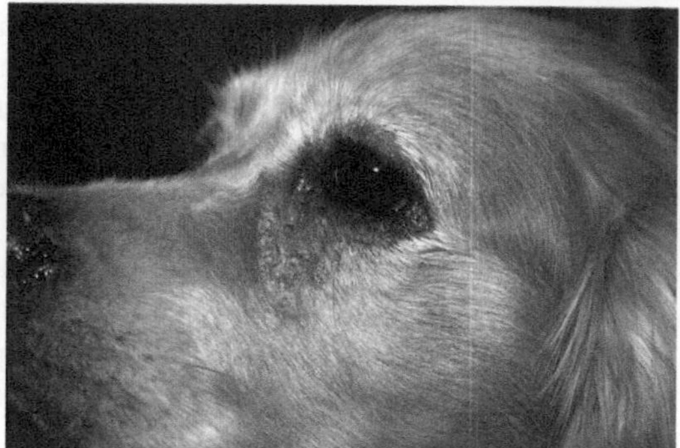

Figure 145a

What are two common causes of epiphora in this breed of dog?

144. i. Cyclosporine is isolated from the fungus *Beauveria nivea* (formerly *Tolypocladium inflatum*).

ii. Cyclosporine is a calcineurin inhibitor that predominantly inhibits T-cell activation. The drug accomplishes this by binding to the intraceullar receptor cyclophilin-1. This complex then inhibits calcineurin, preventing the dephosphorylation and activation of the transcription factor nuclear factor of activated T cells (NF-AT). This prevents the production of several pro-inflammatory cytokines such as IL-2, IL-4, interferon-γ, and tumor necrosis factor-α. The inhibition of IL-2 is thought to play the most critical role and accounts for cyclosporine's main immunomodulating effect (Forsythe and Paterson, 2014). Besides the effects on T cells, cyclosporine also affects B cells, antigen-presenting cells, keratinocytes, mast cells, eosinophils, endothelial cells, and basophils.

iii. Cyclosporine is labeled for dogs in the United States for the control of atopic dermatitis in dogs at least 6 months of age and weighing at least 4 pounds (4 lbs = 1.82 kgs), and for the control of feline allergic dermatitis as manifested by excoriations, miliary dermatitis, eosinophilic skin lesions, and self-induced alopecia in cats at least 6 months of age and at least weighing 3 pounds (3 lbs = 1.36 kgs).

iv. Cyclosporine has been used in the management of canine atopic dermatitis, feline allergic dermatitis, juvenile cellulitis, sterile nodular panniculitis, vasculitis, cutaneous reactive histiocytosis, pemphigus foliaceus (more effective in cats), perianal fistulas, metatarsal fistulas, cutaneous lupus variants, uveodermatologic syndrome, end-stage proliferative otitis externa, erythema multiforme, nasal arteritis, sterile granuloma/pyogranuloma syndrome, feline plasma cell pododermatitis, dermatomyositis, and sebaceous adenitis (Palmeiro, 2013).

v. GI issues (vomiting, diarrhea, and anorexia) are the most common adverse events encountered and are usually mild, occurring in roughly 40% of patients (Nuttall et al., 2014). Papillomatous skin lesions, gingival hyperplasia, and hypertrichosis are occasionally seen and are predominantly cosmetic issues that may improve with dose reductions or cessation of therapy. Rarely, neurologic symptoms may be encountered along with predisposition to uncommon viral, protozoal, bacterial, and fungal infections. At this time, cyclosporine when used at standard doses for atopic dermatitis does not appear to be a risk factor for neoplastic development, nephrotoxicity, or systemic hypertension (Nuttall et al., 2014).

145. The two most common causes of epiphora in this breed are blockage of the nasal lacrimal duct and distichiasis. This dog's nasal lacrimal duct was patent. Careful examination of the patient under mild sedation revealed severe distichia on both the lower and upper eyelids. This case of distichiasis was treated by electroepilation of the cilia.

146. A 3-year-old miniature dachshund presented for examination of intense pruritus of 6–8 weeks' duration. The patient was previously diagnosed with atopic dermatitis a year ago at which time the owners elected supportive care consisting of antihistamines and fish oil supplementation, as they did not want to start drugs or allergen-specific immunotherapy. In the past, pruritus has been a minor dermatologic problem for this dog. The owner reported that the pruritus began shortly after the trees started to bloom this year. Skin scrapings were negative for *Demodex* mites, and no evidence of fleas was found, consistent with the dog's reported year-round use of a monthly oral flea preventative. The dog's ventral abdomen, neck, and distal extremities are alopecic, thickened, and hyperpigmented with some patchy mild crust formation, and exudate from the crevices of the skin is very oily (**Figure 146a, b**).

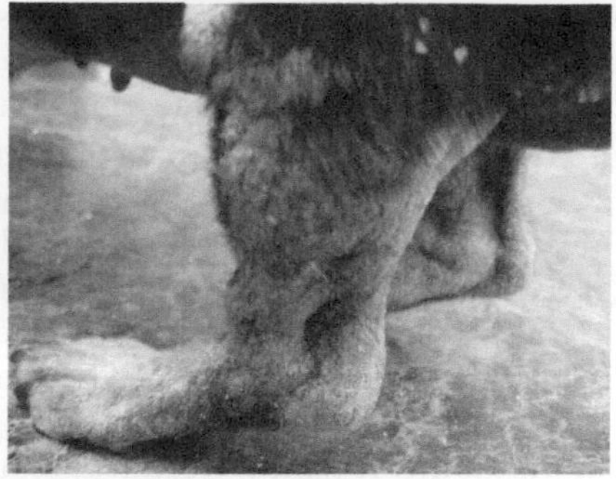

Figure 146a

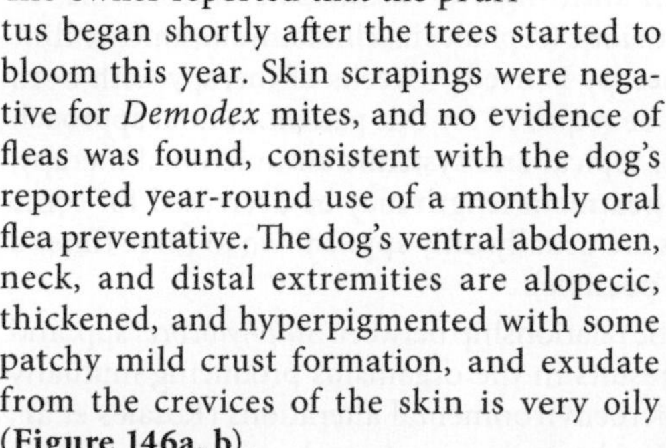

i. What common microbial infections will an impression smear of this dog's skin be expected to show?

ii. Assuming these two common pathogens are found, how should these combined infections be treated?

iii. What is the proposed relationship between these two organisms?

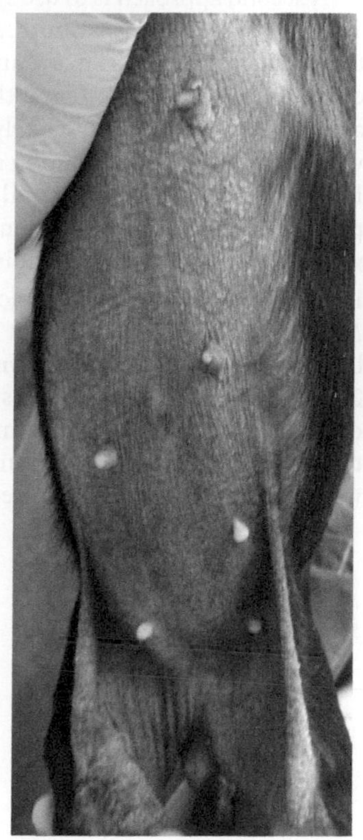

Figure 146b

146. i. Concurrent *Staphylococcus pseudintermedius* and *Malassezia* spp. infections are common in pruritic patients, especially dogs with atopy, disorders of keratinization, or endocrinopathies.

ii. Assuming both are present in this patient as verified by cytology findings, a minimum of 4 weeks of concurrent treatment for both the bacterial and yeast infection is required. There are a couple of different approaches that can be taken in any patient with concurrent infections.

One approach is to treat both infections topically with baths, sprays, lotions, mousse applications, or some combination thereof, with formulations containing miconazole, climbazole, or ketoconazole combined with chlorhexidine. If topical treatment alone is used, it needs to be frequent (at least three to four times per week; if not daily).

A second approach is to use systemic antimicrobials to treat both infections. This requires the use of both an antifungal (ketoconazole, fluconazole, or terbinafine) along with an oral antibiotic (cephalexin, clindamycin, amoxicillin-clavulanate). If only systemic therapy is used, 4 weeks of therapy with both agents concurrently would likely be required for this patient. A final approach would be to use a combination of topical and systemic antimicrobial therapy. If this option is chosen, overall treatment length may be decreased for some patients, and topical applications are usually only applied two to three times a week (although more frequent is possible).

iii. There appears to be a symbiotic relationship between *Staphylococci* spp. and *Malassezia pachydermatis* that results in the organisms producing mutually beneficial growth factors and microenvironmental alterations (Rosales et al., 2005). Clinical evidence of this has been shown where dogs with *Malassezia* dermatitis have increased numbers of *Staphylococcus pseudintermedius* on their skin, frequently concurrent pyodermas, and patients fare better clinically when both organisms are treated as compared to only one.

147. A young kitten presented primarily for "behavioral reasons" as the owners note it is restless and jittery compared to the rest of the litter. The kitten is from a small hobby farm and lives outdoors. The owners also report that the kitten scratches and grooms itself more often than the rest of the kittens. Physical examination of the kitten was normal except for the hair coat, which displayed patchy alopecia and generalized thinning with macroscopic white organisms found along the hairs (**Figure 147a**). Many of the organisms were also observed to move upon parting of the hairs.

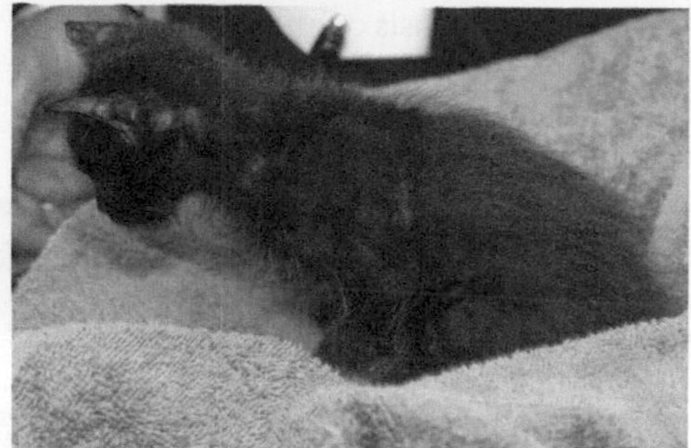

Figure 147a

i. What is the most likely diagnosis, and how can the diagnosis be confirmed?

ii. This parasite is divided into two major subcategories, what are they, and which species affect the dog and cat? What are the key clinical features of each, and what species has most likely infested this kitten?

iii. What other parasites can appear as white and macroscopic in the cat?

148. A 1-year-old neutered male Siamese cat presented for evaluation of progressive hair loss and excessive self-grooming. The owners adopted the patient roughly 6 months ago and have observed an increase in self-grooming since that time. A sample of hair was taken from the periphery of an alopecic patch and is revealed in **Figure 148a**.

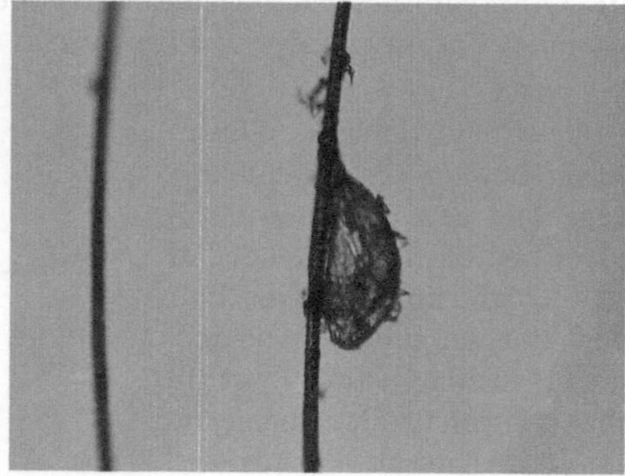

Figure 148a

What is the diagnosis, what species is associated with cats, and how is it differentiated from the other known species observed in companion animal medicine?

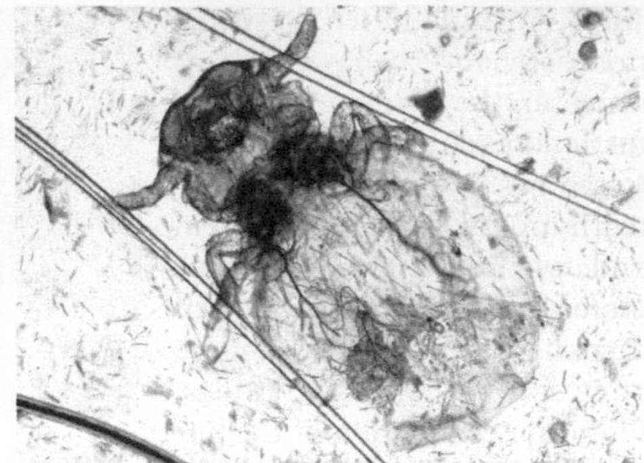

Figure 147b

147. **i.** Pediculosis or an infestation with lice. The diagnosis may be made via visual examination of the hair coat or following flea combing as lice are large parasitic insects. It may also be confirmed following microscopic examination of samples acquired from skin scraping, trichogram, or acetate tape preparations.

ii. Lice are divided into two suborders: consisting of Anoplura (sucking lice) and Mallophaga (biting lice). *Linognathus setosus* is the sucking louse of dogs, which is more likely to be found attached to the skin and can cause anemia in heavily infested patients. *Trichodectes canis* and *Felicola subrostratus* are the biting lice of the dog and cat, respectively. Biting lice move more rapidly than sucking lice and may cause more irritation. Pruritus may range from asymptomatic to severe in affected patients. Additionally, *Trichodectes canis* (**Figure 147b**) may act as an intermediate host for *Dipylidium caninum* (canine tapeworm). Lice are very host specific, and as a result, this cat is infested with *Felicola subrostratus.*

iii. Other parasites that can appear as "white" are *Dermanyssus gallinae* (poultry mite), *Cheyletiella* spp., and *Lynxacarus radovsky.*

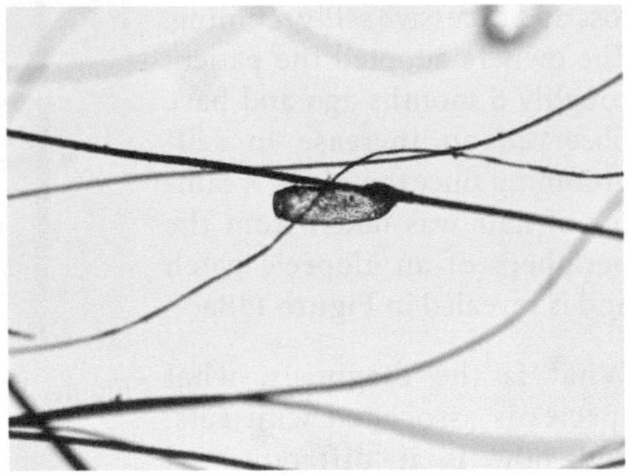

Figure 148b

148. Cheyletiellosis. **Figure 148a** shows a *Cheyletiella* spp. egg. The egg of this mite is identified by its loose, fibrillar strand attachment to the hair and nonoperculated free end. This is in contrast to a louse nit that is larger, firmly cemented to the hair shaft, and operculated at the free end as seen with this photomicrograph of a *Felicola subrostratus* nit (**Figure 148b**). *C. blakei* is the species most commonly associated with cats, while *C. yasguri* and *C. parasitivorax* are associated with the dog and rabbit, respectively. This mite does not exhibit extreme host specificity and poses a zoonotic risk. The species can be identified from each other based on a sense organ found on the anterior-most pair of legs along genu I in adult mites. This structure has a conical shape in *C. blakei*, a heart shape in *C. yasguri*, and a dome/global shape in *C. parasitiovorax.*

149. Images from a 10-year-old castrated male Yorkshire terrier presented for a second opinion are shown (**Figure 149a–d**). The owner's complaint is increasing generalized pruritus, excessive scaling, and pigmentation changes of 5 months' duration. The dog has no prior history of skin disease, and skin scrapings have been negative. The patient has previously received treatment with topical selamectin, cephalexin, and ketoconazole, which failed to provide any benefit. The pruritus is also noted to be nonresponsive to glucocorticoid therapy. Physical examination today reveals generalized erythema, excessive large-scale formation, and mucous membrane (oral, ocular, and anal) depigmentation with crusting. Cytology samples were acquired from the perioral region under one of the crusts. A representative photomicrograph from the patient's cytology sample is shown (**Figure 149e**).

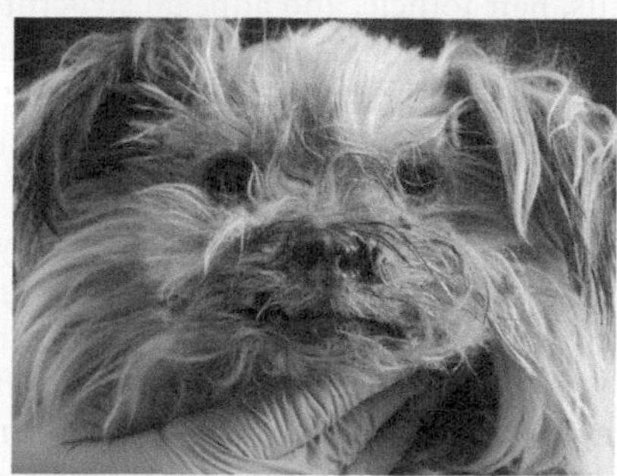
Figure 149a

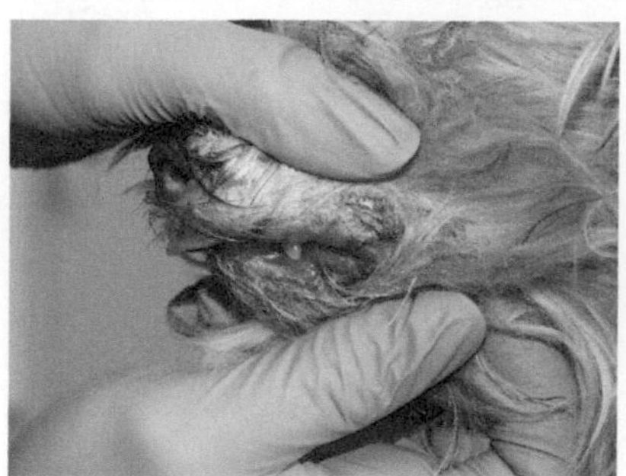
Figure 149b

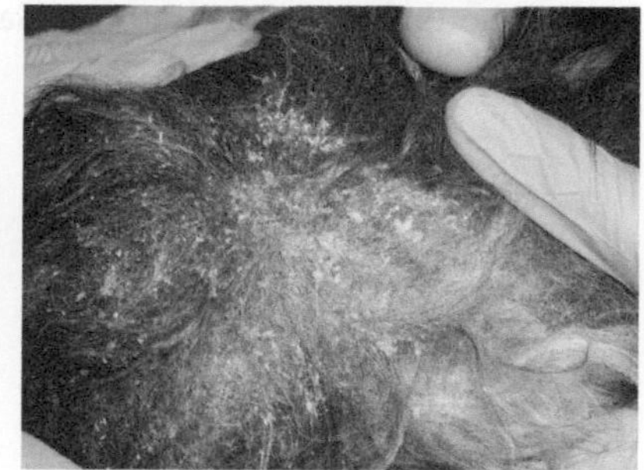
Figure 149c

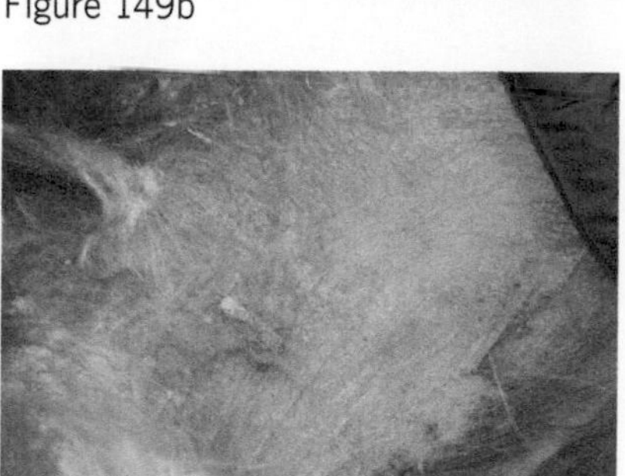
Figure 149d

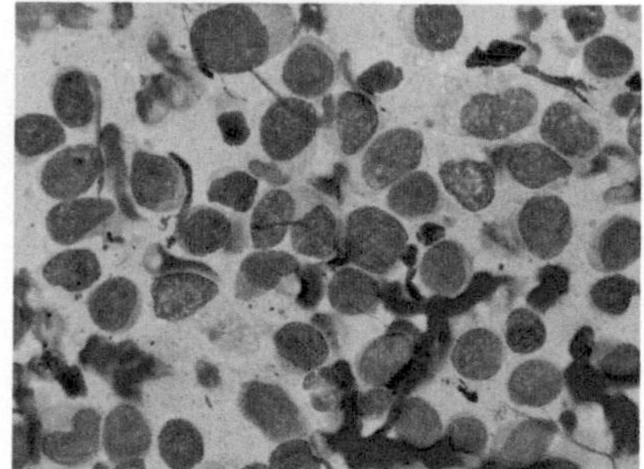
Figure 149e

i. What is the most likely diagnosis for this patient, and how will you confirm your suspicion?

ii. What are the treatment options for this patient?

149. i. Epitheliotropic lymphoma. The age of onset, progressive nature, and simultaneous occurrence of erythroderma (erythema and excessive scaling), mucous membrane depigmentation, nonglucocorticoid responsive pruritus, and presence of neoplastic lymphocytes on cytology are almost pathognomonic for this condition. Epitheliotropic lymphoma is an uncommon variant of lymphoma, where the neoplastic cells infiltrate epidermal structures (epidermis, hair follicle, and adnexal structures). Although cytology findings can be suggestive of epitheliotropic lymphoma, the diagnosis is confirmed via biopsy with histopathology, which demonstrates the characteristic epitheliotropism of the neoplastic cells and differentiates this condition from nonepitheliotropic cutaneous lymphoma.

ii. At this time, treatment is primarily considered palliative, as prognosis for the condition is grave with a median survival time of 6 months following diagnosis (Fontaine et al., 2010). Several therapeutic protocols have been proposed (attesting to the fact none have good efficacy), utilizing high-dose linoleic acid therapy (safflower oil), lomustine, synthetic retinoids, glucocorticoids, combination cytotoxic drugs, phototherapy, and total skin radiation therapy. Currently, the most commonly utilized agent remains lomustine given orally, once every 3 weeks, but a recent case report suggests that total skin radiation therapy should be evaluated further (Santoro et al., 2017).

150. What is a potassium hydroxide (KOH) preparation, and how is it performed?

151. A 3-year-old dachshund presented for bilateral pinnal alopecia (**Figure 151a, b**). The hair loss has been slowly progressive, is limited to the ear pinnae, and the dog is nonpruritic. Skin scrapings are negative, as are fungal cultures. A skin biopsy revealed miniaturization of all hair follicles.

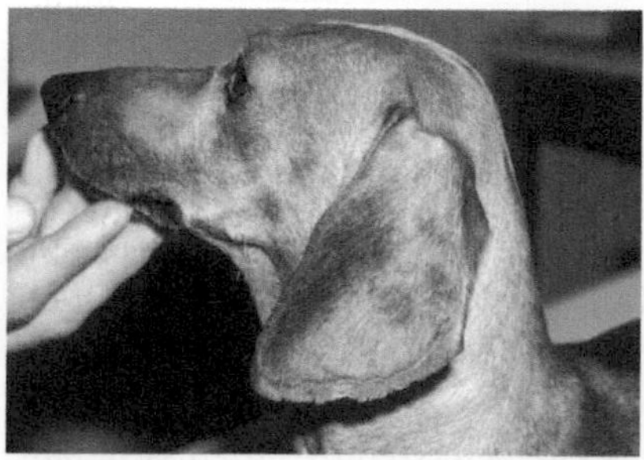
Figure 151a

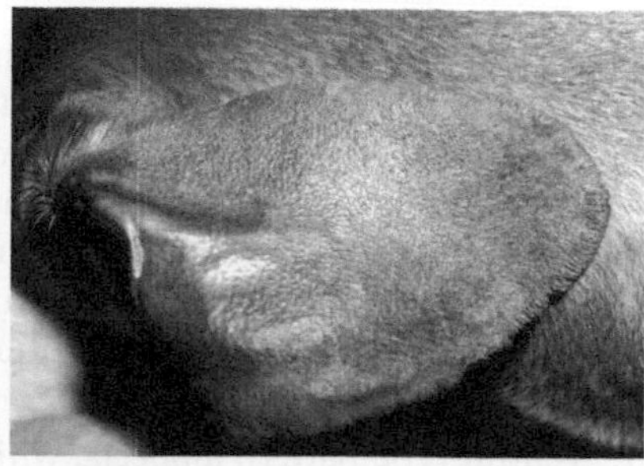
Figure 151b

i. What is the most likely cause for this patient's hair loss?
ii. What is the second recognized form of the condition this patient was diagnosed with?
iii. What treatment recommendations should be made for this patient?

152. Two different dogs are presented for evaluation of a superficial bacterial pyoderma (**Figure 152a, b**). One had an infection caused by a susceptible strain of *Staphylococcus pseudintermedius*, while the other had an infection caused by a methicillin-resistant strain *Staphylococcus pseudintermedius*.

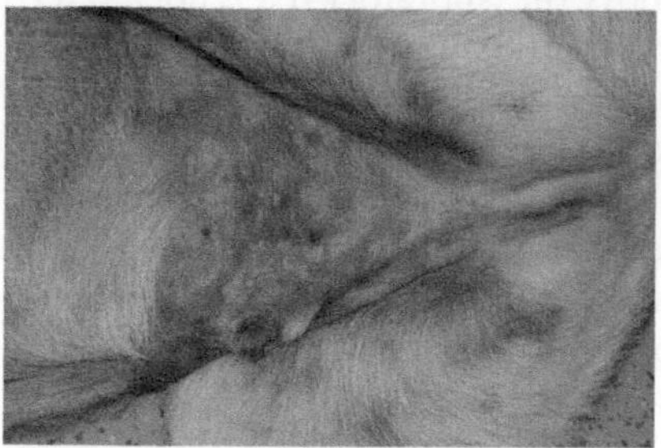
Figure 152a

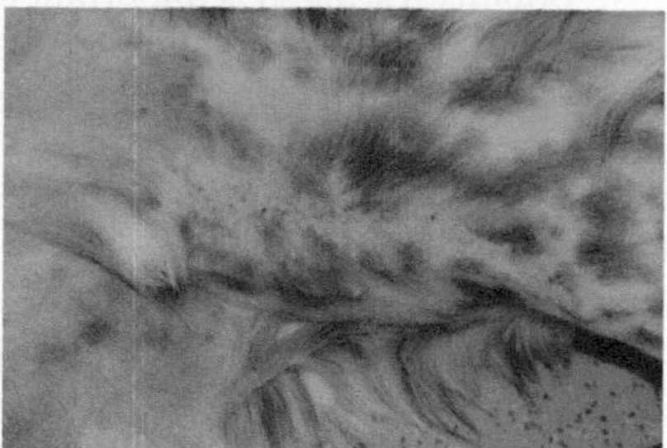
Figure 152b

Which one is which?

150. A KOH preparation is a standard technique used by some veterinary dermatologists to aid in the direct microscopic examination for fungal hyphae and spores in hair, scale, and claws. KOH is used because it "clears" keratin, exposing these structures and making them easier to find. To perform the technique, the keratinized specimen is placed on a slide, and several drops of 10%–20% KOH are added before a coverslip is placed over the sample. The slide is then either gently heated for 15–20 seconds (do not overheat/boil) or allowed to stand for 15–30 minutes prior to microscopic review.

151. **i.** The most likely cause is pinnal-type pattern alopecia. This type of pattern alopecia is observed mainly in smooth-haired and wire-haired dachshunds. The dogs are born with a normal hair coat and at some point after 6–9 months of age develop a progressive alopecia restricted to the pinnae that results in complete hair loss and hyperpigmentation of the ears. Alopecia and melanoderma of the Yorkshire terrier is clinically very similar to this condition and may actually be the same condition seen in a second breed (Mecklenburg et al., 2009).
ii. Ventral-type pattern alopecia, which is characterized by progressive hair loss along the ventral body surfaces, caudomedial thighs, and postauricular regions. Similar to the pinnal type, affected dogs are born with a normal hair coat and then, after 6 months of age, develop progressive alopecia that leaves the affected regions partially to completely bald. This form of pattern alopecia is seen in dachshunds, Chihuahuas, miniature pinschers, whippets, greyhounds, Italian greyhounds, Boston terriers, Manchester terriers, and boxers.
iii. These conditions are cosmetic problems and therefore do not require therapy. Spontaneous hair regrowth is unlikely but has been observed.

152. Clinically, it is impossible to distinguish between a methicillin-resistant and a methicillin-susceptible staphylococcal infection on a simple physical examination. The only way to determine this is with bacteriologic culture and susceptibility testing. It is important to notify the laboratory if it is not a veterinary-specific diagnostic laboratory to speciate the bacteria, as both *S. aureus* and *S. pseudintermedius* are coagulase-positive staphylococcal organisms. The implications for zoonosis are necessary information with regard to client education and patient handling. In general, *S. pseudintermedius* does not readily colonize or cause disease in people, but in some circumstances, infections have been reported in people due to this organism. Colonization with *S. pseudintermedius* may be more common in people within the veterinary community.

153. A dog with discoid lupus erythematosus presented on referral for treatment of refractory disease (**Figure 153a**). This condition is one of many seen in veterinary medicine that is known to be aggravated or caused by exposure to ultraviolet (UV) light.

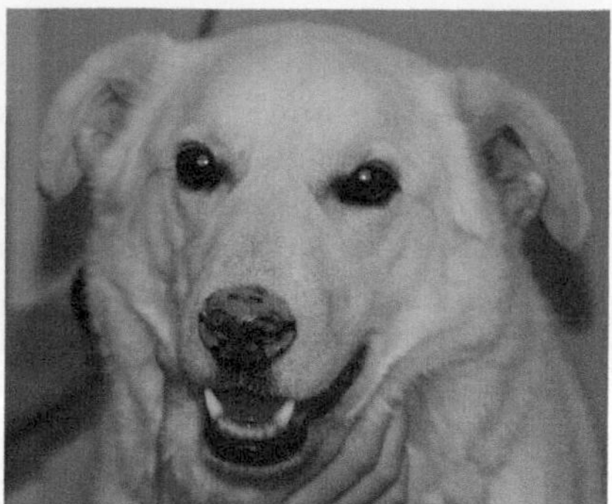
Figure 153a

i. What are the spectrums of UV radiation?

ii. How are UV light–associated diseases classified?

iii. What effect does elevation have on UV exposure?

iv. What does SPF mean?

154. Amitraz is the active ingredient in the products Tactic 12.5% (large animal formulation) and Mitaban 19.9% (small animal formulation). Normally, 10.6 mL of Mitaban is diluted in 2 gallons (9.2 L) of water and then used as a sponge-on treatment for demodicosis in dogs.

If the small animal formulation was unavailable, how should the amount of Tactic to be used in place of the 10.6 mL Mitaban be calculated?

155. A 3-year-old intact female Yorkshire terrier presented for a second opinion due to a persistent right ear infection. The owner notes that the infection first occurred about 5 months ago and that it had been previously treated on several occasions with a topical ointment for 7–10 days at a time. The owner reports that each time the ear is treated, the clinical signs improve, but they recur within 2 weeks after the medication is stopped. Additionally, it is getting more difficult to physically put the medications into the ear. Physical exam reveals a pliable right ear canal with moderate patient discomfort on palpation of the vertical canal. The ear canal opening is markedly stenotic due to hyperplastic changes preventing thorough examination of the canal (**Figure 155a**). No cranial nerve deficits are appreciated, and the left canal is determined to be unremarkable, as is the remainder of the exam. Ear cytology reveals a mixed bacterial population and *Malassezia* spp. along with the presence of white blood cells.

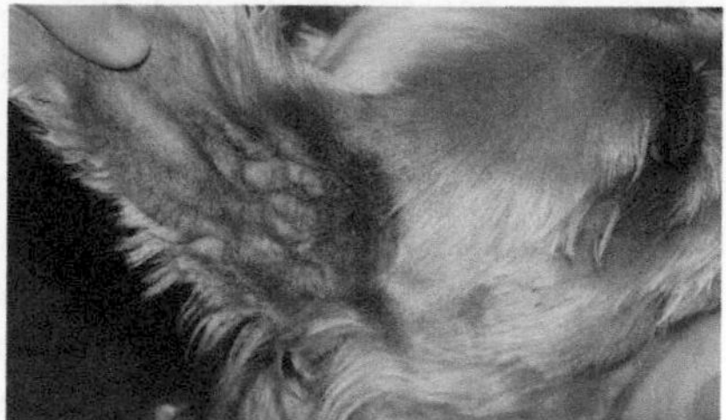
Figure 155a

Given the clinical presentation, what is the most important therapeutic aspect that should be implemented for this patient?

153. i. The effects of UV light on skin are complex, and our understanding of these effects is ever evolving. UV light makes up a small portion of the electromagnetic radiation spectrum and is classically divided into three components. The first is UVC (290–320 nm), which is germicidal and removed prior to reaching the earth's surface by the ozone layer. The second is UVB (290–320 nm), which is considered the erythrogenic region of the spectrum causing sunburns, local skin immune suppression, and DNA damage. Roughly 90% of UVB radiation is absorbed by the ozone layer, but despite this large filtration, UVB is the predominant spectrum that reaches the earth's surface. The final component is UVA (320–400 nm), the "black light" spectrum that is associated with photoaging, aggravating UV-associated dermatoses, and potentiating the effects of UVB immune suppression. UVA is not filtered by the ozone layer but instead is depleted by atmospheric factors (Palm and O'Donoghue, 2007).

ii. Skin diseases caused or aggravated by UV exposure can be classified into one of four main groups: (1) immunologically mediated or idiopathic (i.e., actinic dermatitis); (2) drug-/chemical-induced photosensitivity; (3) defective DNA repair (i.e., carcinogenesis); and (4) photoaggravated dermatoses (i.e., cutaneous lupus variants) (Bylaite et al., 2009). The effect UV light has on an individual is dependent on duration of exposure, intensity, and inherent patient characteristics, such as skin color and coat thickness.

iii. The intensity of UV radiation changes with season (greater during summer months), time of day (greatest around the noon hour), ground surface (snow reflects UVB), and elevation. A 300 m increase in elevation is reported to result in a ~4% increase in intensity, while a 1 km increase in altitude is reported to increase UV radiation by 10%–25% (Palm and O'Donoghue, 2007). Methods for controlling UV radiation exposure include limiting access to the outdoors, using protective clothing (several canine-specific companies out of Australia), or applying sunscreen.

iv. Sun protection factor (SPF) is a concept used to measure protection from sunburn. SPF is a calculated ratio of the minimal erythema dose (time to redness of skin) between sunscreen-protected skin and unprotected skin. What this means is that if it takes an individual 10 minutes of solar exposure to display onset of erythema, then application of a sunscreen with an SPF of 30 would in theory provide 300 minutes of protection against sunburn.

154. First, calculate the number of grams of amitraz needed for the Mitaban dilution:

(19.9% = 19.9 g amitraz/100 mL of solution)

19.9 g amitraz/100 mL of solution × 10.6 mL of solution = 2.1 g amitraz

Then calculate how many milliliters of Tactic is needed to get the same amount:

(12.5% = 12.5 g amitraz/100 mL of solution)

2.1 g amitraz × 100mL/12.5 g of amitraz in the solution = 16.8 mL of Tactic

Therefore, 16.8 mL of Tactic can be used in the dilution in place of 10.6 mL of Mitaban.

155. Given the hyperplastic changes resulting in stenosis of the canal, the most important aspect of treating this patient is to open the canal back up and prevent further chronic inflammatory changes. The most effective therapeutic agents for accomplishing this task are systemic glucocorticoids. Prednisone or its derivatives should be prescribed at or near a 1 mg/kg once-daily dose, which is then tapered over time based on clinical response and the occurrence of drug-related adverse events. In this particular case, methylprednisolone was started at 1.1 mg/kg daily dose that was continued for 10 consecutive days prior to tapering of the medication over the course of a 30-day period. In conjunction, a topical proprietary combination ear medication with a fluoroquinolone as the active antibacterial was started, as the tympanic membrane integrity was not initially known. Topical therapy was discontinued after 21 days of treatment, which also corresponded to cytological resolution of the secondary infections. **Figure 155b** shows the external ear at 30 days post-initial presentation. Following initial therapy, atopic dermatitis was eventually determined to be the cause of the patient's recurrent otitis; this was subsequently managed with allergen-specific immunotherapy.

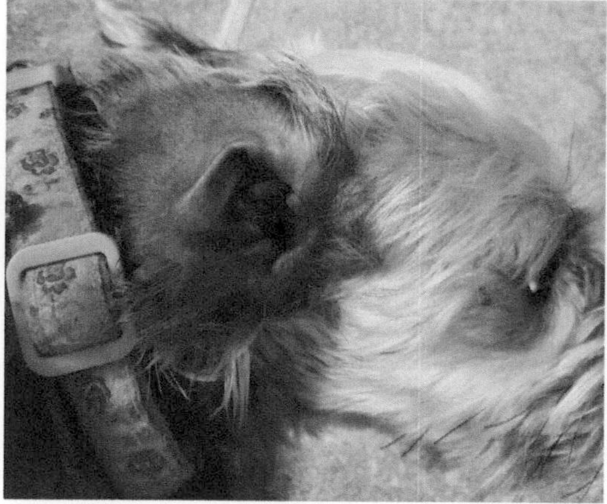

Figure 155b

156. A 10-year-old castrated male shih tzu presented with a 5-month history of progressive swelling, crusting, and hemorrhagic discharge involving all four paws. The owner notes that the patient has been previously treated with systemic antibiotics and antifungals along with topical antiseptics that have provided minimal benefit. On examination, all four paws were markedly affected. Interdigital erythema with increased keratosebaceous debris and edema were present, while multiple small nodules with hemorrhagic draining tracts were also appreciated on the palmar and plantar aspects (**Figure 156a**, **b**). Prescapular and popliteal lymph nodes were prominent, while the rest of the physical exam was fairly unremarkable.

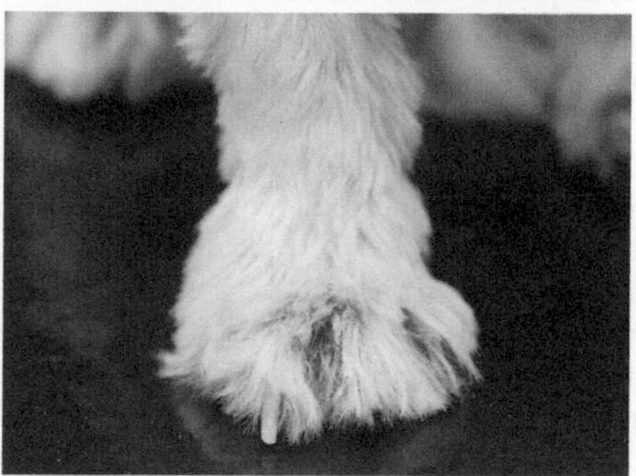

Figure 156a

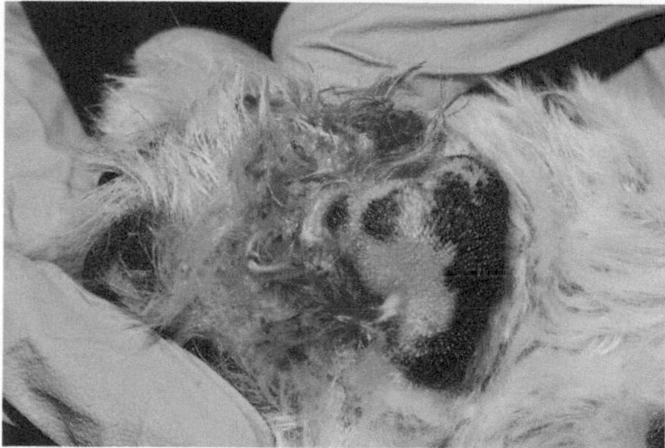

Figure 156b

i. What is the most common cause for this clinical presentation of pododermatitis?

ii. You elect to confirm your clinical suspicion via a trichogram. What diagnostic differences exist between a trichogram and a skin scrape for this purpose?

156. **i.** Canine demodectic pododermatitis. This is a unique presentation of generalized demodicosis, which in the author's opinion is the form of the condition most commonly misdiagnosed. These patients are in pain, diagnostics are often not performed, and many practitioners expect lesions elsewhere. In many cases, lesions may be confined only to the feet, and clinical signs are similar to those recognized with standard generalized demodicosis. In almost all cases, the paw lesions are complicated by secondary bacterial infections that also need to be addressed during therapy, and in this case, is the reason why partial benefit was observe by the owner when systemic antimicrobial therapy was utilized. All cases of pododermatitis should have trichograms or skin scrape samples acquired to eliminate *Demodex* mites as a potential cause.

ii. Trichograms or trichography is a diagnostic modality that is performed by plucking hairs from affected regions. The hairs are then placed on a slide in a drop(s) of mineral oil, covered with a glass coverslip, and examined via light microscopy. This diagnostic method is preferred by the author for evaluation of patients when demodicosis is suspected and lesions are confined to areas that are difficult to scrape (face and paws). A study evaluating the diagnostic utility of trichograms compared to skin scrapes in cases of canine demodicosis found trichograms to have a sensitivity of roughly 85% (Saridomichelakis et al., 2007). The same study also demonstrated trichograms to be more accurate in cases of generalized demodicosis and when disease was complicated by secondary infections. As a result, when using only trichgrams, it is important to take an adequate number of hairs and samples to lower the likelihood of missing parasitic elements. Given the lower sensitivity though, it is also important to realize that negative results may not necessarily rule out *Demodex* spp. as a potential cause.

157. A 3-year-old spayed female coonhound presented for progressive worsening of nonseasonal scratching and chewing for the past 1.5 years. On physical exam, marked generalized erythema with alopecia of the craniomedial forelimbs, ventral neck, axillary, and inguinal regions were appreciated (**Figure 157a–e**). In addition, papules were noted on the ventral neck along with salivary staining of the dorsal paws. Skin scraping and trichogram samples from the patient revealed no significant findings. Impression cytology samples taken from all affected areas demonstrated the presence of *Malassezia* spp. and coccoid-shaped bacteria forming pairs and quartets.

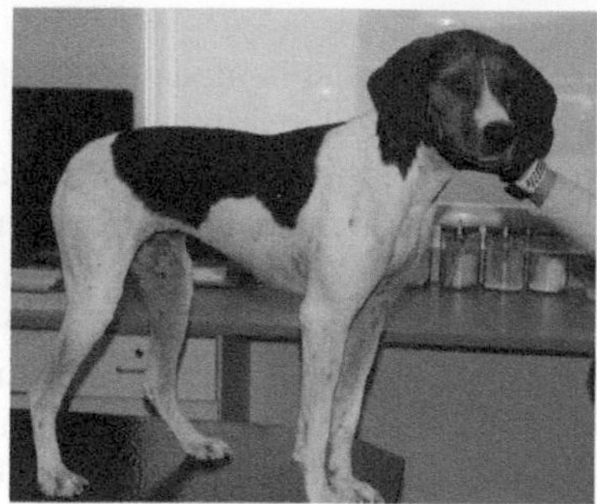

Figure 157a

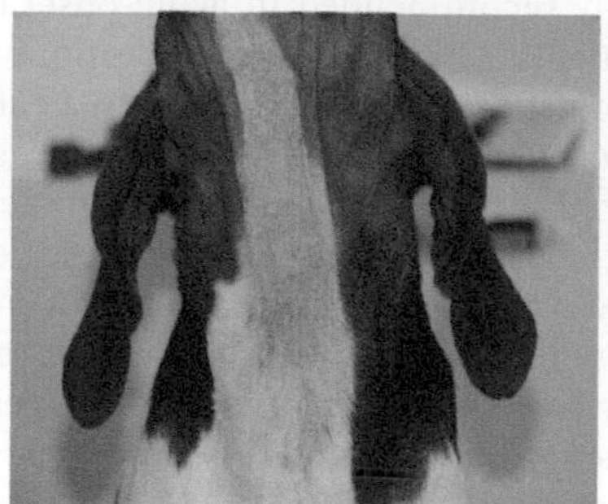

Figure 157b

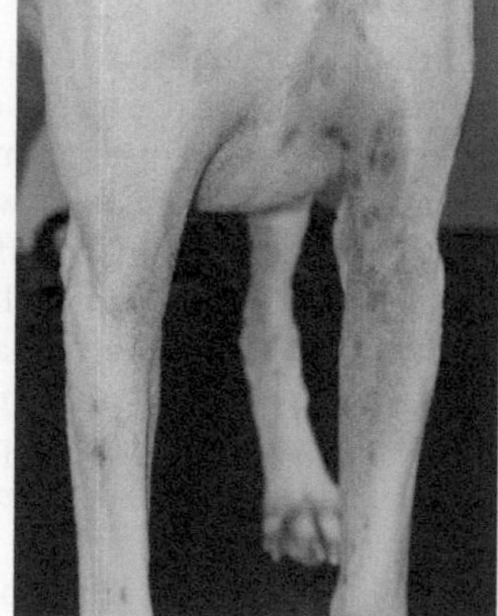

Figure 157c

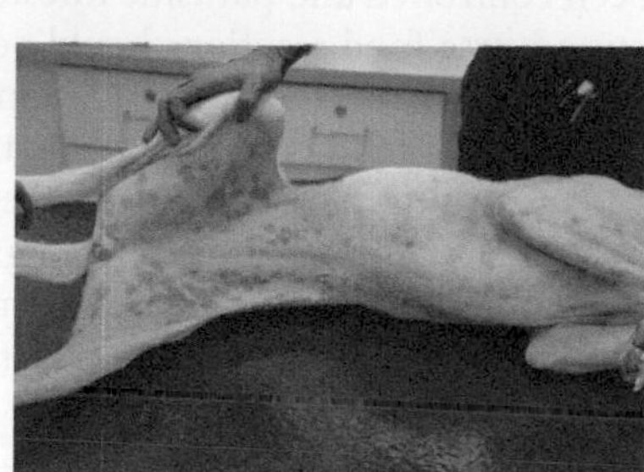

Figure 157d

i. How should this patient be treated initially?

ii. If this patient is suspected to have canine atopic dermatitis, how is that diagnosis be made?

iii. What are the clinical manifestations of atopy in this dog?

iv. What is the major route of allergen exposure in atopic patients?

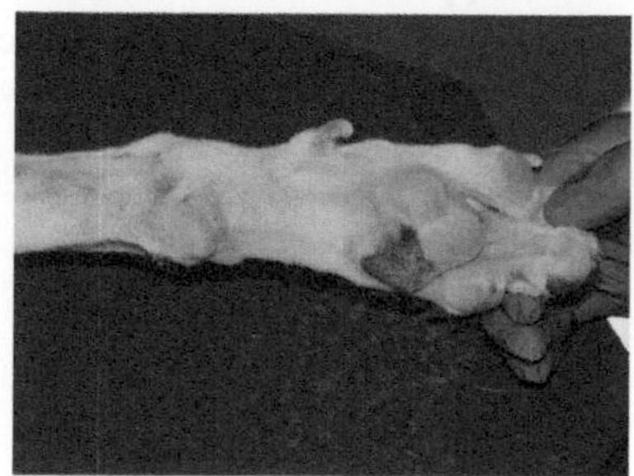

Figure 157e

157. **i.** This patient has secondary skin infections that are most likely the result of an underlying allergic condition. These infections should first be treated to determine the extent to which they are contributing to the patient's clinical symptoms. To treat the infections, either topical therapy by itself or in combination with systemic antibiotics and antifungals would be acceptable given the diffuse nature of the lesions. Regardless of therapeutic protocol, this patient should be treated for 3–4 weeks and then reevaluated to determine if the secondary infections have resolved. Once the secondary issues have been resolved, the patient's baseline symptoms can be evaluated to determine if further intervention is warranted, and if so, the efficacy of those therapies can be better monitored.

ii. Canine atopic dermatitis is a clinical diagnosis that is made based off the history, a patient's clinical features, and ruling out other skin conditions with compatible or overlapping symptoms. In this case, the age of onset and clinical symptoms are consistent along with lesion distribution. If pruritus persists despite resolution of secondary infections, the first differential to consider would be flea allergy dermatitis. Depending on the patient's geographical location, fleas could potentially be a year-round issue. Prior to proceeding, it should be verified that the owner is practicing effective adulticidal flea control. The length of this therapy prior to proceeding with workup is geographically dependent. In addition to fleas, other ectoparasites should be considered, such as *S. scabiei* and *Cheyletiella* spp., regardless if they are not found via skin scraping. Trial treatments are strongly recommended in acute-onset cases and those with extremely pruritic patients. Once secondary infections have been controlled and parasitic infestation eliminated as a possibility, a cutaneous adverse food reaction should be considered in patients with nonseasonal symptoms. A strict diet elimination trial should be fed for at least 8 weeks to determine if food is playing a role in the patient's symptoms. If the patient is still pruritic despite these efforts, then and only then in this particular scenario, the patient can be definitively diagnosed as atopic. One important caveat to remember though, is that patients may have more than one allergic hypersensitivity. In these rare instances, all issues will need to be simultaneously controlled to resolve a patient's clinical symptoms.

iii. Dogs with atopic dermatitis may present for pruritus, alopecia (self-inflicted), recurrent pyoderma or *Malassezia* dermatitis, recurrent otitis externa, pyotraumatic dermatitis, acral-lick dermatitis, and conjunctivitis.

iv. The most important route of allegern presentation in dogs with atopic dermatitis is percutaneous exposure (Marsella et al., 2012).

158. A 4-year-old male beagle presented for nonresolving lesions associated with pyoderma despite appropriate systemic antimicrobial therapy with cephalexin for the past 3 weeks. Physical exam reveals pustules and epidermal collarettes, while cytology verifies the presence of intra- and extracellular coccoid-shaped bacteria. A sample for bacterial culture was acquired and submitted with the sensitivity report revealing heavy pure growth of a methicillin-resistant strain of *Staphylococcus pseudintermedius*.

How do treatment guidelines and expected clinical outcomes of a methicillin-resistant versus a methicillin-susceptible staphylococcal infection compare?

159. A 5-month-old female Labrador retriever presented for examination of multiple raised hairless lumps along her face and her front distal extremities (**Figure 159a**). Upon questioning, it is reported by the owner that the lumps were first observed as small crusts 2 weeks ago and that the areas are getting bigger. Palpation of the lesions reveals that they are painful, and a serosanguineous discharge is easily expressible. Skin scrapings and trichograms did not reveal the presence of mites or fungal organisms, while skin cytology also showed an absence of infectious agents. As a result, a fine-needle aspiration from one of the nodules was performed, and the results are shown in **Figure 159b**.

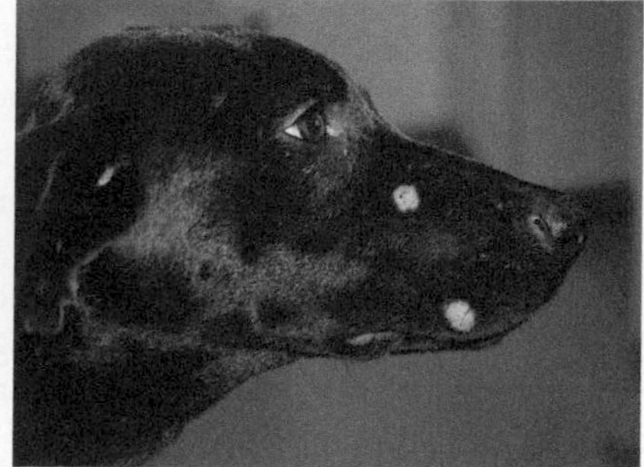

Figure 159a

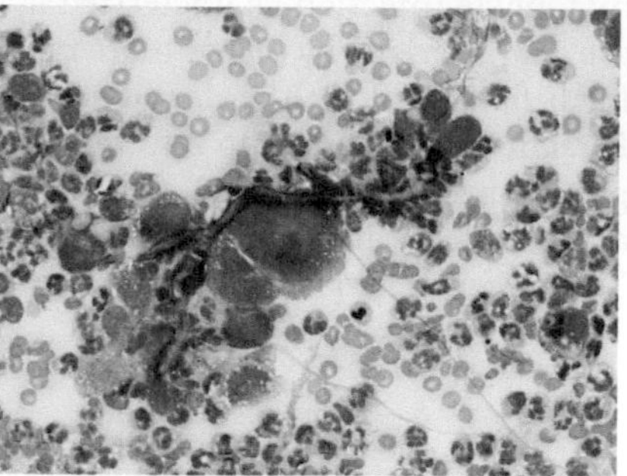

Figure 159b

i. What is your diagnosis?

ii. What is the name of these lesions, what are they, and what causes them?

iii. Cats rarely develop this type of lesion. However, a similar but more severe type of lesion has been described in cats. What is the name of that condition, and what breed is it most commonly observed in?

158. Treatment duration guidelines are the same for methicillin-susceptible or methicillin-resistant staphylococcal pyoderma. For superficial infections, treatment duration should be for 3–4 weeks or 1 week past clinical resolution and for deep pyoderma 6–8 weeks or 2 weeks past clinical resolution regardless of methicillin-resistance status. Additionally, clinical outcome between the two is similar with the prognosis being good, depending on the underlying cause and comorbidities. However, clinical resolution of a methicillin-resistant staphylococcal infection may take longer but is likely a consequence of infection chronicity or cutaneous pathologic changes and not the result of methicillin-resistant strains being more virulent (Cain, 2013).

159. i. Dermatophytosis. The FNA results show pyogranulomatous inflammation with the presence of septated, nonpigmented fungal hyphae.

ii. This lesion is known as a kerion. A kerion is well-demarcated, exudative, inflammatory, nodular type of furunculosis that may develop draining tracts with chronicity. They are most often associated with *M. gypseum* or *T. mentagrophytes* and commonly found along the face and distal extremities. In this particular case, the causative agent was determined to be *T. mentagrophytes* via culture results. The dog had access to a farm and was routinely observed to chase rabbits and rodents. Thus, the source of exposure was presumed to be from these species on the farm.

iii. Dermatophytic pseudomycetoma. These lesions represent a chronic dermatophyte infection characterized by tumor-like growth. Pseudomycetomas are characterized by one or more raised, firm subcutaneous nodules that may form fistulas along the dorsal trunk and have been observed primarily in Persian cats secondary to infection with *M. canis*. Treatment of dermatophyte pseudomycetomas can be difficult, potentially requiring surgical excision and long-term antifungal therapy. Similar lesions have also been described in Yorkshire terriers.

160. A 2-year-old castrated male boxer presented for evaluation of the small, roughly 1 cm diameter dome-like mass on the ventral neck as shown in **Figure 160a**. The owners of this dog have owned several other boxers, all of which died from one type of neoplasm or another. The owners are very concerned because this lesion developed very rapidly in their young dog. The dog is otherwise healthy. A fine-needle aspiration of the mass was performed and yielded the cytology shown in **Figure 160b**.

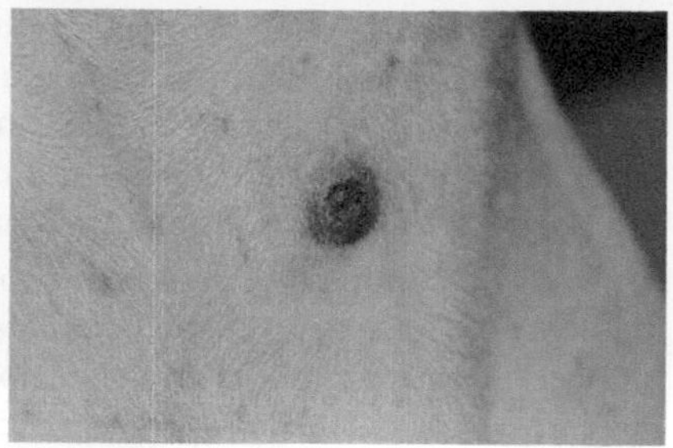

Figure 160a

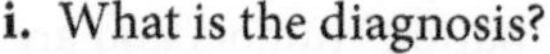

i. What is the diagnosis?

ii. What prognosis should be discussed with the clients, and what is the treatment of choice?

iii. This disorder represents a spectrum of conditions. Briefly describe them.

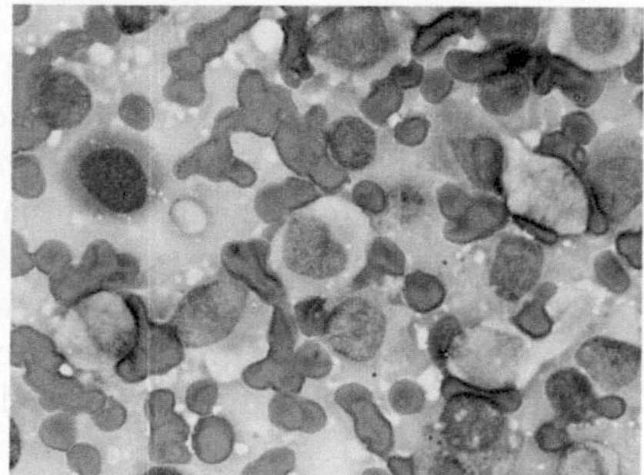

Figure 160b

161. What is leflunomide, what dermatologic conditions has it been used for, and what are the major adverse events encountered with use of the drug?

160. **i.** Histiocytoma. Cytology reveals a monomorphic population of large round cells that exhibit a moderate nuclear:cytoplasmic ratio, contain abundant basophilic cytoplasm, and have smooth-to-scalloped cell margins. Nuclei vary from round to oval in shape and may be indented, imparting a reniform appearance. Nuclei contain fine chromatin and indistinct nucleoli.

ii. This is a common benign tumor of young dogs seen most frequently in the boxer and dachshund (Moore, 2014). The tumor normally spontaneously regresses within 3 months and does not require any specific treatment. In the cases where lesions become problematic (pruritic, ulcerated, or infected), surgical excision is often curative but seldom warranted.

iii. There are multiple documented histiocytic syndromes that affect dogs and cats, but several are well recognized in the dog (Moore, 2014). The most common is the *histiocytoma* seen in young dogs. These are usually single, benign tumors that can occur in any age of dog but are normally observed before 3 years of age. They are described as dome-shaped or "button" tumors and are commonly seen along the head, pinna, or limbs. The tumor usually appears quite rapidly and is known to normally spontaneously regress within 3 months. *Cutaneous histiocytosis* is an inflammatory proliferative disorder that affects the skin and subcutis of middle-aged to older dogs that on rare occasions may extend to involve local lymph nodes. Lesions commonly present as multiple erythemic plaques or nodules that may ulcerate and tend to be found along the trunk and extremities. However, lesions may be limited to the nasal planum giving the dog a "clown nose" appearance. Lesions tend to wax and wane with most dogs benefiting from immune-modulating therapy. *Systemic histiocytosis* is similar to cutaneous histiocytosis, sharing many clinical similarities with respect to cutaneous findings. Significant differences between the syndromes include an onset in young to middle-aged dogs, palpably enlarged lymph nodes, and involvement of multiple organ systems. It is a slowly progressive disease with clinical signs dependent on lesion extent and location, which may include anorexia, weight loss, conjunctivitis, and breathing difficulty. Lesions and symptoms tend to wax and wane but do not spontaneously resolve. Treatment usually involves aggressive immunosuppressive therapy with azathioprine, leflunomide, or cyclosporine. *Histiocytic sarcoma* is a rare form of neoplasia that can occur as localized or disseminated disease. Clinical symptoms are dependent on the tissue or organs involved. Histiocytic sarcomas can occur in the skin, spleen, stomach, liver, lymph nodes, lungs, bone marrow, CNS, and the periarticular/articular tissues of the limbs. Neither form carries a very favorable prognosis, with the disseminated form displaying a rapid and fatal progression.

161. Leflunomide (Arava) is a prodrug whose metabolite teriflunomide is an immunomodulatory agent. The drug is thought to exert its effect primarily via two mechanisms of action. The first is through inhibition of dihydroorotate dehydrogenase, which is involved with pyrimidine synthesis causing arrest of lymphocyte activation and expansion. The second is inhibition of cytokine production and tyrosine kinase–mediated signal transduction. The drug is rarely used as a primary or sole therapeutic agent but is instead used as an adjunctive or alternative immunosuppressive agent when standard therapies fail. It has been primarily used in autoimmune conditions such as pemphigus foliaceus or in cases of histiocytic disease. Ideal dosing and therapeutic monitoring protocols have not been established, and adverse events such as profound bone marrow suppression (anemia, leukopenia, and thrombocytopenia), bone marrow necrosis, and severe GI symptoms (hematemesis and hematochezia) have been reported.

162. A 7-year-old spayed female boxer presented with the complaint of "hard skin." The owners report the dog has developed "rock-hard skin lumps" over the last 6 months. Most of the lesions do not seem to bother the dog; however, a few are exudative and pruritic, and the dog chews at these lesions. Physical examination reveals a depressed, panting, pot-bellied patient with a thinning truncal hair coat and a history of polyuria, polydipsia, and polyphagia. On dermatologic examination, there are numerous well-demarcated, firm, erythematous plaques and other areas of hair loss with accumulation of white particulate material (**Figure 162a, b**). These raised plaques are generalized but seem to be most numerous on the dorsum and caudal rear legs. The dog traumatizes all of the sites it can reach, suggesting that the dog is pruritic.

i. What is the most likely diagnosis for the skin lesions?

ii. How can the dog's pruritus be accounted for?

iii. What other diseases can cause these lesions in the skin?

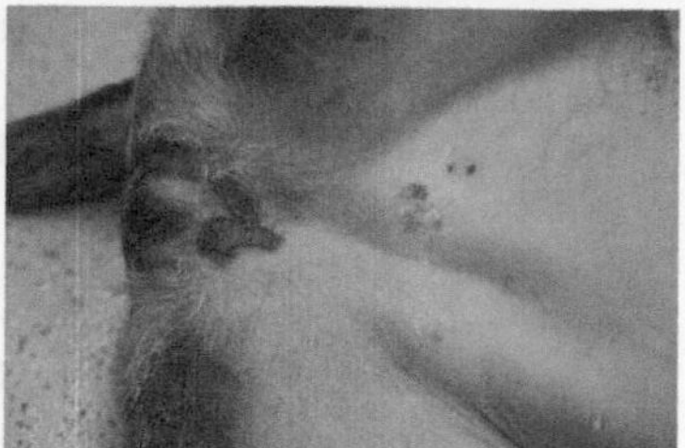

Figure 162a

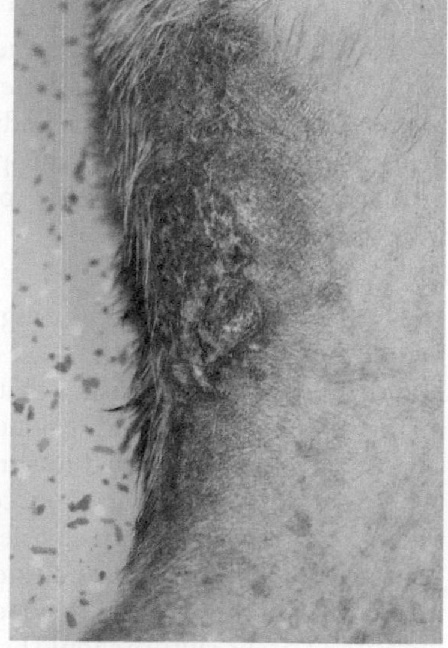

Figure 162b

163. A 4-year-old female spayed mixed breed dog presented for multiple cutaneous masses of 4 months' duration. Physical examination revealed multiple 1–2 cm raised, firm, erythemic cutaneous nodules (**Figure 163a**). The lesions were nonpruritic and haired. According to the owner, the lesions tend to wax and wane. The dog is otherwise healthy.

i. Nodules and tumors in dogs are classified as inflammatory (infectious and noninfectious) or neoplastic. What initial diagnostic tests are indicated in this case?

ii. List the noninfectious differential diagnoses for this dog's lesions.

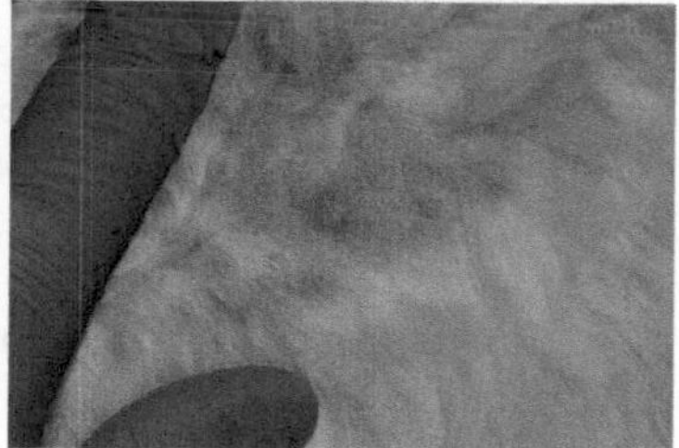

Figure 163a

162. **i.** Calcinosis cutis. This patient had hyperadrenocorticism.

ii. Lesions of calcinosis cutis can be very inflammatory and may cause pain and pruritus. It is usually assumed that dogs with calcinosis cutis secondary to hyperadrenocorticism will not be pruritic; however, this is not always the case. Often the sites resemble areas of deep pyoderma and are pruritic to the patient. There is no specific treatment for calcinosis cutis. Lesions resolve when the underlying cause is addressed and treated (iatrogenic or spontaneously occurring hyperadrenocorticism). Resolving lesions of calcinosis cutis can become very pruritic and often develop a secondary infection. When secondary infections are present, topical or systemic antimicrobial therapy is required, which may lessen the patient's pruritus. Depending on the cause of the calcinosis cutis, it may take weeks to months to resolve.

iii. Calcinosis cutis can be classified as dystrophic or metastatic calcification. The most common cause of the latter is chronic renal disease. Dystrophic causes include inflammatory (foreign body, demodicosis, systemic fungal infections), degenerative (follicular cysts), neoplastic, endocrine related (hypercortisolism or diabetes mellitus), iatrogenic (percutaneous calcium administration), and idiopathic.

163. **i.** Initial diagnostic testing should start with a FNA. The purpose of beginning with an FNA in a case presented for evaluation of any cutaneous nodule in the dog is to ensure that it is not a mast cell tumor. Given the case history of waxing and waning nodules, an FNA is very appropriate as mast cell tumors have been observed to shrink and swell. Additionally, FNA samples provide initial information about cell populations within the lesion and potentially could reveal diagnostic infectious agents. Finding either one of these components may alter what additional tests are pursued. Once an FNA is performed and determined to be nondiagnostic, further diagnostics such as skin biopsy and tissue culture should be performed. Neoplasia is unlikely due to the age of the dog and overall good health. Thus, the most likely cause is an infectious or sterile disease. Cultures should be done on aseptically collected surgical specimens and submitted for aerobic, fungal, and mycobacteria cultures.

ii. Noninfectious causes of cutaneous nodules include urticaria, angioedema, eosinophilic granulomas, arthropod bite granulomas, calcinosis cutis, calcinosis circumscripta, xanthoma, panniculitis, hematomas, seroma, cutaneous amyloidosis, histiocytic diseases, nodular dermatofibrosis, sterile nodular granuloma/pyogranuloma, erythema multiforme, dermoid/follicular cysts, multiple cutaneous/follicular tumors, and foreign-body reactions. This was a case of idiopathic sterile nodular panniculitis. The dog was treated with oral prednisone (2 mg/kg PO q24h) until the lesions resolved and then tapered slowly over a couple of months. Although not seen in this case, relapse is common in this disorder, and affected dogs may require lifelong therapy. Cases prone to relapse upon medication withdrawal can be managed with cyclosporine (5 mg/kg PO q24–48h).

164. Imidacloprid is a commonly used insecticide that was brought to the veterinary marketplace in the early 1990s by Bayer for the treatment and prevention of flea infestations.

What is the mechanism of action of this drug, in what formulations is the drug found for use in small animal medicine, and what are the labeled indications of those products?

165. A 3-year-old spayed female boxer presented for annual examination and vaccination. While in, the owner also notes that the patient has been chewing at her paws constantly. On examination you observe alopecia, marked erythema, and swelling of all four paws predominantly affecting the ventral and lateral aspects along with hyperkeratosis of the pads. Other than the changes affecting the paws, the skin is fairly unremarkable. As part of the patient's annual examination, a fecal floatation was performed, and the following was found **(Figure 165a)**.

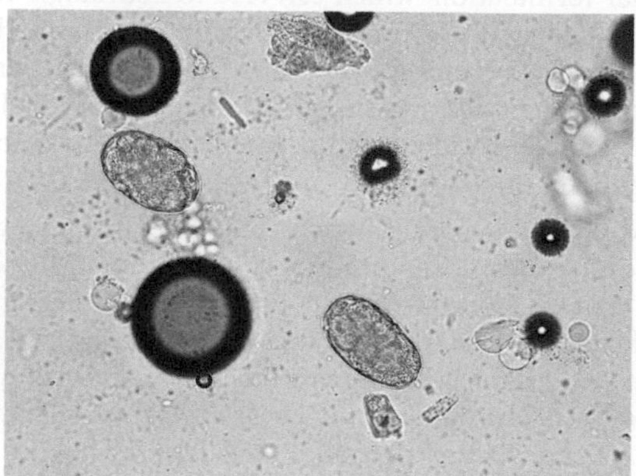

Figure 165a

i. What is the patient's likely diagnosis, and what nematode species causes this condition in dogs?

ii. What treatment recommendations should be given for this patient?

164. Imidacloprid is a neonicotinoid insecticide, which is also the same family of chemicals that include nitenpyram and dinotefuran. These drugs work as nicotinic acetylcholine receptor agonists with a preference/selectivity for insect receptors. Binding of neonicotinoids to the receptor on postsynaptic membranes (found predominantly in the CNS of insects) leads to rapid neural depolarization and inhibition of the insect nervous systems that results in paralysis (Vo et al., 2010). Imidacloprid in found in the following formulations for dogs and cats along with the labeled indications:

- Advantage II (imidacloprid and pyriproxyfen) is available as a spot-on for both dogs and cats and is indicated for the treatment and prevention of flea infestations in dogs along with the treatment of lice infestation in dogs. The advantage of this particular product is that it can be applied up to weekly if needed.
- K9 Advantix II (imidacloprid, pyriproxyfen, and permethrin) is available as a spot-on for use in dogs only due to the presence of permethrin in this particular formulation, which can lead to neurologic toxicity and death in cats. In a survey of practitioners from Australia, this spot-on formulation was the second most commonly implicated product that resulted in permethrin toxicity in cats (Malik et al., 2010). The product is labeled for the prevention and treatment of fleas, ticks, biting fleas/mosquitos, and lice on dogs.
- Advantage Multi (imidacloprid and moxidectin) is available as a spot-on for use in dogs and cats. The product is labeled for the prevention of heartworm disease, treatment and prevention of flea infestations, treatment of chewing lice, treatment of sarcoptic mange, treatment and control of ear mites, along with the treatment and control of *Ancylostoma caninum*, *Ancylostoma tubaeforme*, *Uncinaria stenocephala*, *Toxocara canis*, *Toxocara cati*, *Toxascaris leonine*, and *Trichuris vulpis*. A similarly formulated product marketed as Adovcate is available in many countries with additional label indications for the treatment of lungworms (*Eucoleus aerophilus*), treatment of notoedric mange, and treatment and control of demodicosis.
- Seresto (imidacloprid and flumetrhin) is available as a collar for use in both dogs and cats. The product has a labeled indication for the prevention of tick infestations, treatment and prevention of flea infestations, killing of chewing lice, and treatment and control of sarcoptic mange. The unique aspect of this product is that it is intended to be worn continuously for up to 8 months before needing to be replaced.

165. i. Hookworm dermatitis, as hookworm eggs were observed from the fecal float. This condition is caused by contact with third-stage larvae of *Ancylostoma braziliense, A. caninum*, or *Uncinaria stenocephala* that are present on grass or contaminated soil and percutaneously invade the skin that is in contact with the ground. Areas of the body that have been observed to be affected in dogs with hookworm dermatitis are the distal limbs, caudal rear legs, sternum, ventral abdomen, perineum, tail, and over boney prominences (elbows, hocks). *Ancylostoma* spp. are more likely to be encountered in warmer climates, while *U. stenocephala* is found in cooler climates.

ii. The patient should be treated with an appropriate anthelmintic (fenbendazole or pyrantel pamoate) to clear the current infection and placed on a monthly heartworm preventative with activity against intestinal parasites to help prevent recurrence. Short-term use of a systemic or topical glucocorticoid can be beneficial in alleviating the pruritus. This parasitic disease requires cleaning of the premises once diagnosed but can be prevented by good sanitation (daily removal of feces), routine use of heartworm preventatives, and exercising the patient in a clean area. In some circumstances, treatment of dirt areas with sodium borate may be required.

105 i. Hookworm dermatitis, as hookworm eggs were observed from the fecal float. This condition is caused by contact with third-stage larvae of *Ancylostoma braziliense*, *A. caninum*, or *Uncinaria stenocephala* that are present on grass or contaminated soil and percutaneously invade the skin that is in contact with the ground. Areas of the body that have been observed to be affected in dogs with hookworm dermatitis are the distal limbs, caudal rear legs, sternum, ventral abdomen, perineum, tail, and over boney prominences (elbows, hocks). *Ancylostoma* spp. are more likely to be encountered in warmer climates, while *U. stenocephala* is found in cooler climates.

ii. The patient should be treated with an appropriate anthelmintic (fenbendazole or pyrantel pamoate) to clear the current infection and placed on a monthly heartworm preventative with activity against intestinal parasites to help prevent recurrence. Short-term use of a systemic or topical glucocorticoid can be beneficial in alleviating the pruritus. This parasitic disease requires cleaning of the premises once diagnosed but can be prevented by good sanitation (daily removal of feces), routine use of heartworm preventatives, and exercising the patient in a clean area. In some circumstances, treatment of dirt areas with sodium borate may be required.

166. A second opinion is requested on a cat with nonhealing, draining nodules on the face and limbs for 6 weeks. Another veterinarian suspected a bacterial infection and prescribed 21 days of oral antibiotics at the correct dose and dosage. The cat did not respond, and the owner reports that the infection seems to be spreading. On physical examination, multiple ulcerative draining nodules of varying size are appreciated on the face, pinnae, and distal extremities (**Figure 166a**). An impression smear of the exudate was performed. The impression smear (**Figure 166b**, green arrow) shows severe pyogranulomatous inflammation and numerous intracytoplasmic organisms.

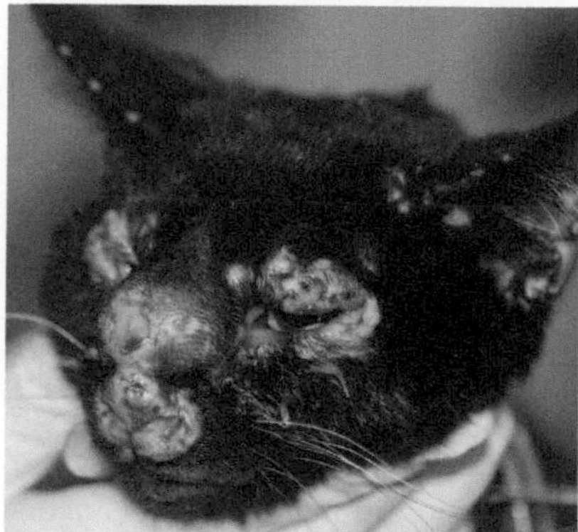
Figure 166a

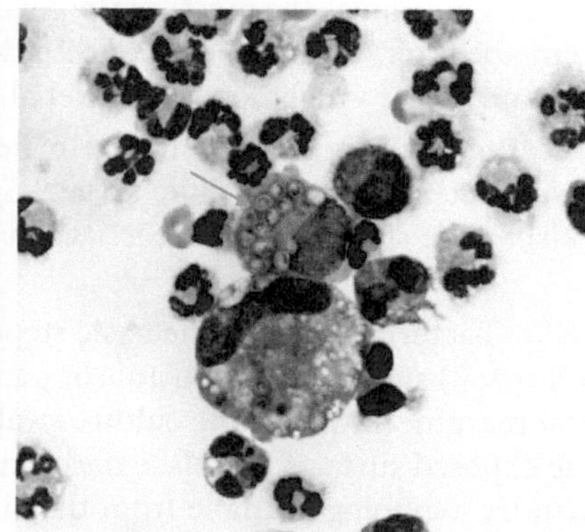
Figure 166b

i. What is the diagnosis, and what is the treatment of choice?
ii. What unique clinical manifestation of this disease is seen in dogs?
iii. What infectious organisms are likely to be observed within macrophages on cytology?

167. What diagnostic procedure is being performed in **Figure 167a**, and what are the basic steps for performing this procedure?

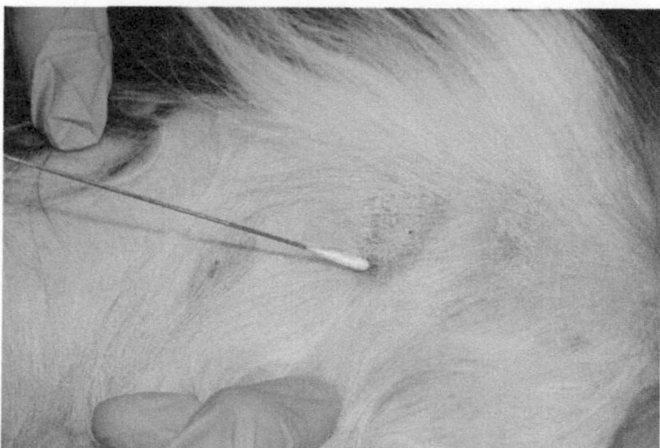
Figure 167a

166. i. Histoplasmosis is a subcutaneous fungal disease caused by the dimorphic fungus, *Histoplasma* spp. The organism is found worldwide and exists as three distinct species: *H. capsulatum* (New World pathogen), *H. farciminosum* (Old World pathogen), and *H. duboisii* (African pathogen). The organism is associated with soil containing nitrogen-rich organic matter such as bird and bat excrement. Household potted plants may also be a source of exposure (Reinhart et al., 2012). At this time, itraconazole is considered the treatment of choice, but recent investigations have suggested that fluconazole may be a possible alternative (Reinhart et al., 2012; Wilson et al., 2018).

ii. In dogs, GI signs can predominate and may occur without detectable respiratory symptoms. The most common GI symptom is large bowel diarrhea with hematochezia. The severity of GI disease can lead to a protein-losing enteropathy and severe weight loss (Blache et al., 2011).

iii. Infectious organisms likely to be found within macrophages include mycobacteria, dermatophyte spores, *Sporothrix schenckii*, *Histoplasma* spp., *Leishmania* spp., and *Rhodococcus* spp.

167. Bacterial culture. The basic steps for performing this procedure are as follows: (i) sterilely lance pustule or papule/lift crust/expose exudative peripheral margin; (ii) insert the culture swab into the lanced lesion or roll it along the exposed surface; (iii) place the culture swab into the transport system; (iv) acquire a cytology sample from the cultured lesion (done to ensure concordance between the two tests); and (v) submit the collected sample to a laboratory capable of identifying *Staphylococcal* spp. relevant to veterinary medicine. A brief patient history and results of cytology findings should be provided to the reference laboratory at the time of sample submission.

168. The concave aspect of the left pinna of a Dogo Argentino is shown in **Figure 168a**. The owners arrived home to find the dog shaking and scratching its left ear. On examination, the dog wants to keep its head tilted to the left, and there is a soft, fluctuant swelling on the medial aspect of the left ear pinna.

i. What is the most likely diagnosis?

ii. The owners do not believe the diagnosis. How can it be confirmed?

iii. What are the treatment options?

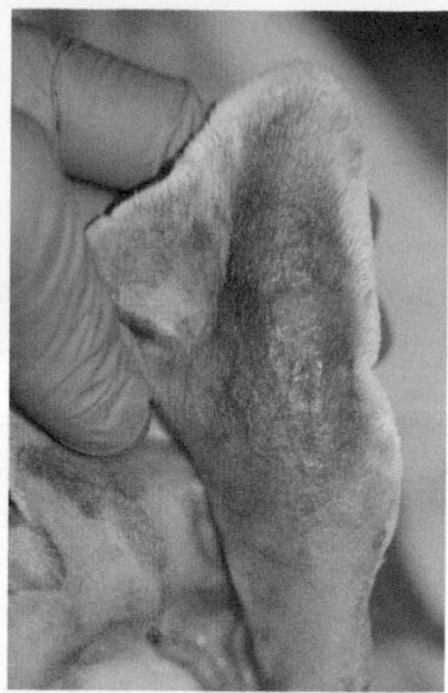
Figure 168a

169. A 4-year-old Labrador retriever presented for evaluation of recurrent nodules between the toes that eventually rupture and drain a blood-tinged fluid. The owners report that the patient licks at the feet only when lesions are present. Physical exam revealed painful, fluctuant swellings with draining tracts on the dorsal aspect of both front paws between the fourth and fifth digits. Examination of the corresponding ventral aspects revealed marked erythema, swelling, follicular plugging, and expression of keratosebaceous debris upon light manipulation of the dorsal surface (**Figure 169a, b**).

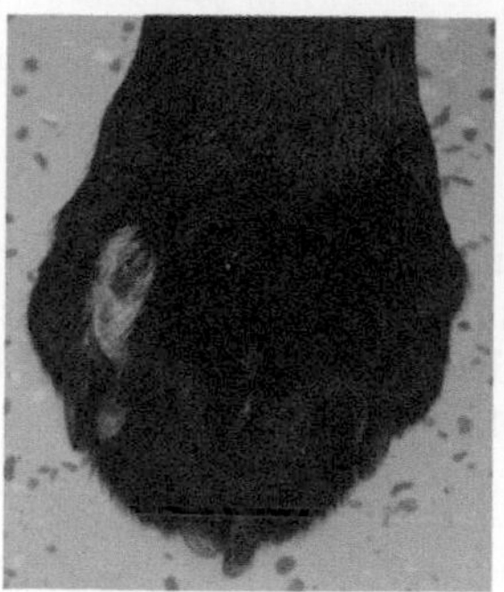
Figure 169a

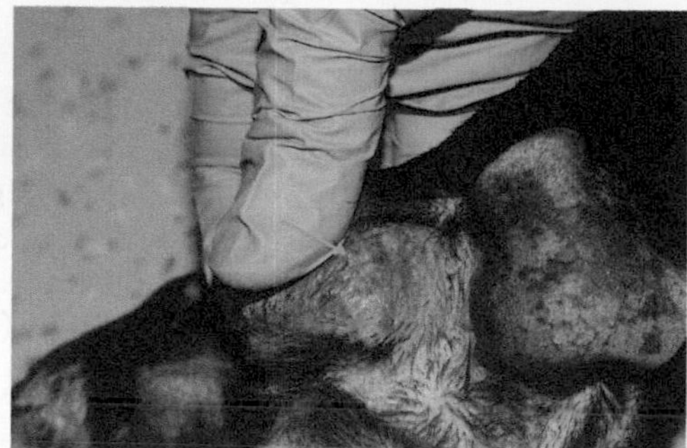
Figure 169b

i. What is the name of this condition?

ii. What is the preferred treatment option for this condition?

170. A 6-month-old stray puppy found in Texas, near the U.S.–Mexico border, presented for painful feet. Physical examination revealed a febrile puppy with significant digital hyperkeratosis, a small amount of nasal hyperkeratosis, along with ocular and nasal discharge.

i. What are the differential diagnoses for dogs with footpad lesions?

ii. Which of these differential diagnoses is the most likely cause of the digital hyperkeratosis in this case?

168. i. Aural hematoma.

ii. The diagnosis can be confirmed by aspirating fluid (i.e., blood) from the swelling. This should be done with a small-gauge needle because it is painful, and the pressure within the hematoma will cause it to ooze blood.

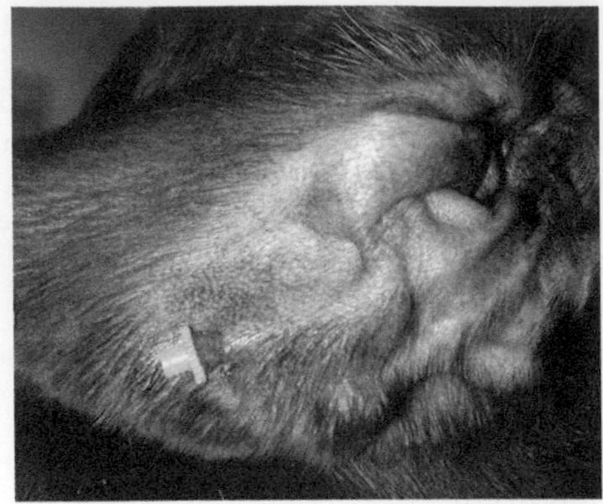

Figure 168b

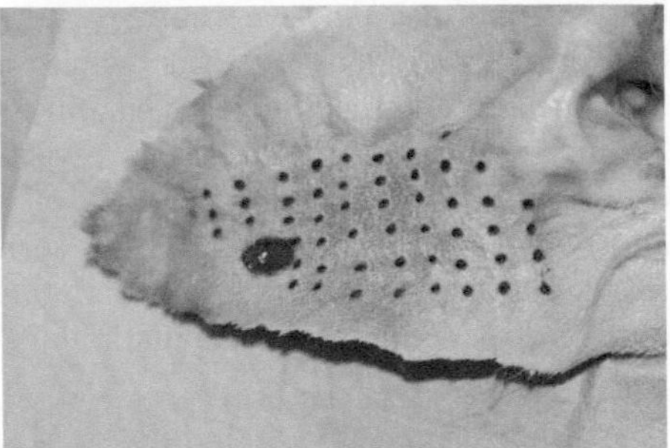

Figure 168c

iii. There are numerous treatment options to address aural hematomas, but recognizing and treating the underlying ear disease (otitis externa, *Otodectes cynotis*, etc.) is essential to minimize the chance of recurrence. Aural hematomas, although uncomfortable for the patient, are not life-threatening and will resolve without treatment in most cases but with scarring. Optimal intervention requires one of the following treatment options: simple needle aspiration, teat cannula placement (**Figure 168b**), Penrose drain, closed-suction drain, intralesional or systemic glucocorticoids, surgical correction with an S-shaped incision and placement of full-thickness staggered sutures, the creation of circular fenestrations with a punch biopsy, or surgical correction via a CO_2 laser technique in which a circular partial-thickness defect is created followed by multiple full-thickness incisions (**Figure 168c**) (MacPhail, 2016).

169. i. Canine interdigital follicular cysts. Lesions are usually first noted in young adult dogs and present as dorsal interdigital nodules, hemorrhagic bullae, or draining tracts. Interdigital follicular cysts most often occur on the front paws between the fourth and fifth digits but may occur anywhere, affect more than one interdigital space, or occur symmetrically. The current understanding for why this condition occurs is that cysts form secondarily to abnormal friction or trauma to the ventral interdigital webbing associated with congenital (varus or valgus deformity) or acquired anatomic deformities (Duclos et al., 2008). The abnormal friction or wear creates changes to the interdigital skin that results in plugged follicular openings. Keratin production within the follicular lumen continues and results in follicular dilation and cyst formation. Cyst rupture results in keratin, hair, and bacteria being released into the dermis that then incites an infectious and foreign-body response. Repeated rupture of the follicular cysts results in fistulous tract formation and dorsal lesion formation.

ii. The preferred treatment method for interdigital follicular cysts is surgical ablation with a CO_2 laser. The method for performing this procedure is well documented and results in roughly a 70% first-time success rate (Duclos et al., 2008). Recurrence is not uncommon, and repeat procedures may be needed to permanently address the condition. Medical management can be attempted in cases of early lesion development or when surgical intervention is not an option, but this tends to be of limited efficacy. Use of products containing benzoyl peroxide, salicylic acid, or Epsom salt soaks may be beneficial because of their follicular flushing and keratolytic properties. Antimicrobial and systemic glucocorticoid therapy may be beneficial in resolving secondary infections and inflammation associated with ruptured cysts, but neither resolve the condition nor prevent further episodes. If medical management is attempted, duration of antimicrobial therapy should be sufficiently long to address the deep infection.

170. i. Diseases associated with footpad lesions include contact dermatitis, canine distemper, leishmaniasis, pemphigus foliaceus and vulgaris, bullous pemphigoid, systemic lupus erythematosus, vasculitis, hepatocutaneous syndrome, zinc-responsive dermatosis, familial footpad and idiopathic nasodigital hyperkeratosis, and paw pad corns.

ii. The vaccination history of this puppy is unknown, and the dog is showing signs of systemic illness; therefore, distemper is the most likely cause.

171. A 2.5-year-old castrated male standard poodle presented with a complaint of hair color and texture change (**Figure 171a, b**). Close examination of the skin revealed the affected regions were excessively dry, with increased scale formation and the presence of follicular casts. Previous diagnostics and treatments included skin scrapings, impression smears, fungal cultures, flea control, and 30 days of oral cephalexin (30 mg/kg PO q12h). There was no response to treatment, and all previous diagnostic testing was negative. A skin biopsy was performed that revealed a lack of sebaceous glands, a mild lymphocytic perifollicular infiltrate, hyperkeratosis, and follicular plugging.

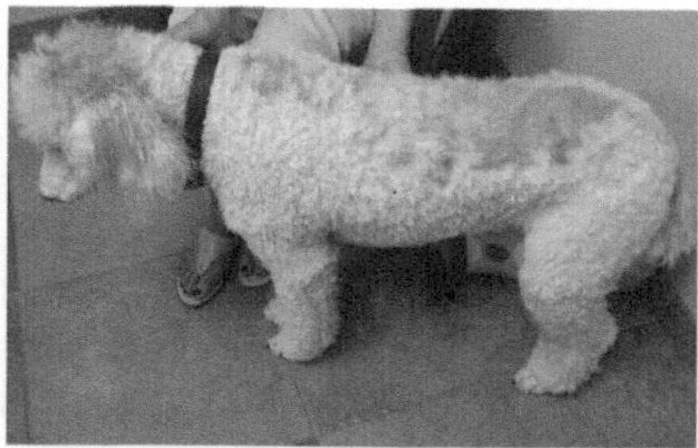
Figure 171a

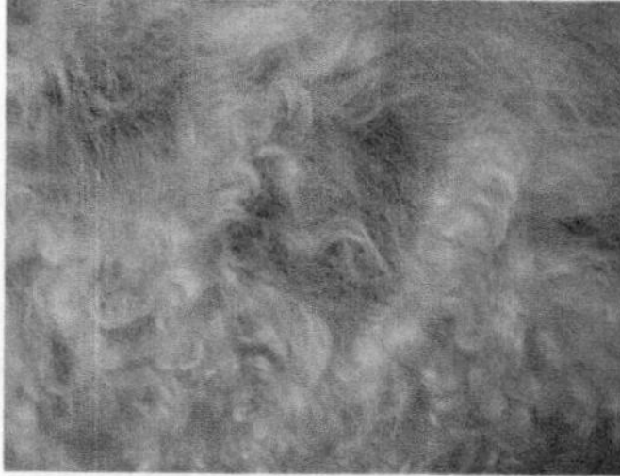
Figure 171b

i. What is the diagnosis?
ii. What breeds are overrepresented for this condition?
iii. What are the primary goals for treatment of this condition?

172. A 5-month-old male DSH presented for matting of the hair coat and a small swelling with an associated draining lesion on the ventral neck (**Figure 172a**). The owner reported that the hair coat changes and lesion were first noted 2 days prior to presentation. The kitten was not febrile, and the swelling was nonpainful upon palpation. During manipulation of the swelling, a moving object was observed in the opening of the draining lesion. The object was removed from the swelling (**Figure 172b**).

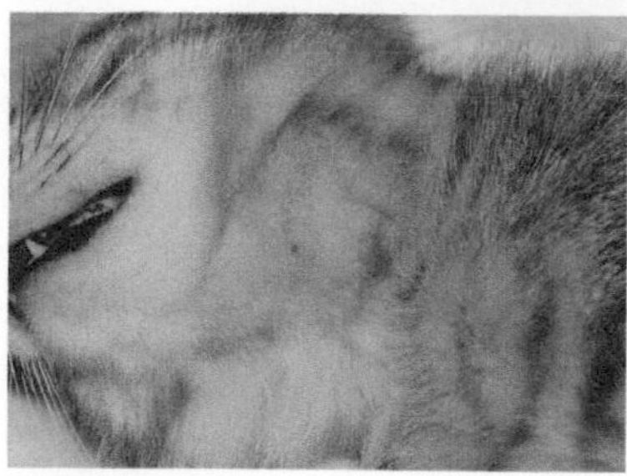
Figure 172a

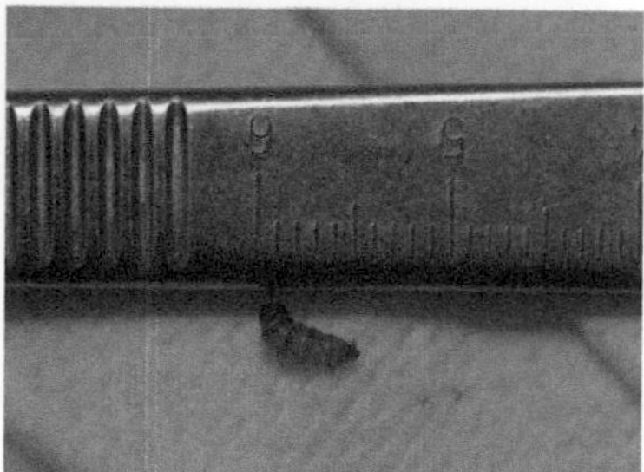
Figure 172b

i. What is the object?
ii. How should this condition be treated?
iii. What are the primary hosts for this parasite?

171. **i.** Sebaceous adenitis.

ii. Standard poodles, Akitas, Samoyeds, vizsla, Havanese, beagles, and golden retrievers.

iii. The primary goals of therapy are to (1) prevent further gland destruction if active inflammation and glands are present in biopsy specimens (cyclosporine, glucocorticoids, retinoids); (2) replenish oils to the skin (baby oil soaks and topical humectants) and improve barrier function (ceramide-/phytosphingosine-containing shampoos and fatty acid supplementation); and (3) prevent and manage secondary infections.

172. **i.** *Cuterebra* spp. larvae.

ii. Treatment consists of careful removal of the larva. This may require surgical enlargement of the wound to facilitate removal of the entire parasite (**Figure 172c**). Leaving retained portions of a larva could result in foreign-body reactions, irritant reactions, and in rare cases, allergic/anaphylactic reactions. The wound should then be flushed and managed as an open wound. A broad-based systemic antimicrobial should be prescribed for 10–14 days depending on the extent of secondary infection. Analgesics may be required.

iii. Rabbits and rodents act as the natural hosts for *Cuterebra* spp., with the species affecting rabbits having less host specificity.

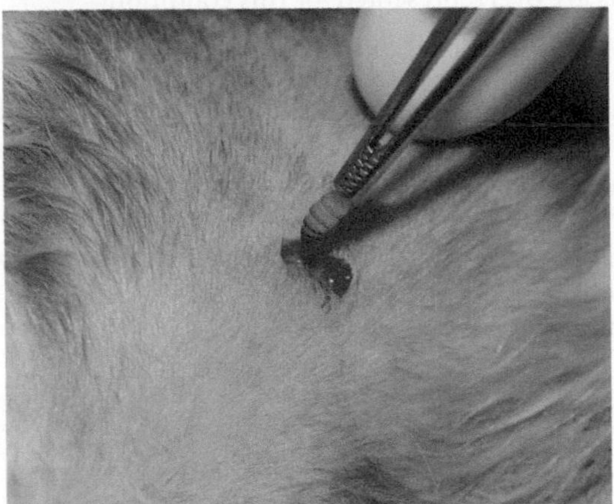

Figure 172c

173. What procedure is demonstrated in **Figure 173a**, and what can it be used to help identify?

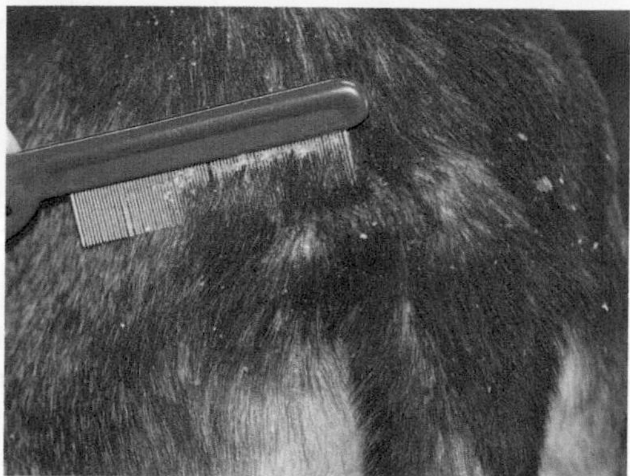

Figure 173a

174. A 7-month-old dog presented for the first time with the complaint of "bumps." **Figure 174a** shows the tufted hairs appreciated on examination that are commonly described as "hive"-like on the skin.

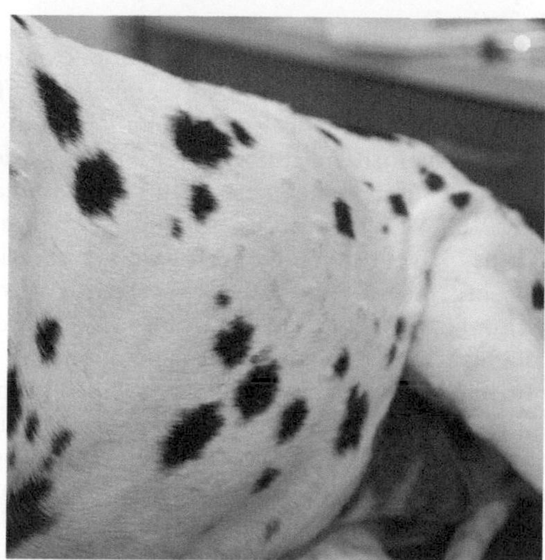

Figure 174a

i. What is the name of this condition, and what is seen upon close examination of the skin?

ii. What differential diagnoses and diagnostic tests should be performed to confirm the diagnosis?

iii. What is the mechanism of action of fluoroquinolone antibiotics, and why would this drug class not be an appropriate antibiotic choice in this dog?

173. Flea combing. This procedure can be helpful in trying to directly collect parasitic elements that can be grossly identified such as fleas, flea feces, or lice. It can also be used to enhance detection of *Cheyletiella* spp. mites. When used for the latter purpose, a large area of the patient's body is combed to collect scale and surface debris. The collected material can then be placed in either a Petri dish to examine under a dissecting microscope or a fecal floatation device and treated similarly to looking for intestinal parasites in fecal material.

174. **i.** This is an example of superficial bacterial folliculitis. Close examination of the skin would reveal small folliculocentric papules or pustules at the base of the hairs. These papules/pustules may then progress, causing the formation of tiny epidermal collarettes, which may be seen encircling the base of the hairs. In short-coated dogs, these lesions are often mistaken/mistreated as urticaria ("hives") due to the fact that hairs stand erect secondary to folliculitis, giving the illusion of "hives" from afar. The presence of crusts, however, should rule out this differential.

ii. The major differential diagnoses for folliculitis are demodicosis, dermatophytosis, and pyoderma. However, the most common reason for this presentation in short-coated dogs is bacterial folliculitis or pyoderma. Skin scrapings should be performed to rule out demodicosis, impression smears to look for the presence of neutrophils and bacteria, and dermatophyte cultures where there is a suspicion of infection.

iii. Fluoroquinolone antibiotics impair bacterial topoisomerase enzymes, specifically topoisomerase II (bacterial DNA gyrase) and IV. These enzymes are involved with bacterial DNA replication, and inhibition of DNA gyrase is associated with activity against Gram-negative bacteria, while inhibition of topoisomerase IV confers activity against Gram-positive organisms (Pallo-Zimmerman et al., 2010). Although this class of antimicrobials is classified as "broad spectrum," they have historically been used for infections associated with Gram-negative organisms. Fluoroquinoles currently used in veterinary medicine include ciprofloxacin, difloxacin, enrofloxacin, marbofloxacin, orbifloxacin, and pradofloxacin. Although newer generations are more effective against Gram-positive organisms, they should be avoided in the treatment of pyoderma unless the organism is determined to be resistant and results of a culture and sensitivity report show they are the safest remaining option due to growing concerns that this class of antimicrobials may contribute to methicillin resistance in *Staphylococcus* spp. Additionally, fluoroquinolone antibiotics would be contraindicated in this particular patient because they are known to cause an erosive arthropathy in young, growing dogs.

175. An 8-month-old kitten presented for raised, firm, pencil-like lesions on the caudal aspects of both hind legs. The owner reports that the lesions developed rapidly but do not seem to bother the kitten. Dermatologic examination reveals hard, linear lesions in the superficial dermis (**Figure 175a**). Skin biopsies reveal eosinophilic granulomatous inflammation and collagen degeneration.

i. What is the diagnosis, and what are other clinical presentations of the same "syndrome?"

ii. What are the treatment options?

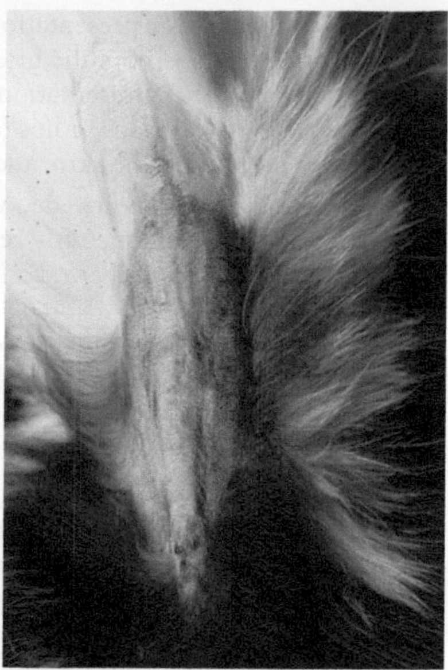

Figure 175a

176. An owner presents his dog for hair loss along the cranial elbows and cranial thighs. The owner is adamant that the patient is not pruritic or chewing at the areas and insists that the hair must be falling out. You elect to perform a skin scraping, trichogram, and impression smear from the affected areas. The skin scraping and trichogram revealed no significant findings, but the impression smear demonstrated numerous organisms in multiple fields similar to that shown in **Figure 176a**. What is the organism, and what is the significance of recovering it from the lesional areas of this patient?

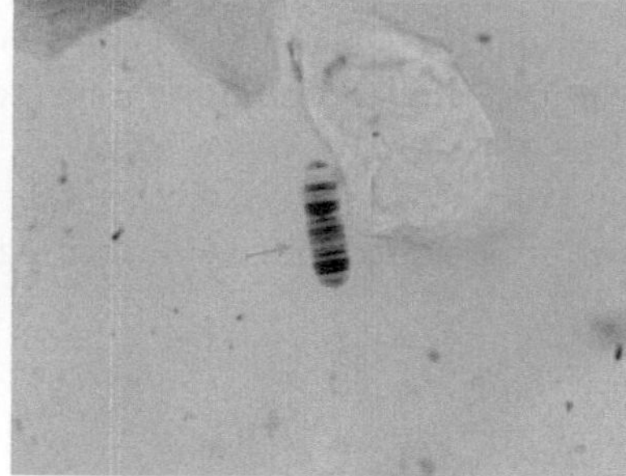

Figure 176a

177. A 7-year-old spayed female DSH presented for the problem of acute onset of hair loss in the last 3–4 days (**Figure 177a**). The cat is nonpruritic, and the skin shows no signs of inflammation. Large amounts of hair can be pulled from the coat with normal petting. Trichogram of the shed hairs reveals they were all in the telogen phase of the hair cycle. Skin biopsy reveals large numbers of hairs in anagen. Two months prior to presentation, the cat had a dental procedure performed under general anesthesia.

i. What is the diagnosis?

ii. How should this disorder be treated?

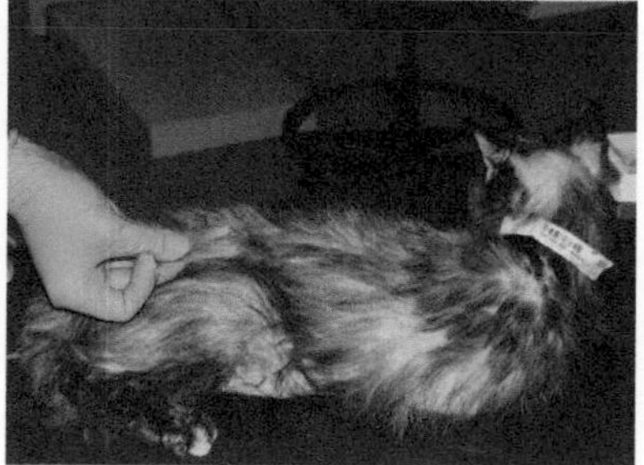

Figure 177a

175. **i.** This is a classic presentation of a feline eosinophilic granuloma. This is the lesion of the eosinophilic granuloma complex that is most variable in its presentation. Other presentations include firm swellings on the chin (fat chin syndrome), swollen lower lips (pouting cat syndrome), oral lesions in the mouth, firm nodules in the skin, and nodules on the ear pinnae.

ii. Treatment is not always needed when lesions occur in cats less than 1 year of age as they may spontaneously resolve in 3–5 months. In cases that do not spontaneously resolve, daily oral administration of glucocorticoids ([methyl] prednisolone) can be administered until the lesions improve, and then the dose is tapered. In cases where glucocorticoid administration is not possible, treatment with cyclosporine may be beneficial (Vercelli et al., 2006).

176. *Simonsiella* sp. This is a normal bacterial inhabitant of the oropharynx. The recovery of this organism from the alopecic areas is indicative of oropharyngeal contamination of the regions. This implies that the patient is licking or chewing at the affected areas causing traumatic alopecia, even though the owner is not observing their pet displaying these behaviors.

177. **i.** This is a case of telogen effluvium. This is a unique syndrome in which a severe illness, drug, high fever, shock, surgery, anesthesia, or other stressful event causes a disruption of the hair growth cycle and synchronization of the hair follicles followed by a sudden loss of hair 1–3 months later. Anagen effluvium is a similar condition except that the hair loss occurs shortly after (within days to a week) the event.

ii. Specific treatment is not required for this condition, and hair should regrow within several months if the inciting factor has been corrected.

178. Chlorhexidine solution (8 oz [240 mL] of 0.05%) is to be dispensed for wound flushing. The stock solution is 2%.

How is this prescription compounded?

179. A 3-year-old indoor-outdoor cat presented for a second opinion. The owner had been to several veterinarians with the complaint that the cat frequently shook its head and scratched at its ears. Previous diagnostics included ear swabs for mites (negative), cytological examination of ear debris (no bacteria or yeast observed), flea combing (negative), and fecal float (no parasites seen). The owner practiced intermittent flea control. Systemic glucocorticoids provided relief, but the cat's symptoms always returned within several days of discontinuing therapy. On this occasion, the cat presented for severe self-trauma of the head and neck. Upon examination, severe linear excoriations were present on the cat's head and neck. The ear canals appeared normal upon otoscopic examination and were free of debris. Ear swabs were negative for mites and microbial organisms. Further examination of the skin revealed erythemic claw beds and interdigital erythema. Skin scrapings of the head and interdigital region revealed the organism shown in **Figure 179a**.

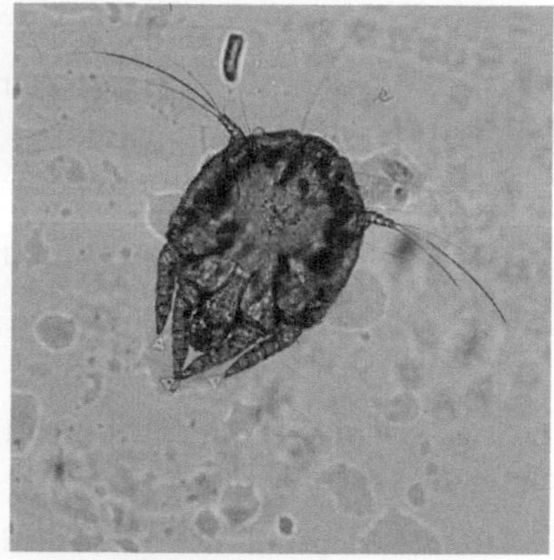

Figure 179a

i. What are the diagnosis and treatment options for this patient?

ii. What are the identifying characteristics of this mite?

iii. What is the life cycle of this parasite?

180. What procedure is demonstrated in **Figure 180a**?

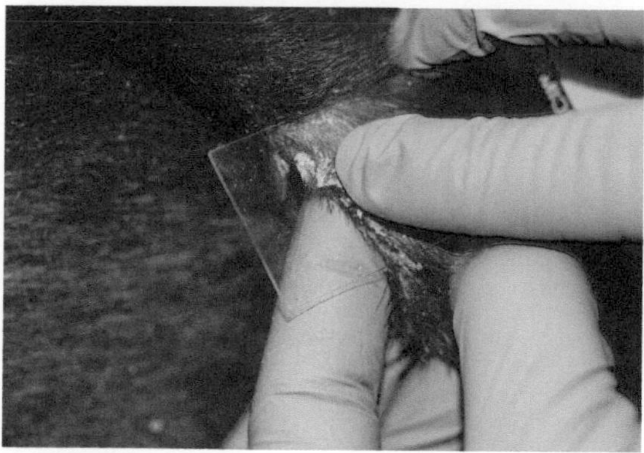

Figure 180a

178. First convert both strengths from percentage (%) to milligrams per milliliter (mg/mL):

Available: 2% = 2 g/100 mL = 2000 mg/100 mL = 20 mg/mL

Needed: 0.05% = 0.05 g/100 mL = 50 mg/100 mL = 0.5 mg/mL

Then, calculate the number of milligrams of chlorhexidine needed in 240 mL of solution:

0.5 mg/mL × 240 mL = 120 mg

Next, calculate how many milliliters of chlorhexidine 2% (20 mg/mL) are needed to get that amount:

120 mg ÷ 20 mg/mL = 6 mL

Then, calculate the quantity of distilled water to add to get a 240 mL solution of chlorhexidine 0.05%:

240 mL − 6 mL = 234 mL of distilled water

Therefore, 6 mL of 2% chlorhexidine solution would be diluted in 234 mL of distilled water to obtain 240 mL (8 oz) of 0.05% chlorhexidine solution.

179. i. The organism is *Otodectes cynotis* (ear mite). Although more commonly just associated with otic disease, the mite can cause ectopic symptoms that resemble other pruritic conditions such as fleabite hypersensitivity, cutaneous adverse food reaction, or atopy. Given the presentation of the disease in this patient, treatment with a systemic acarcidal is preferred. Available therapeutic options for this patient are topical selamectin, a topical imidacloprid/moxidectin combination product, topical fipronil, injectable ivermectin or doramectin, and the newer isoxazoline products (flurolaner, selamectin/sarolaner) approved for use in cats (Becskei et al., 2017; Taenzler et al., 2017). Short-term use of a systemic glucocorticoid (orally administered prednisolone or methylprednisolone at a 0.5–1 mg/kg dose) would also be recommended and appropriate for this patient to alleviate the intense pruritus while mite-specific therapy is instituted.

ii. The mite is usually easily identified by its large size and short, unjointed pedicles with suckers. The adult form of the mite displays sexual dimorphism. In male mites, four pairs of legs that extend beyond the body are visible, and all contain pedicles and suckers. Meanwhile, in female mites, the fourth pair (posterior set) of legs is rudimentary, and only the first two sets of legs have pedicles and suckers.

iii. The life cycle of *O. cynotis* is similar but slightly unique compared to the other mites that affect cats and dogs. *Otodectes* live on the surface of the skin where they feed on cellular debris and tissue fluid. The life cycle takes approximately 3 weeks with adults surviving for roughly 2 months. The mite can survive off the host for 1–2 weeks with this time span dependent on the environmental temperature and relative humidity. Females lay eggs that produce a six-legged larva, which then hatches to form a protonymph with eight legs that then molts to a deutonymph. A male then approaches the deutonymph with the two becoming attached end to end. If a female mite is produced from the deutonymph, copulation occurs immediately, and the female mite becomes egg bearing.

180. This is an example of a skin impression smear. The target skin area is gently "lifted" toward the glass slide to enhance sample collection. The glass microscope slide is then pressed onto the site. In order to obtain a sample of the exudate, it is very important to apply pressure directly over the target area. Using digital pressure from the index finger or thumb easily accomplishes this, minimizing the chance of breaking the glass slide during the impression smear. Enough pressure has been applied if there is an impression of cell debris on the unstained slide. Heat fixation of these samples is not needed, and heat fixing may damage cellular architecture. Following sample collection, the slide is simply stained with a Romanowsky-type stain variant (i.e., Diff-Quik).

181. A 3-year-old cat presented for evaluation of a solitary lesion that had been present for several months (**Figure 181a, b**). Except for this lesion, the cat is otherwise healthy. The lesion is raised and a FNA was obtained (**Figure 181c**).

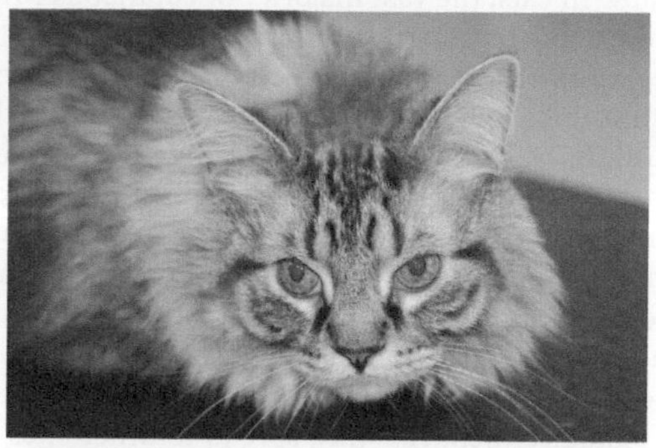

Figure 181a

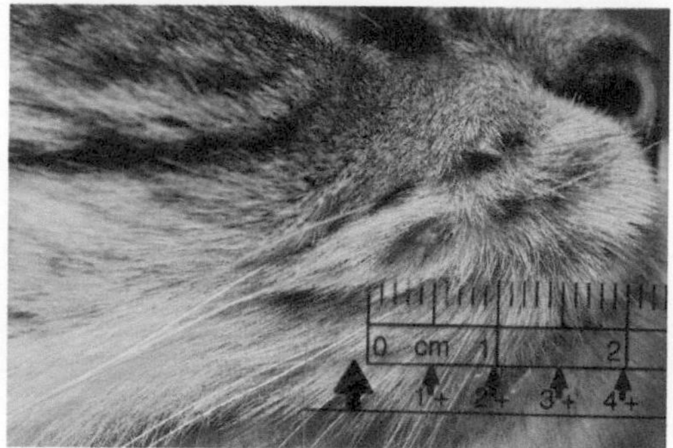

Figure 181b

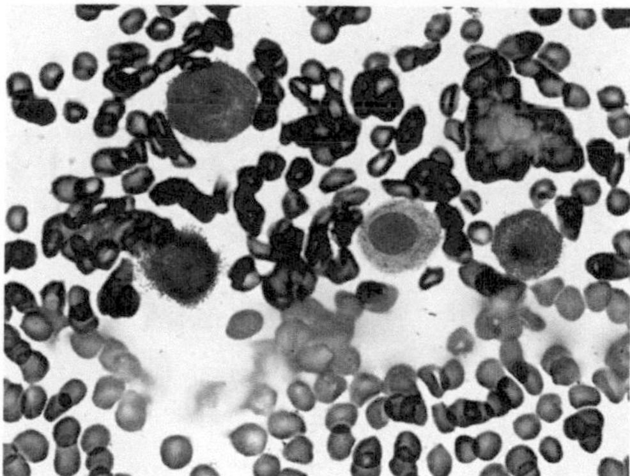

Figure 181c

i. What is the diagnosis?

ii. What is the prognosis for this cat?

181. i. The aspirate shows several mast cells along with numerous red blood cells (RBCs). This finding is consistent with a cutaneous mast cell tumor.

ii. The prognosis for a cat with a solitary lesion is good following surgical excision or cryotherapy. In cats, the vast majority of cutaneous MCTs are benign, unlike their canine counterpart. In addition, unlike in dogs, it is not possible to predict the degree of malignancy based on the histological type. The extent of staging prior to surgical intervention in the cat also tends to be significantly less, but at a minimum evaluation of a buffy coat should be performed. The reasoning for this is that cutaneous MCTs in cats can represent metastatic lesions from visceral forms of the disease, which carry a worse prognosis. Following surgical excision, the cat should be monitored for recurrence and/or development of new lesions. Feline cutaneous MCTs tend to occur most commonly on the heads of younger cats and along the trunks of older cats. Multiple tumors with a generalized distribution over the body are more likely to be associated with malignant biological behavior (i.e., spread to other sites and/or organs) than solitary tumors (Melville et al., 2015).

182. A 5-year-old spayed female American Staffordshire terrier presented for a recent onset of moderate pruritus. The owner describes an increase in licking and scratching behavior particularly along the ventral abdomen, inner rear legs, and flanks. The owner believes a similar thing occurred last year but to a much milder degree. On physical exam, you notice these lesions on the ventral abdomen (**Figure 182a**). No other lesions are appreciated on the patient.

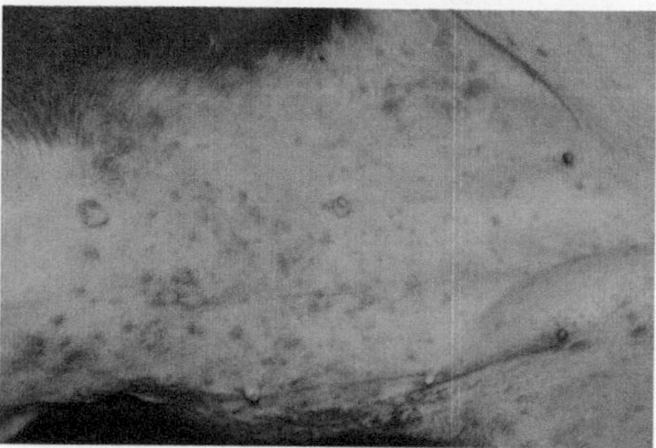

Figure 182a

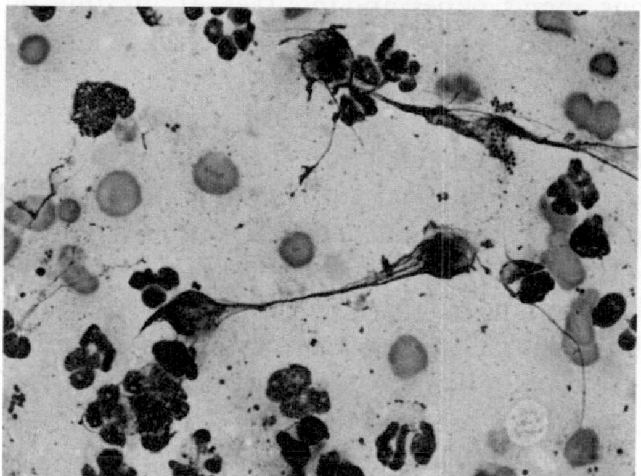

Figure 182b

i. Describe the lesions seen on this patient.

ii. This is a common presentation of dermatologic disease in the dog. These lesions are consistent with what process, and what initial diagnostics should be performed?

iii. Cytology from one of the lesions is shown (**Figure 182b**). What is this patient's diagnosis?

iv. This patient's condition is confined to the ventral abdomen, and given the increasing concern surrounding resistant infections, you recommend that the patient be treated topically. What active ingredients should the products contain, and what treatment recommendations should be provided to the owner?

182. i. There are multiple papules, pustules, crusts, and epidermal collarettes present along the ventral abdomen.

ii. These findings along with patchy, moth-eaten alopecia are common clinical lesions indicating the presence of folliculitis. Frequent causes of folliculitis in the dog include demodicosis, superficial bacterial folliculitis, and dermatophytosis. In a patient with this presentation, initial diagnostics should consist of skin scraping, skin cytology, and trichogram. If mites and bacteria are not seen on the initial samples or if suspicion is high for dermatophytosis, a fungal culture should be acquired.

iii. The image shows neutrophilic inflammation with the presence of coccoid-shaped bacteria. These cytological findings are consistent with superficial bacterial folliculitis.

iv. To date, the best evidence of efficacy for the topical treatment of pyoderma in veterinary medicine exists for chlorhexidine. To a lesser degree, products containing benzoyl peroxide have also been shown to be effective. The concentration of these two active agents should ideally be 2%–3% (or more [4%] for chlorhexidine) for both in any formulation. Other agents that are recommended but have weak efficacy data are ethyl lactate, acetic acid/boric acid combinations, fusidic acid, hypochlorous acid, sodium hypochlorite, nisin, and silver compounds. These ingredients are found in various formulations such as shampoos, lotions, sprays, wipes, and mousses. At this time, numerous protocols have been described, but the common theme is that more frequent application is needed when topical therapy is used as the sole treatment. A recent study showed the use of a combination chlorhexidine shampoo and spray protocol was as effective as systemic amoxicillin-clavulanic acid for the treatment of superficial pyoderma (Borio et al., 2015). In this study, patients were bathed twice weekly and sprayed once daily on nonbathing days. Regardless, for any protocol to be effective, the owner must be able and willing to treat their pet topically, and they should have a say in formulation selection to maximize outcome success. Until optimal protocols are described, the treatment guideline for superficial bacterial folliculitis is to continue therapy for 7 days beyond clinical resolution (Hillier et al., 2014).

183. A 3-year-old spayed Australian shepherd presents for acute severe generalized pruritus. On examination, there is pinnal hypotrichosis with excoriations and scaling along the outer margins (**Figure 183a, b**). The ventral abdomen was also erythemic with scattered papules present (**Figure 183c**). The patient has a positive pinnal-pedal reflex. The owner notes the dog spends roughly 50% of her time outdoors and that they have seen foxes in the area recently. The patient is treated monthly with topical fipronil and oral ivermectin for flea and heartworm prevention. You perform skin scrapes that are negative for mites.

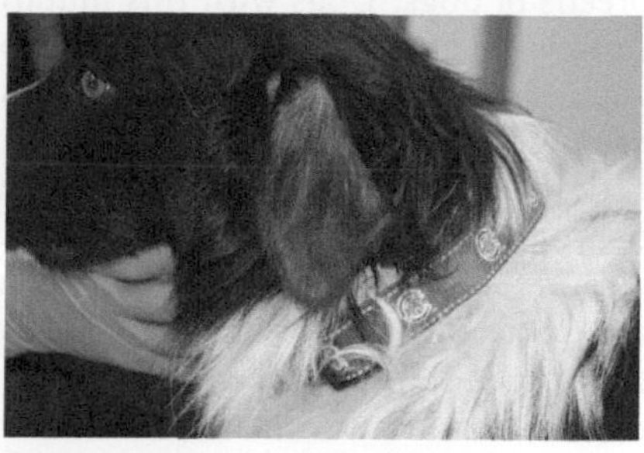
Figure 183a

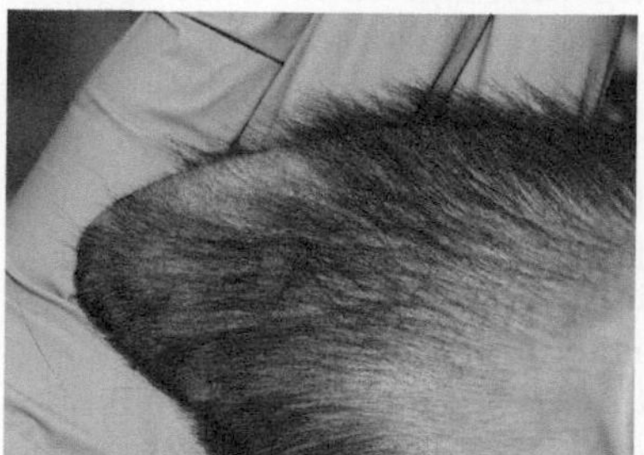
Figure 183b

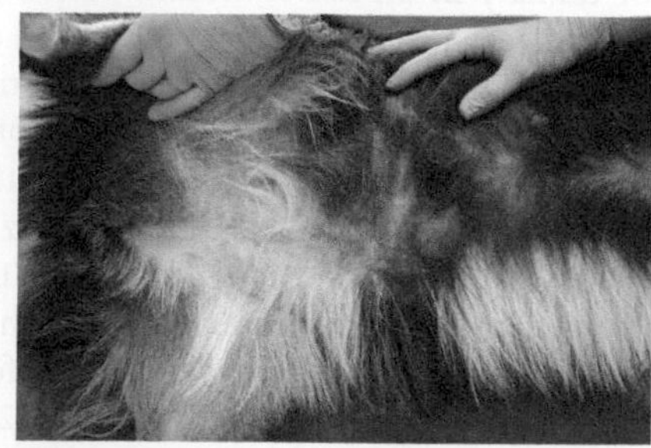
Figure 183c

i. Based on your suspicion, you elect to treat empirically for what disease?

ii. What concerns do you have related to the breed of dog, and what treatment options are available for this patient?

iii. What new diagnostic test is available for this condition, and what are the limitations of the test?

184. A golden retriever presented for examination because the dog's nose had changed color (**Figure 184a**). The owner reported that the dog's nose and skin were normal until a couple of months ago. At that time, she noticed a small patchy loss of color that has progressed to the lesion depicted. No other abnormalities were found on examination.

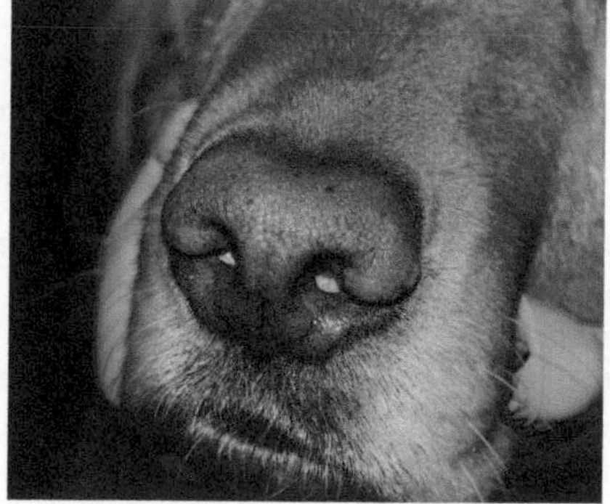
Figure 184a

What condition does this patient have?

183. i. Sarcoptic mange.

ii. Australian shepherds are one of the breeds that are overrepresented for MDR-1 gene mutations that are encountered most commonly with herding breeds of dogs. Dogs with this mutation have compromised P-glycoprotein function that results in severe neurological toxicity when treated with exaggerated doses of avermectins. This class of drugs works through potentiation of GABA-gated chloride channels, which results in inhibition of neurologic activity. GABA-gated chloride ion channels exist throughout the peripheral nervous system of arthropods and nematodes, but in mammals are found within the CNS. P-glycoprotein is a major component the blood-brain barrier that protects mammals from toxicity by pumping drugs out of the CNS. Due to this fact and the unknown MDR-1 status of this patient, ivermectin and doramectin should be avoided for treatment, as scabicidal doses are much higher than what is used for heartworm prevention (leading to increased potential for toxicity in an MDR-mutant patient). Regardless, given the wide array of available treatment options, finding an effective option for these breeds is not as challenging as it has historically been. It should always be remembered that lime sulfur dips are a safe, effective option, which may also be soothing and provide pruritus relief for this or any patient with scabies. Additional treatment options for this patient include amitraz dips applied biweekly for three treatments; selamectin 6–12 mg/kg applied topically every 2 weeks for three doses; a topical moxidectin/imidacloprid combination product (AdvantageMulti or Advocate) applied at 2-week intervals for three doses; fipronil spray 3 mL/kg applied as a pump spray to the body at 2-week intervals for three doses; or one of the newer isoxazoline antiparasitics (afoxolaner, fluralaner, lotilaner, and sarolaner) at standard flea preventative dosages (Becskei et al., 2016).

iii. Recently, *in vitro* serum antibody ELISA tests have been marketed for the serological diagnosis of sarcoptic mange in dogs. These tests have been evaluated in a couple of different studies. The results of these studies have shown a specificity ranging from 89.5% to 93% and a sensitivity of 84.2%–94%. Both of these investigations concluded that the tests have usefulness, but when atopy is a potential diagnosis, positive results are of little diagnostic value likely due to cross-reactivity of the test in dogs who are sensitized to house dust mite antigens (Buckley et al., 2012; Lower et al., 2001).

184. Idiopathic nasal depigmentation. In this condition, dogs are born with a pigmented nasal planum that later loses its color. The condition may wax and wane, but only the nose is affected, with no changes in the nasal planum architecture (i.e., the cobblestone-like appearance is maintained). Other variants of this condition that are seen in practice are the layperson terms *snow nose* and *Dudley nose*. Snow nose is a seasonal decrease in nasal pigmentation commonly observed in Arctic breeds and retrievers. Dogs with Dudley nose have no nasal pigmentation and are generally affected from birth. All of these examples are cosmetic defects and do not warrant further investigation or therapy. The major differential for this condition is vitiligo. Vitiligo is a rare acquired disease associated with melanocyte destruction that affects multiple sites simultaneously, not just the nasal planum.

185. An adult Chinese shar-pei presented with the complaint of "blisters." The axillary region of the dog is shown, and numerous vesicles ranging in size from 0.5–1 cm are present (**Figure 185a**). The vesicles are firm to the touch, and the contents are a clear, viscous exudate (**Figure 185b**).

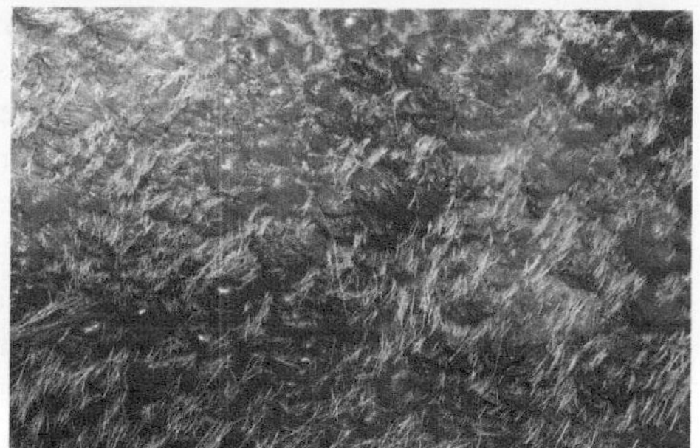
Figure 185a

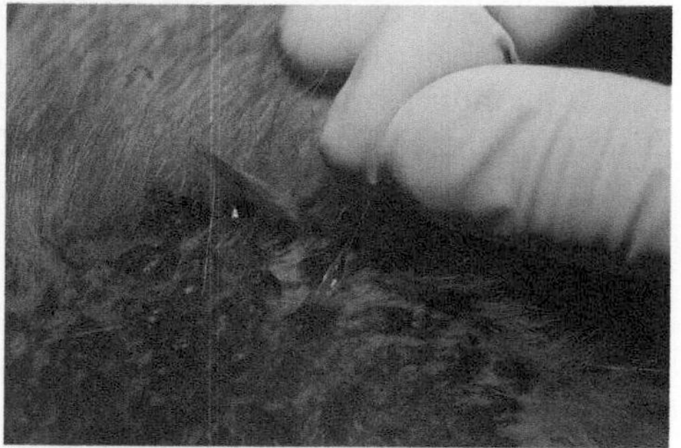
Figure 185b

i. This is a common skin condition in this breed. What is it?

ii. How can it be diagnosed and managed?

iii. What causes this condition in Chinese shar-peis?

186. A 6-year-old spayed female dachshund presented for a complaint of anorexia, lethargy, and crusts along her dorsal and ventral trunk that first began 1 week ago. Close inspection of the skin revealed matting of the hair coat along the dorsal thoracic region with large yellow to golden crusts. Crusts were also noted on the ventral abdomen along with the presence of numerous intact pustules. A photomicrograph from the cytologic examination of a ruptured intact pustule is shown in **Figure 186a**.

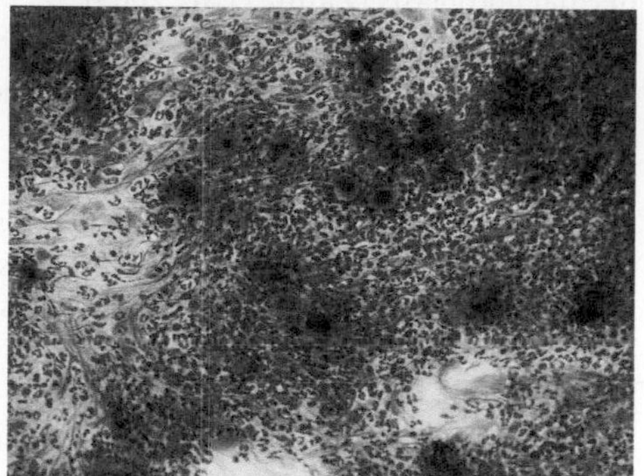
Figure 186a

i. What is present in the image?

ii. Given the presentation, what is your primary differential, and what infectious condition(s) may cause similar cytologic findings?

iii. What recommendations should be made to the owner to confirm your clinical suspicion?

iv. What are the hallmark body locations in a dog that, when affected, should raise your suspicion for this condition?

185. i. Although this resembles an autoimmune vesicular disease, it is actually cutaneous mucinosis. Chinese shar-peis have an excessive amount of dermal mucin, which gives them their characteristic "wrinkled" appearance. The vesicles contain dermal mucin that has percolated from the dermis through the basement membrane and into the epidermis, creating a subcorneal "vesicle." They commonly occur in frictional areas.

ii. The condition is normally diagnosed based on signalment and clinical findings of exaggerated folds with mucin-containing vesicles. The easiest way to diagnose cutaneous mucinosis is to gently puncture one of the vesicles with a sterile needle and express the contents. The mucin is thick, clear, and stringy as shown in **Figure 185a, b**. The condition can also be confirmed via biopsy with histopathology demonstrating excessive dermal mucin with no other abnormalities. This is a cosmetic problem and requires no treatment. In some cases, the lesions can become large and pendulous, especially when they occur on the hocks. The more wrinkled the dog, the more likely for these cosmetic lesions to be large. Oral prednisone (2 mg/kg) for 7–10 days followed by a slow reduction over 30–45 days will decrease mucin production. However, this will occur over the dog's entire body, not just in focal areas, and owners should be warned that their dogs will lose some of their wrinkled appearance. Owners often refer to this as "deflating" their Chinese shar-pei.

iii. Primary idiopathic cutaneous mucinosis of the Chinese shar-pei is the result of massive accumulations of hyaluronic acid within the dermis. Investigations have shown that this increase in hyaluronic acid production is most likely the result of a regulatory mutation with hyaluronan synthase-2 in dermal fibroblasts (Zanna et al., 2009).

186. i. The image shows predominantly neutrophilic inflammation with the presence of acantholytic keratinocytes and the absence of obvious infectious etiologic agents.

ii. A dog presenting with systemic clinical signs and cytologically sterile pustules containing acantholytic keratinocytes is suggestive of pemphigus foliaceus. Both *Staphylococcus pseudintermedius* and dermatophytosis (specifically *Trichophyton mentagrophytes*) are known to cause formation of acantholytic cells.

iii. At this time, a biopsy of one or more intact pustules should be collected and submitted for histopathology. In addition, a sample from an intact pustule should be collected and submitted for bacterial and fungal culture to verify the lesions are sterile. The documentation of intracorneal pustules with acantholytic keratinocyte formation that are culture negative, is the definitive diagnosis of pemphigus foliaceus.

iv. Symmetric lesions affecting the "3P's" in a dog should raise a clinician's suspicion of pemphigus foliaceus. The 3P's are the nasal planum, pinnae (specifically the nonhaired concave aspect), and pads. Not all three areas need to be affected, but if pustules or crusts are observed at any of these sites, pemphigus foliaceus should be a differential diagnosis consideration.

187. **Figure 187a** shows the four strengths in which Zoetis's new product Cytopoint is currently available.

i. What is this product, and how is it classified with regard to pharmaceuticals?

ii. What is the labeled dosing for this product?

iii. What is the labeled indication for this product?

iv. How is this product metabolized and excreted?

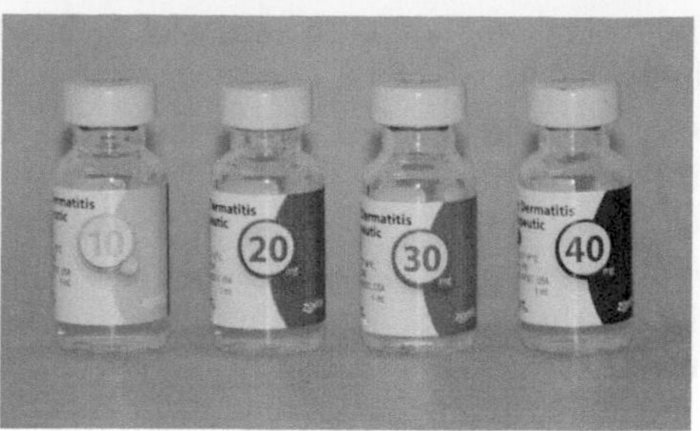

Figure 187a

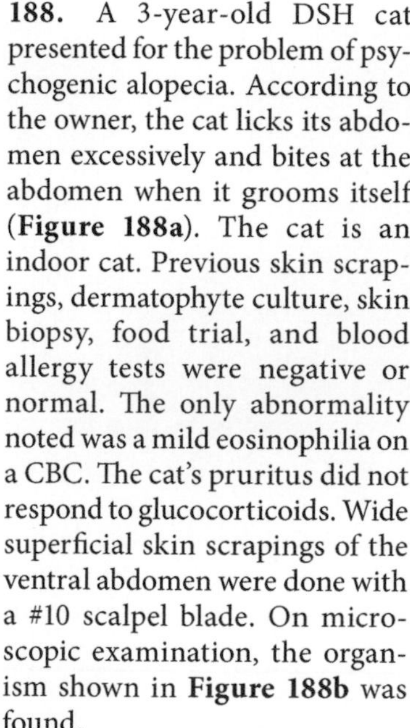

188. A 3-year-old DSH cat presented for the problem of psychogenic alopecia. According to the owner, the cat licks its abdomen excessively and bites at the abdomen when it grooms itself (**Figure 188a**). The cat is an indoor cat. Previous skin scrapings, dermatophyte culture, skin biopsy, food trial, and blood allergy tests were negative or normal. The only abnormality noted was a mild eosinophilia on a CBC. The cat's pruritus did not respond to glucocorticoids. Wide superficial skin scrapings of the ventral abdomen were done with a #10 scalpel blade. On microscopic examination, the organism shown in **Figure 188b** was found.

i. What is present, and how is it treated?

ii. How does this relate to the psychogenic alopecia?

iii. What other diagnostic test(s) can be used to identify ectoparasites in cats?

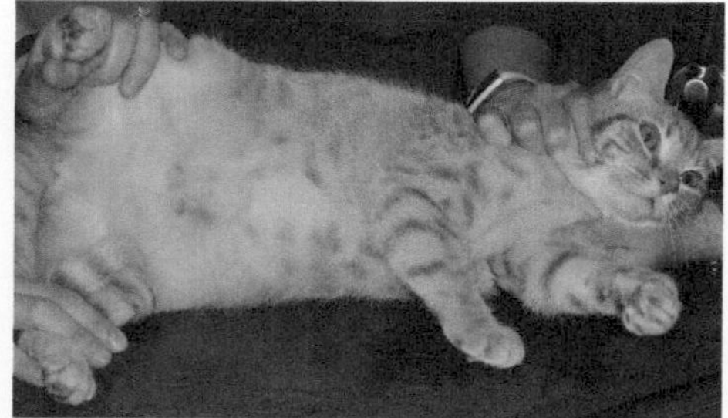
Figure 188a

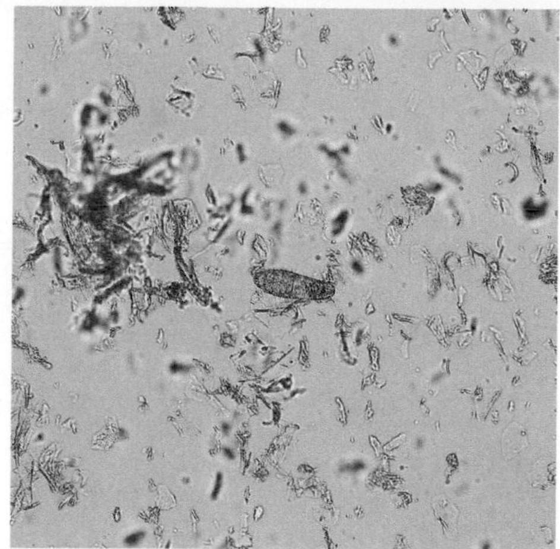
Figure 188b

187. **i.** Cytopoint is a caninized anti-interleukin-31 (IL-31) monoclonal antibody (mAb). mAbs are classified as biotherapeutics and should not be considered similar to classic pharmacotherapy (i.e., the use of drugs).

ii. Labeled dosing for Cytopoint in the United States is 2 mg/kg administered by subcutaneous injection every 4–8 weeks as needed. In the European Union and elsewhere, the product is labeled for use at 1 mg/kg once a month.

iii. In the United States, the labeled indication for Cytopoint is that lokivetmab has been shown to be effective for the treatment of allergic dermatitis and atopic dermatitis in dogs, while elsewhere it is labeled for the treatment of clinical manifestations of atopic dermatitis in dogs.

iv. Monoclonal antibodies are not metabolized and excreted like normal pharmaceutical agents. Monoclonal antibodies are eliminated via intracellular catabolism within the lysosome, where they are broken down to peptides or amino acids that can either be recycled for protein synthesis or excreted by the kidneys.

188. i. *Demodex gatoi* mite. This is the most common form of feline demodicosis encountered, which has also demonstrated some geographic variability in its occurrence. The mite is unique with respect to other variants of *Demodex* spp. in that it is (i) contagious; (ii) causes pruritus without the presence of a secondary infection; (iii) is surface dwelling, not follicular; and (iv) standard treatment recommendations are different from other forms of demodicosis. The preferred treatment at this time is weekly 2% lime sulfur dips. In the case of a confirmed *D. gatoi* infestation, the affected cat and all in-contact cats should be treated weekly for a minimum of 6 weeks. In cases of suspected infestation, the affected cat should be treated weekly for three applications, and if clinical improvement is observed, then an additional three treatments at weekly intervals should be performed along with treating all in-contact cats as previously described (Beale, 2012). Additionally reported options include oral ivermectin at a dose of 0.2–0.3 mg/kg daily to every other day, topical amitraz, and topical moxidectin (Short and Gram, 2016). Anecdotally, the use of isoxazolines at monthly preventative doses has also been reported to be effective. At this time, treatment with lime sulfur appears to be the most reliable, however, treatment failures are encountered with all options.

ii. Feline demodicosis as a result of *D. gatoi* is a cause of pruritus in cats. It should be considered in the differential diagnosis of any and all feline skin diseases associated with excessive grooming, such as atopy, food allergy, "feline scabies," FAD, and contact dermatitis. It is important to remember that *D. gatoi* dwells superficially and, as a result, can be easily removed during overgrooming, making it difficult to find. Psychogenic alopecia is a term used to describe a self-induced hair loss condition believed to represent a compulsive or behavioral disorder observed in cats. The pattern of alopecia commonly observed with both *D. gatoi* and psychogenic alopecia is similar and affects the ventral abdomen, flanks, medial rear legs, and forelimbs. Psychogenic alopecia is a diagnosis of exclusion, which can only be made if primary dermatologic and other medical conditions (cystitis, urinary tract infection, arthritis, etc.) have been thoroughly ruled out. This process of exclusion requires a comprehensive medical workup that can be expensive and may not be pursued due to owner financial constraints. This lack of medical workup likely leads to many cases being given a presumptive diagnosis of psychogenic alopecia, rather than a definitive diagnosis. It is important to note that psychogenic alopecia is significantly overdiagnosed, and any such diagnosis should be rightfully questioned (Waisglass et al., 2006).

iii. *D. gatoi* can be difficult to find via skin scrapings in affected patients. When used, superficial scrapings should be performed over large, expansive regions including areas that are nonalopecic and hard for the patient to groom. Due to the fastidious grooming nature of cats, the author has found fecal flotation to be a reliable method to yield positive results in suspected cases even when mites could not be recovered via scrapings. Additionally, some authors have suggested other nonaffected household cats undergo skin scraping, as although they may appear normal, mites can be easily recovered in high numbers from these individuals. Regardless, as is the case with canine scabies, when *D. gatoi* is suspected, patients should be treated for the condition even if mites are not observed.

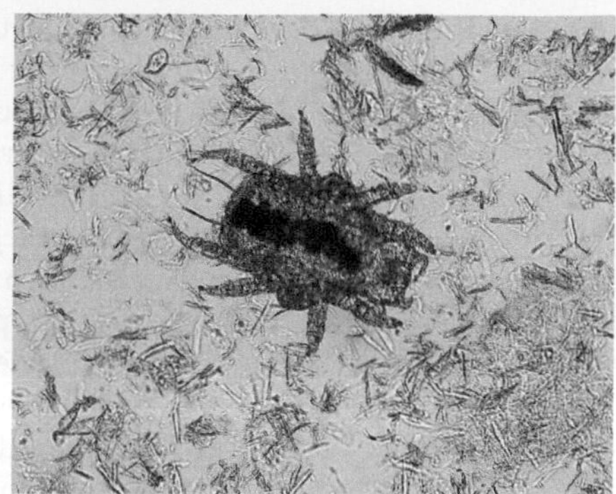
Figure 189a

189. A long-term client comes to your clinic and brings in a small container filled with scale and debris recovered from along the dorsum of his dog. The owner notes that his dog has had a significant increase in debris along his back over the last several weeks. You agree to look at the material under the microscope, and the organism shown in **Figure 189a** was found in the debris.

i. What is present, and how is it differentiated from other mites that cause disease in dogs and cats?

ii. What clinical signs does this parasite cause in dogs and cats?

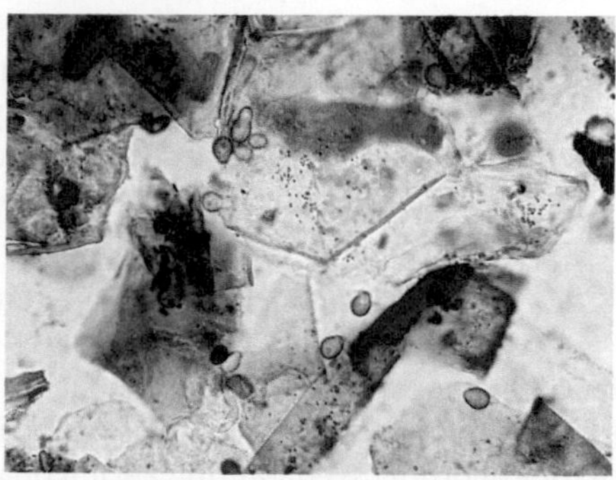
Figure 190a

190. A 3-year-old castrated male black Labrador retriever presented for a history of chronic nonseasonal pruritus for the last 1.5 years. The owners felt that the severity of disease had been progressing but remained confined primarily to the paws. The patient was reported to be moderately pruritic with a fair amount of time spent licking and chewing the paws. Salivary staining and moderate interdigital erythema with mild paronychia were noted on all four paws.

i. A photomicrograph from an acetate tape impression is shown (**Figure 190a**). What are these organisms?

ii. With regard to treatment recommendations, what agents have been shown to be efficacious?

189. i. This is a *Cheyletiella* spp. mite that is commonly referred to as the "walking dandruff mite." The diagnostic features that help identify this as a *Cheyletiella* spp. are its large size and accessory mouthparts (palpi) that terminate in hooks ("Viking helmet" appearance). *Otodectes* mites are large and highly motile on samples. They are most likely to be found in or near the ears. The anus is terminal, and they have four legs that extend beyond the body wall, except for the fourth pair in females, with short, unjointed stalks with suckers on all four legs in males and the first two pairs in females. *Sarcoptes* mites and *Notoedres* are very difficult to differentiate. Both are very small (200–400 μm) and oval. In *Sarcoptes,* the first two pairs of legs are short with long unjointed stalks containing suckers. In *Notoedres,* the stalks are of medium length, and the caudal legs have long bristles. The anus is terminal in *Sarcoptes,* while it is dorsal in *Notoedres.*

ii. Clinical signs are quite variable and may range from asymptomatic to an intensely pruritic dermatitis. In dogs, initial lesions are reported to be excessive scaling that is more pronounced along the dorsum. With chronicity and increased mite numbers, generalized erythema and traumatic alopecia are seen. In cats, clinical signs are reported to vary as well from asymptomatic to excessive barbering alopecia or miliary dermatitis.

190. i. *Malassezia* spp., most likely *M. pachydermatis.* The dark brown to black coccoid- to elliptical-shaped materials present are melanin granules.

ii. Numerous studies have been published evaluating various treatment options for *Malassezia* dermatitis in dogs. There is strong evidence to support the use of topical products containing 2% miconazole with 2% chlorhexidine (Mueller et al., 2012b). There is growing evidence for topical products containing solely chlorhexidine at concentrations greater than 3%, combination chlorhexidine with climbazole, 2% climbazole-containing products, and enilconazole. In cases where topical therapy treatment is impractical or not possible, there is fair evidence for systemic use of ketoconazole and itraconazole (Negre et al., 2009). At this time, there is growing evidence for the use of fluconazole and terbinafine, but these agents require further controlled studies to validate their therapeutic use.

191. A 10-month-old spayed female dalmatian presented for hair loss and "sores" along the legs, face, and lateral chest. The lesions shown in **Figure 191a, b** are characteristic of others present over the dog's body. The patient lives predominantly outdoors, and symptoms began shortly after the dog dug multiple holes in the ground. The patient is bright, alert, and responsive with no systemic signs of illness. The patient is also not pruritic at this time.

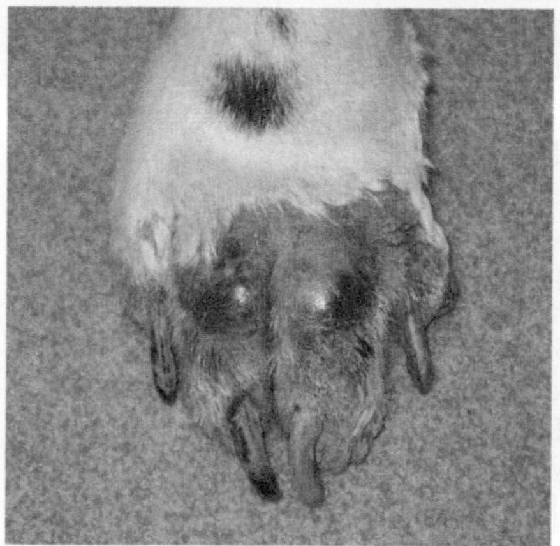

Figure 191a

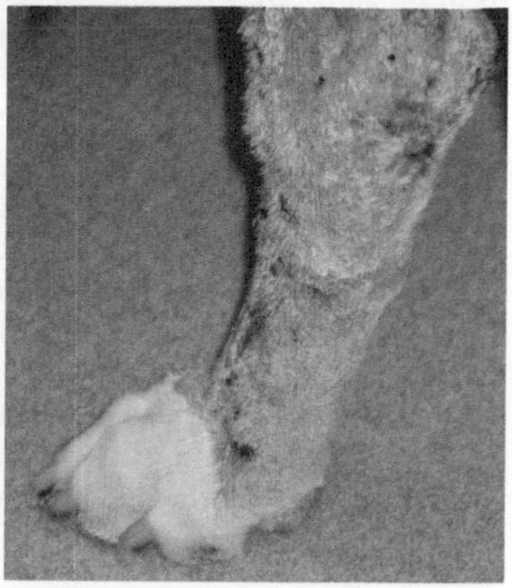

Figure 191b

i. What are the differential diagnoses?

ii. Initial diagnostics tests (skin scraping and cytology) do not reveal a diagnosis, and the owner declines treatment pending further results. A cytologic preparation from a pending diagnostic test is shown in **Figure 191c**. What is the diagnosis, and how do you explain where the dog got this condition?

iii. What systemic therapy options can be recommended for this condition with confidence at this time?

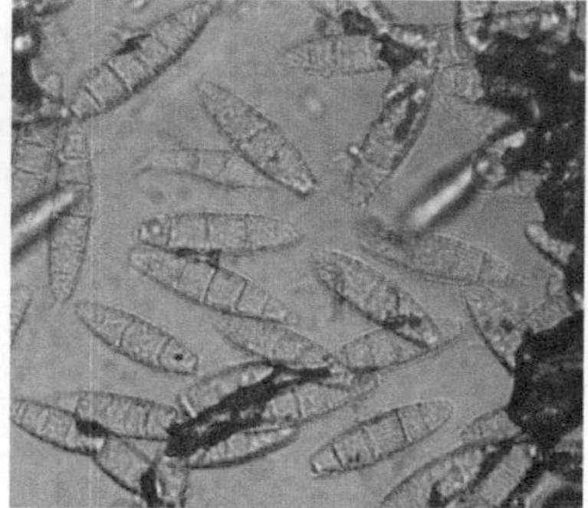

Figure 191c

192. A trichogram sample is prepared by plucking a group of hairs from the skin, placing them in mineral oil, and covering the sample with a coverslip. The hairs are then examined under a microscope with a 4× or 10× objective.

For what conditions involving the hair or hair follicle can a trichogram provide diagnostic information?

191. i. Given the patient's age, demodicosis, dermatophytosis, and bacterial pyoderma with or without secondary *Malassezia* overgrowth are most likely.

ii. Dematophytosis caused by *Microsporum gypseum*. Numerous spindle- or canoe-shaped macroconidia are present with thin walls, rounded ends, and up to six cells. These are all characteristics of *M. gypseum*. The thin walls and lack of a terminal knob are the features most helpful at distinguishing this species from *M. canis*. *M. gypseum* is a geophilic dermatophyte species that inhabits the soil and is found worldwide. This infection was likely acquired while digging holes in the ground.

iii. At this time, a recent published consensus guideline for treatment of dermatophytosis in dogs and cats concluded that itraconazole and terbinafine are the safest and most effective systemic treatments for the condition. Fluconazole and ketoconazole are also possibilities, but available data suggest they are less effective, and ketoconazole has more potential adverse events associated with its use. Although griseofulvin is effective, adverse effects associated with its use and the advent of newer, safer options have relegated this medication to a treatment of historical significance except in geographic regions where it is the only available therapeutic option. Lufenuron is a chitin synthesis inhibitor, which at this time provides absolutely no benefit in the treatment or prevention of dematopytosis and should not be recommended (Moriello et al., 2017).

192. Dermatophytosis (presence of fungal hyphae or ectothrix spores), self-inflicted/barbering alopecia (broken but normal hairs), demodicosis (all life stages of the mite), lice (nits), cheyletiellosis (eggs), telogen or anagen effluvium (hairs predominantly in one phase), sebaceous adenitis (follicular casting), color dilution alopecia (melanosome aggregates and distorted hair shafts), nutritional disorders (malformed/misshapeded hairs), and alopecia areata.

193. A 2-year-old spayed female giant schnauzer presented for evaluation of a rash on her inner leg. Physical examination revealed the lesions shown in **Figure 193a** affecting the left inguinal region.

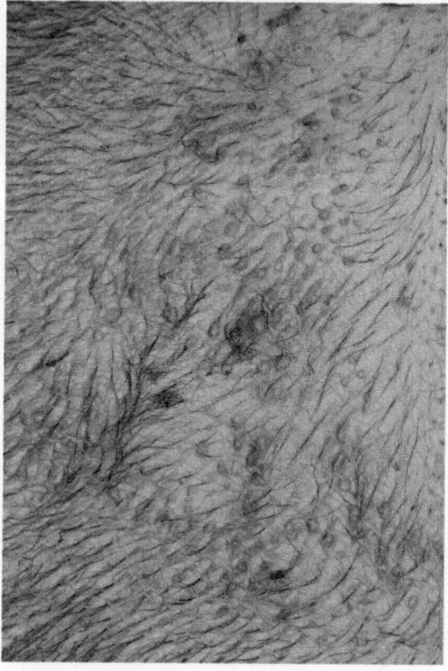

Figure 193a

i. Describe the clinical findings.
ii. What further questions do you have for the owner?

193. **i.** There are multiple milia and ingrown hairs present along with a couple of papules/pustules and small comedones at the periphery. In addition, there appears to be cutaneous atrophy as demonstrated by the thinning and wrinkling or crepe paper appearance to the skin. Milia are thin-walled keratin-filled cysts that appear just under the skin, which are commonly misidentified as "whiteheads" or pustules.

ii. When cutaneous lesions similar to this are observed, the owner should be questioned as to whether or not they are applying any topical product to the site. These cutaneous lesions are common in dogs with a steroid excess that may be the result of endogenous overproduction or exogenous application/administration. Upon further questioning in this case, the owner reported they had been applying a topical ointment to the area (contained betamethasone) that had been prescribed for their own use by their physician.

194. A Labrador retriever puppy presented for acute onset of facial swelling, crusting, and erosive exudative lesions affecting the ears (**Figure 194a–c**). The owners noted that the patient was nonpruritic and had become progressively lethargic with a decreased appetite since the lesions were first observed 1 week ago. On physical examination, the patient was febrile with a marked submandibular and prescapular lymphadenomegaly (**Figure 194d**). A representative photomicrograph of cytology taken from one of the intact pustules on the rostral muzzle is shown in **Figure 194e.**

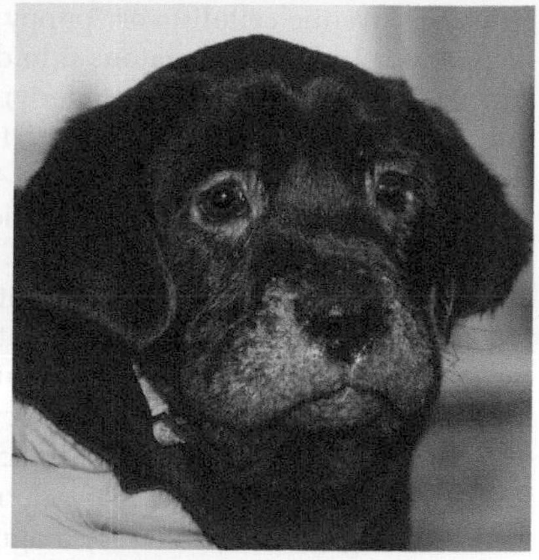
Figure 194a

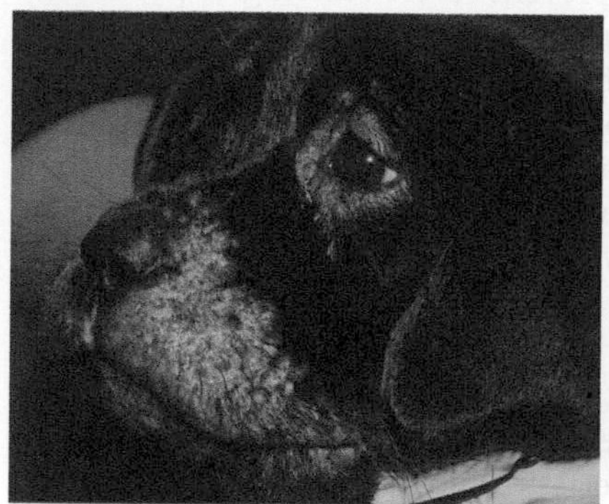
Figure 194b

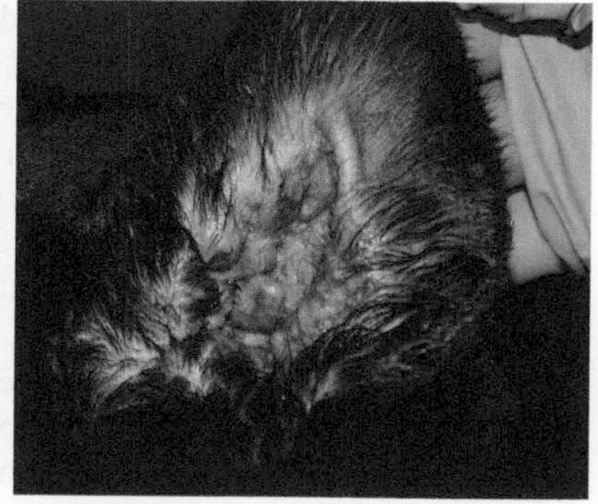
Figure 194c

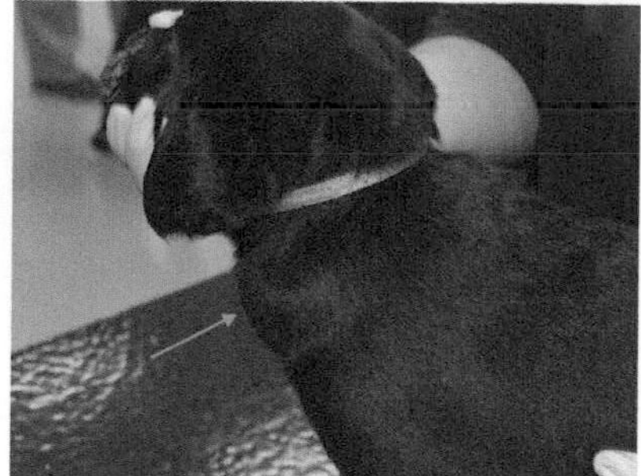
Figure 194d

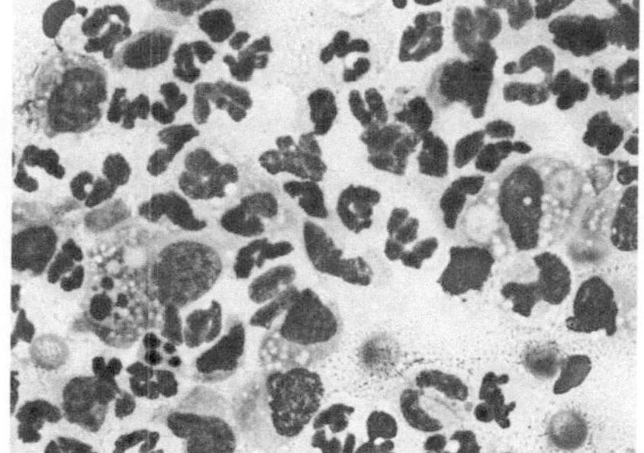
Figure 194e

i. This is a classic presentation of what disease?

ii. What is the treatment of choice for this condition?

iii. What are the less common presentations of this disease?

194. i. Juvenile cellulitis or "puppy strangles." This is an uncommon sterile pustular and granulomatous skin disease that affects the face, pinnae, and lymph nodes of puppies. The underlying cause for development of this condition is unknown but believed to be the result of immune dysfunction. The condition normally develops prior to 4–6 months of age, and although no sex predilection is observed, golden retrievers, dachshunds, and Gordon setters have been reported to be predisposed. Cytology samples from intact pustules, bullae, or nodules will primarily contain a mix of neutrophils and activated macrophages with no infectious agents. Specimens acquired from older, ruptured lesions are more likely to contain a mixture of inflammatory cells that may include eosinophils and lymphocytes along with the presence of bacterial organisms that are not present in intact lesions. Primary differential diagnoses for this condition include deep pyoderma, demodicosis, and adverse drug reaction. Although not necessary for diagnosis, skin biopsy findings are consistent with granulomatous panniculitis.

ii. Systemic glucocorticoids are the treatment of choice for this disease. Early and aggressive treatment is needed to prevent severe scarring or potentially death. Oral prednisone or methylprednisolone (2 mg/kg PO q24h) is administered until the lesions resolve and is then gradually tapered over time based on response. If glucocorticoids are discontinued too rapidly, relapse will occur. Topical therapy with warm antibacterial soaks may be used to remove debris and exudates. Systemic antimicrobials may also be needed if a secondary bacterial infection is present. Therapy with cyclosporine may be beneficial in refractory cases or those where adverse events secondary to systemic glucocorticoids are deemed excessive.

iii. This disease can develop in older dogs (>6 months age) as periocular granulomatous dermatitis. Also, puppies may present with edematous pinnae or nodular panniculitis alone or with classic lesions. In rare instances, dogs presenting with lameness, paresis, or neurologic symptoms have also been described (Park et al., 2010).

195. A 9-month-old spayed female Labrador retriever was referred for the complaint of persistent pruritus. The owners practice flea control, and the other dog in the household is normal. The dog sleeps with the family's children, and none of them have skin lesions. The dog was treated for *Sarcoptes scabiei* mites with topical selamectin (q2 weeks, three doses total). The pruritus did not respond to a 4-week course of oral antibiotics (cephalexin) and ketoconazole at the appropriate dose and dosage for this patient. Skin scrapings, flea combings, and a dermatophyte culture were negative. The only other piece of historical information obtained was the owners reported the dog defecates three to four times a day, even though it is fed only once daily. The feces vary in consistency from firm to soft. Dermatologic examination reveals hair lodged between the dog's teeth and gums, generalized thinning of the hair coat, and a mild oiliness to the coat.

i. What differential diagnoses have been ruled out by the previous diagnostics?

ii. What are the most likely differential diagnoses at this time, and what diagnostic tests should be performed at this time?

iii. What is the relationship between intestinal parasitism and cutaneous adverse food reactions?

196. A dog presented for evaluation of a nodular swelling over his distal right front extremity. The owner reported that the mass was progressively enlarging over the past 2 months and was observed to be draining a blood-tinged fluid within the last week. As an initial diagnostic, you elect to perform a fine-needle aspiration of the mass, the result of which is shown in **Figure 196a**.

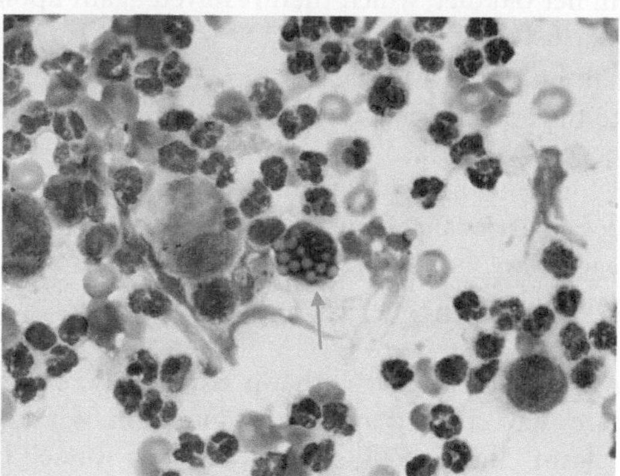

Figure 196a

What is present at the end of the green arrow?

195. **i.** The negative skin scrapings make demodicosis unlikely. The topical selamectin therapy helped rule out lice, *Sarcoptes* and *Cheyletiella* mites. In addition, these are highly contagious mites, and the other dog in the house is normal, and the people in contact with this dog have no unexplained rashes. The negative fungal culture and 4-week treatment with antimicrobials also make infections an unlikely cause. Additionally, the distribution of clinical lesions and routine use of flea preventatives makes a flea infestation or lice infestation unlikely.

ii. The most likely differential diagnoses are a cutaneous adverse food reaction and/or atopy. Given the nonseasonal nature and young age of onset, a cutaneous adverse food reaction should be suspected first, although the historical findings do not exclude atopy as a possibility. The frequent bowel movements could be related to the skin disease, since some dogs with food allergies have concurrent GI issues. At this time, the most logical step is to proceed with a diet elimination trial. To perform this trial, a prescription limited ingredient diet or hydrolyzed protein diet should be fed exclusively to the patient for 8 weeks. A recent review investigating the results of elimination diet trials concluded that greater than 90% of dogs with cutaneous adverse food reaction had improvement or remission of clinical symptoms by this time point (Olivry et al., 2015). Although home-cooked elimination diets are ideal, they should be avoided in young growing dogs unless they are adequately balanced. If the diet elimination trial fails to provide any or limited clinical benefit, the dog should be evaluated for atopy and allergy tested. This dog was diagnosed with a food allergy following improvement while fed a prescription hydrolyzed diet and experienced flaring of clinical symptoms (pruritus) within 48 hours of recheallenge with her old diet, which then resolved again upon being fed the hydrolyzed diet exclusively.

iii. The intestinal mucosa is a protective barrier that does not permit antigens to cross into the body. It has been proposed that one of the mechanisms by which dogs become sensitized to various food antigens is via a damaged mucosal barrier. Intestinal parasites (roundworms, hookworms, giardia, etc.) damage the mucosal barrier and allow antigens into the submucosa, leading to sensitization. In addition, viral diseases of the gut may also play a similar role in predisposing animals to food allergies.

196. This is an activated plasma cell that is commonly referred to as a Mott cell. These cells are characterized by the accumulation of large, pale vacuoles within the cytoplasm. These vacuoles are known as Russell bodies and are packets of immunoglobulin secretions. These vacuoles may be mistaken for fungal spores or intracellular parasites by the untrained observer. Mott cells can be encountered in numerous conditions characterized by chronic inflammation. Russell bodies can also be observed extracelluarly if a Mott cell lysis, as seen by the free vacuole to the right of the highlighted cell in the image.

197. A 10-year-old spayed female DSH cat presented for facial changes observed by the owner 1 hour after the instillation of ear medications into the right ear (**Figure 197a**).

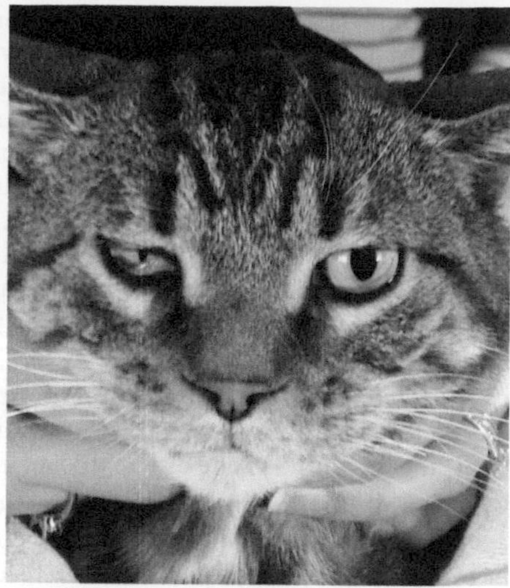
Figure 197a

i. What is your diagnosis for the facial changes, and what are the classic clinical signs of this syndrome in dogs and cats?

ii. How is the syndrome classified?

iii. What pharmacologic test has been proposed to help with lesion localization?

198. A 3-year-old spayed female standard poodle presented for lameness and sloughing (onychomadesis) of her claws. The owner reported that the problem started on one paw, and then gradually developed on all four paws over 3 months. Examination revealed the claws were separating at the claw bed and that previously sloughed claws that had regrown were misshapen, soft, and brittle (**Figure 198a, b**). The footpads were normal, and there were no other signs of skin disease. Previous fungal cultures were negative, and the condition did not respond to a 4-week course of oral antibiotics.

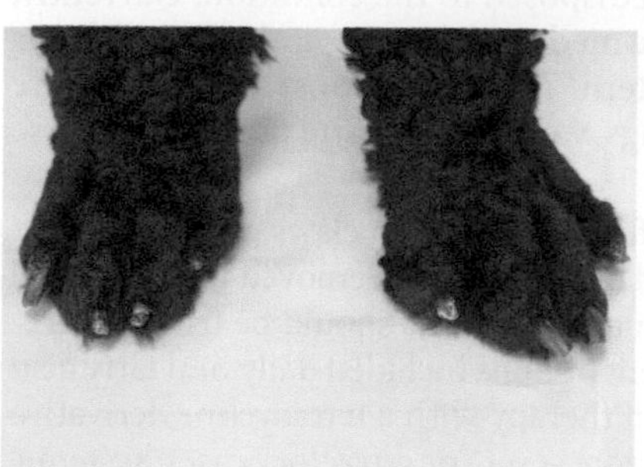
Figure 198a

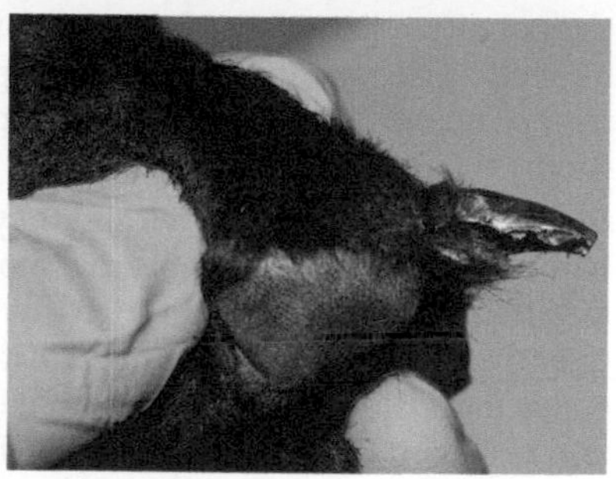
Figure 198b

i. What is the most likely diagnosis?

ii. How should this be treated?

iii. What conditions may present with only claw abnormalities?

197. i. Horner syndrome. This condition is the result of a loss of sympathetic innervation to the ocular/facial region, which can be seen as a result of otitis media/interna, cranial, cervical or thoracic trauma, thoracic neoplasia, CNS inflammation or neoplasia, brachial plexus trauma, and retrobulbar neoplasia (Simpson et al., 2015). The syndrome is characterized by a quartet of clinical signs that include miosis (small pupil), dropping of the upper eyelid (ptosis), enophthalmos or retraction of the eyeball, and protrusion of the third eyelid. In other species including humans, a fifth clinical sign of facial anhidrosis (little or no sweating) may be observed on the affected side.

ii. Horner syndrome is classified according to where the lesion occurs along the sympathetic tract. Lesions are therefore classified neuroanatomically as central, preganglionic, or postganglionic. Preganglionic fibers run from the T1–T3 spinal cord to the tympanic bulla, while postganglionic fibers run from the tympanic bulla to the eye (Garosi et al., 2012).

iii. Topical instillation of phenylephrine, a direct-acting sympathomimetic agent, onto the eye and monitoring for pupil dilation can be used to help with lesion localization. To perform the test, dilute (0.25%–1%) phenylephrine is instilled into both eyes, and the time required for the pupils to dilate is recorded. If pupil dilation occurs in under 20 minutes, the lesion is likely post-ganglionic. It is important to remember that this test is not 100% accurate and that using more concentrated formulations of phenylephrine can lead to false positives (Garosi et al., 2012; Simpson et al., 2015).

198. i. Given the clinical signalment and findings, the most likely diagnosis is symmetric lupoid onychodystrophy. Other reasonable differentials would include onychomycosis, adverse drug eruption, and vasculitis. Gordon setters and German shepherds appear to be predisposed to the condition. Currently, the condition is suspected to be immune mediated, but it is unknown if this is a specific disease entity or a reaction pattern. The latter is most likely, and there may be numerous triggers including drugs, vaccinations, and potential adverse food reactions (Mueller et al., 2003).

ii. These dogs are very lame, and they often snag avulsed claws on carpeting or while walking. The sloughing claw should be avulsed and removed under general anesthesia, if necessary. Additionally, nonavulsed claws should be trimmed frequently to avoid further trauma. Treatment options included daily oral fatty acid supplementation, vitamin E, combination therapy with a tetracycline derivative and niacinamide, and pentoxifylline. In more severe or refractory cases, systemic glucocorticoids, cyclosporine, or azathioprine may be required initially prior to transitioning to a more conservative form of therapy. The author uses a combination of glucocorticoids and pentoxifylline until the sloughing halts, and then continues with pentoxifylline in combination with oral fatty acids and vitamin E supplementation. The requirement of long-term therapy is variable, and some cases require lifelong therapeutic intervention to maintain remission.

iii. Trauma, bacterial infection, dermatophytosis, *Malassezia* infection, leishmaniasis, hookworm dermatitis, symmetric lupoid onychodystrophy, pemphigus vulgaris, subepidermal bullous dermatoses, adverse drug eruption, vasculitis, and neoplasia (squamous cell carcinoma, melanoma, soft-tissue sarcoma, and subungual keratinizing acanthoma).

199. The owners of a 9-year-old spayed female Maltese presented her for the problem of symmetrical nonpruritic hair loss (**Figure 199a, b**). Upon examination, the skin was thin, and the superficial vasculature on the ventral abdomen was more prominent than expected (**Figure 199c**). The dog likes to sunbathe, and the owner reported no changes in the dog's water consumption, urination, defecation, or behavior. A CBC, serum chemistries, and urinalysis panels were initially ordered, and all values were within normal limits.

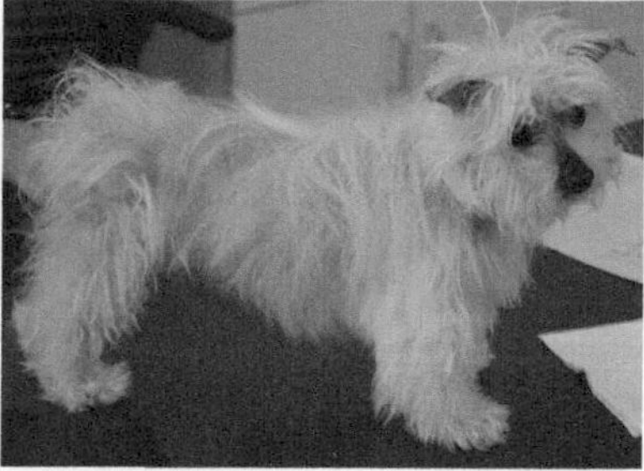

Figure 199a

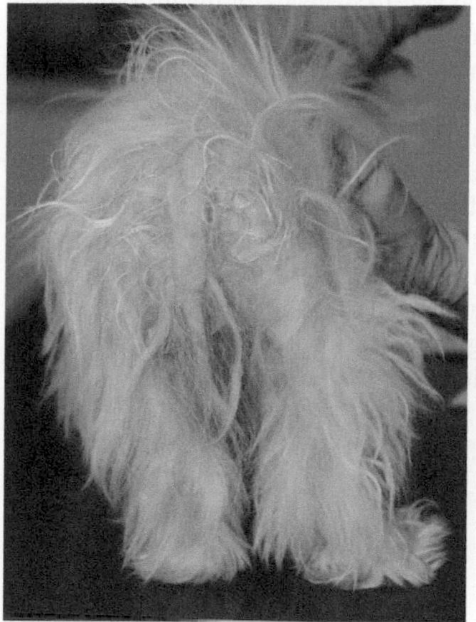

Figure 199b

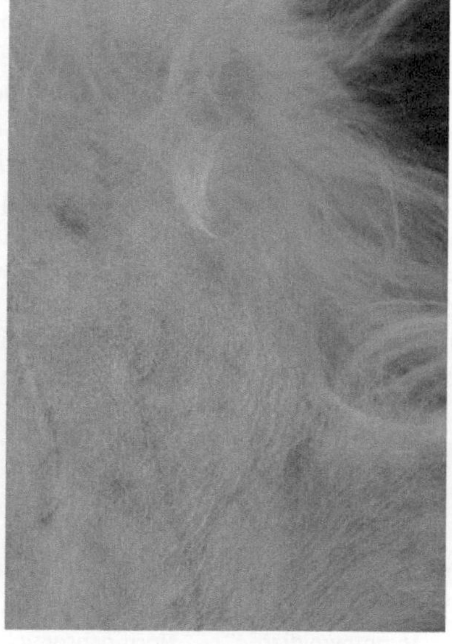

Figure 199c

i. What are the differential diagnoses for nonpruritic symmetrical alopecia in this breed?

ii. Why were the screening diagnostic tests ordered for this patient? Additional diagnostic testing is indicated in this patient. What tests should be ordered?

iii. What is a UCCR, and how might the information be useful in treating this patient?

200. What is azathioprine, what dermatologic condition(s) has it been used for, and what are the major adverse events encountered with use of the drug?

199. **i.** The differential diagnoses include hypothyroidism, hyperadrenocorticism, pattern alopecia, and sex hormone alopecia (endogenous and exogenous). Hyperadrenocorticism is the most common endocrine disorder in this breed, while hypothyroidism would be the next most likely cause of endocrine alopecia. In the early stages when hair loss is the only clinical symptom, the two diseases can look very similar. Pattern alopecia is a hereditary disorder that is seen more commonly in other breeds and begins earlier in life. It usually presents with bilaterally symmetrical hair loss over the head, ears, ventrum, and caudal thigh. Sex hormone alopecia is very rare, and it would be a diagnosis of elimination.

ii. The most likely cause of this patient's hair loss is an endocrine disorder with the dog's clinical signs suggestive of hyperadrenocorticism. However, the patient is not showing any other symptoms (polyuria, polydipsia, polyphagia, panting) except for hair loss and thin skin. In addition, upon further questioning, the owner also stated that the dog was able to sleep all night without having an accident or waking the owner up to go outside to urinate. The history of sunbathing suggests heat-seeking behavior, which could be due to hypothyroidism. However, the heat-seeking behavior could be due to the fact the dog is simply cold because it has lost its hair due to a nonendocrine follicular disorder.

A CBC, serum chemistries, and urinalysis, are indicated to help differentiate causes of endocrine alopecia and help direct selection of further more specific endocrine function testing. A chart of the possible changes observed with the endocrine causes of alopecia is shown in **Figure 199d**. A thyroid screening panel and low-dose dexamethasone suppression test (LDDST) would be the next series of tests. A thyroid screening panel was ordered first in this patient and was found to be normal. The results of LDDST (0.01 mg/kg IV) revealed

Disease	CBC	Serum Chemistries	Urinalysis
Hypothyroidism	Normocytic Normochromic Nonregenerative Anemia	Hypercholesterolemia Hypertrigylceridemia ALT and CK elevations +/- ALP	Normal
Cushing's	Leukocytosis Neutrophilia Lymphopenia Eosinopenia Thrombocytosis	Elevated ALP +/- ALT Hypercholesterolemia Hypertrigylceridemia hyperglycemia Decrease BUN hypophosphatemia	Low Sp. Gravity (<1.020) Bacteriuria Proteinuria Elevated UCCR ratio
Hyperestrogenism	Nonregenerative Anemia Leukopenia Thrombocytopenia	Normal	Normal

Figure 199d

an elevated basal cortisol at 0 hours, marked suppression of cortisol at 4 hours post-dexamethasone, and an elevated cortisol concentration at 8 hours post-dexamethasone. These findings not only answer the question of whether or not the dog has hyperadrenocorticism but also were compatible with PDH. In a normal dog, the 8-hour cortisol concentration would be suppressed, but in this case, it was not.

iii. A UCCR is a screening test that excludes hyperadrenocorticism as a possible disease as the negative predictive value approaches 100% (i.e., if the test is normal, the patient does not have hyperadrenocorticism). Dogs with spontaneous hyperadrenocorticism have an elevated UCCR, but most dogs with an elevated UCCR do not have hyperadrenocorticism. If the test is elevated, dynamic adrenal function tests (ACTH stimulation test or LDDST) are indicated to answer the question of whether or not the dog has hyperadrenocorticism. An abnormal UCCR test would have signaled that adrenal function testing is needed, saving the owner the cost of the thyroid function testing or potential biopsy as is done in some cases of noninflammatory alopecia.

200. Azathioprine (Imuran) is a prodrug whose active metabolite 6-mercatopurine and further metabolites are responsible for the medication's immunomodulatory activity. Azathioprine antagonizes purine synthesis through incorporation of thiopurine analogs in DNA synthesis, which results in chain termination and cytotoxicity. This drug has a particular effect on lymphocytes as they lack a salvage pathway for purine biosynthesis. This results in arrested lymphocyte activation and expansion. Azathioprine is rarely used as a sole therapeutic agent but is most commonly utilized as an adjunctive agent in combination with glucocorticoids to lessen the need for and adverse events encountered with the latter. It has been primarily used for pemphigus foliaceus but has also been advocated for many other autoimmune dermatoses (supepidermal blistering dermatoses, refractory discoid lupus erythematosus or symmetrical lupoid onychodystrophy, and uveodermatologic syndrome). Hepatotoxicosis is reported to occur in roughly 15% of patients with German shepherds potentially overrepresented. Elevated liver values, if they are to be observed, appear to occur within the first 4 weeks of therapy (Wallisch and Trepanier, 2015). The other major adverse event seen with azathioprine use is bone marrow suppression (neutropenia and thrombocytopenia). Bone marrow toxicity is directly related to thiopurine methyltransferase (TPMT) activity, which is responsible for the metabolism of 6-mercatopurine. Dogs have been shown to have variable TPMT activity with giant schnauzers having lower activity and Alaskan malamutes having elevated activity (Kidd et al., 2004). Cats also have significantly decreased TPMT activity, which is why they are more susceptible to the toxic effects; the use of this drug should be avoided in the species.

201. A 7-year-old castrated male domestic longhair presented for a 3-month history of progressive hair loss and pruritus (**Figure 201a**). The patient is the only cat in the household and is allowed unsupervised access to the outside for extended periods of time. Review of the records indicates the patient was current with recommended vaccinations, and the owner reports that they have been using a topical fipronil spot-on for flea prevention on a monthly basis that they are getting from one of the local retail stores. Examination revealed an alert patient whose vitals were unremarkable. Alopecia of the dorsal thoracic and cervical regions were appreciated along with erythema, papules, crusts, and excoriations in the affected region. Additional patchy areas of alopecia were noted along the caudal rear legs, ventral abdomen, and medial aspect of the front legs. During the exam, an organism was observed scurrying across the alopecic region (**Figure 201b**).

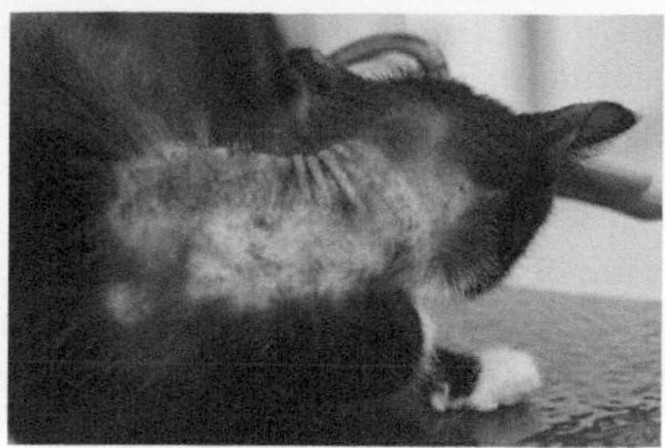
Figure 201a

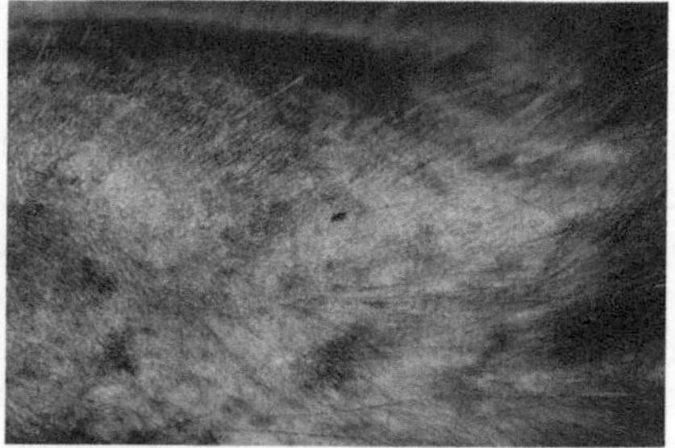
Figure 201b

i. What is the organism and your diagnosis for the patient's clinical presentation?

ii. Describe in detail the life cycle of this organism.

iii. What household products have been used as "natural" or "holistic" repellents for this condition, and what issues can arise due to their use?

202. A 9-month-old German shorthaired pointer presented for examination of its chin. The owners report that the dog develops "pimples" in this area. Upon physical examination, the dog has hair loss, papules, and furuncles on the lips, chin, and muzzle (**Figure 202a**). Many of the hair follicles are plugged with keratin, and purulent material and hairs can be expressed from within these follicles.

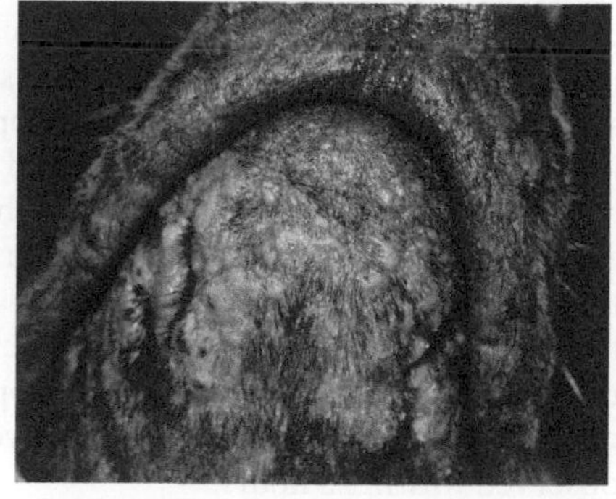
Figure 202a

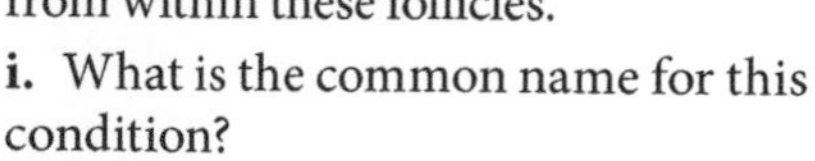

i. What is the common name for this condition?

ii. How is this treated?

201. i. *Ctenocephalides felis* (cat flea) and flea allergy dermatitis. Further questioning about the product the owner had been applying to the patient revealed it was the wrong formulation size for the cat's weight, which led to underdosing and treatment failure in this case. It is important to keep in mind that when apparent treatment failure is observed, the cause is probably the result of treatment deficiency as opposed to insecticide resistance.

ii. The cat flea's life cycle consists of an egg, three larval stages, a pupal stage, and the adult. The cycle can be completed in as little as 12 days or prolonged up to 174 days (or more) with the length of time being predominantly dependent on environmental ambient temperature and humidity. Under normal household conditions, most fleas complete their life cycle in 3–8 weeks (Blagburn and Dryden, 2009). Once an adult flea finds a host, it will consume a blood meal within minutes, which must occur prior to mating. Adult fleas mate within 8–24 hours and lay eggs within 24–36 hours of consuming a blood meal. Adult fleas lay eggs on their host that then fall off into the environment. Female fleas can lay 40–50 eggs per day and continue egg production at a declining rate for more than 100 days. Eggs hatch in 1–10 days (this stage is very temperature sensitive) with larvae displaying negative phototactism and positive geotropism (they move down into things). Larvae feed on organic debris, infertile eggs, other larvae, and flea feces. The larval phase is completed usually in 5–10 days and is the least hardy of all the flea life stages (only ~25% survive). Following the third larval stage, pupation occurs, which is the most resilient life stage demonstrating resistance to desiccation and insecticides. This stage can be prolonged for up to 140 days depending on environmental stimuli. Emergence can occur rapidly and is triggered by factors such as physical pressure, vibrations, carbon dioxide, and temperature (e.g., factors that indicate/mimic the presence of a potential host).

iii. Products such as garlic, thiamine, brewer's yeast, sulfur, Avon Skin So Soft, and various plant-derived herbal products or essential oils have been touted as "natural" remedies or repellents for fleas over the years. Although a few have anecdotal reports describing minimal efficacy, most lack data and any clinical evidence that they are effective. With the rise of marketed "natural" products for use in dogs and cats, specifically essential oils, there have been increased reported adverse events. Essentials oils associated with reported adverse events include tea tree oil, peppermint oil, thyme oil, cinnamon oil, lemongrass oil, and clove oil. Reported adverse events range from weakness, hypersalivation, hyperactivity, and lethargy to vomiting, ataxia, respiratory effects, and seizures (Budgin and Flaherty, 2013; Genovese et al., 2012). At this time, the exact mechanism of toxicity is unknown but thought to be related to terpenes contained in the oils. Toxicity is reported more often in cats and is observed with appropriate and inappropriate applications. In most cases, dermal decontamination and supportive care are sufficient, with full recovery observed within 72 hours.

202. i. Chin pyoderma or canine acne. Chin pyoderma is a bacterial infection. This is not true acne but rather a traumatic furunculosis. Chin pyoderma is almost exclusively seen in short-coated dogs such as the German shorthaired pointer. The exact cause of this condition is unknown, but it is speculated to be associated with trauma (lying on hard floors, friction from chew toys, and rough play or fetching balls) to the chin that forces short, stiff hairs backward through the follicle resulting in a foreign-body reaction that may become secondarily infected.

ii. The most critical step in managing these cases is to identify behaviors that are resulting in chin trauma and have them modified by the owner. In mild cases, topical therapy (benzoyl peroxide, salicylic acid, or mupirocin) may be sufficient to resolve lesions. In moderate to severe cases, oral antibiotics should be administered for 4–6 weeks along with daily cleansing of the lesions. In some recurrent cases, hair removal via tape-stripping to eliminate the inciting "ingrown" hairs may be beneficial. It is important to treat the condition aggressively; the use of systemic glucocorticoids may be required when the inflammatory response is exaggerated to prevent scarring.

203. The abdomen of a 6-year-old female cat is shown (**Figure 203a**). The cat was originally presented for a suspect abscess in this region. The abscess was surgically drained, flushed, and the cat was treated with 14 days of oral amoxicillin-clavulanate. Over the last 7 months, the surgical drainage site has failed to heal and progressed to the lesions shown in the image. Repeated surgery to remove granulation tissue and close the wound has failed to resolve the problem.

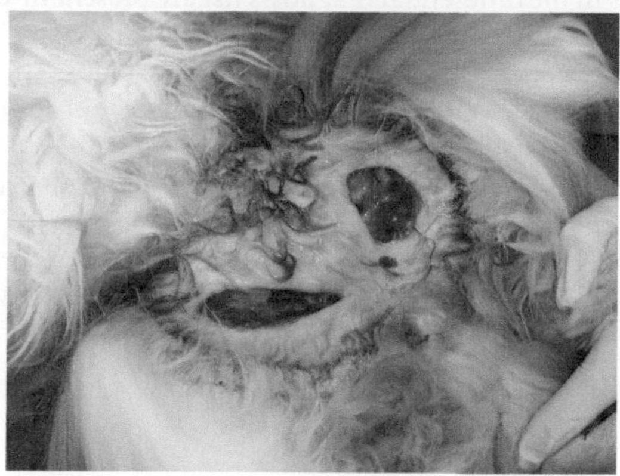

Figure 203a

i. What is this cat's "dermatologic problem," and what differential diagnoses should be considered?

ii. What diagnostic tests are indicated?

iii. An acid-fast stain of an impression smear taken from one of the biopsy samples is shown in **Figure 203b**. What is the most likely cause for this cat's presentation?

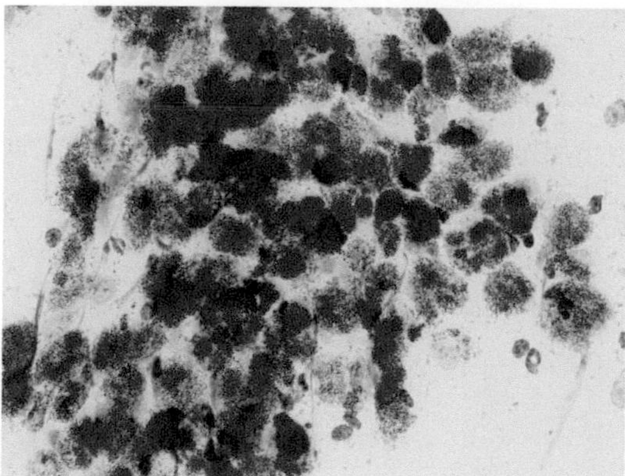

Figure 203b

203. **i.** Nonhealing wound. The differential diagnoses include foreign body, immunosuppression, subcutaneous mycoses, sterile panniculitis, atypical mycobacteria, feline leprosy, actinomycosis, and nocardiosis.

ii. Complete blood work, urinalysis, fungal titers, and FeLV/FIV serologic test should be performed. Additionally, the patient should be anesthetized, and tissue biopsies should be collected for histopathology, bacterial culture, and fungal culture. It is important to obtain deep sections for biopsy and culture. Many of the organisms in the differential diagnosis list are present in small numbers and/or are found in or near the subcutaneous fat. Furthermore, it is important to tell the laboratory processing the cultures and skin biopsy specimens which organisms are suspected, as this will influence the choice of culture media and tissue stains, respectively.

iii. Intracellular acid-fast bacilli are present. Atypical mycobacteria and feline leprosy (*Mycobacterium lepraemurium*) are both acid-fast bacilli. *Nocardia* spp. organisms are only partially acid-fast branching filamentous organisms. This was a case of an atypical mycobacterial infection secondary to *M. fortuitum*.

204. Dogs and cats are often presented by their owners for evaluation of cutaneous nodules because of concern about potential neoplasia. In many instances, fine-needle aspirations are performed to determine whether or not the mass is infectious, benign, or malignant. Specifically, these growths are aspirated to ensure they are not a round cell tumor. **Figure 204a–d** are photomicrographs of aspirates from the four most common round cell tumors.

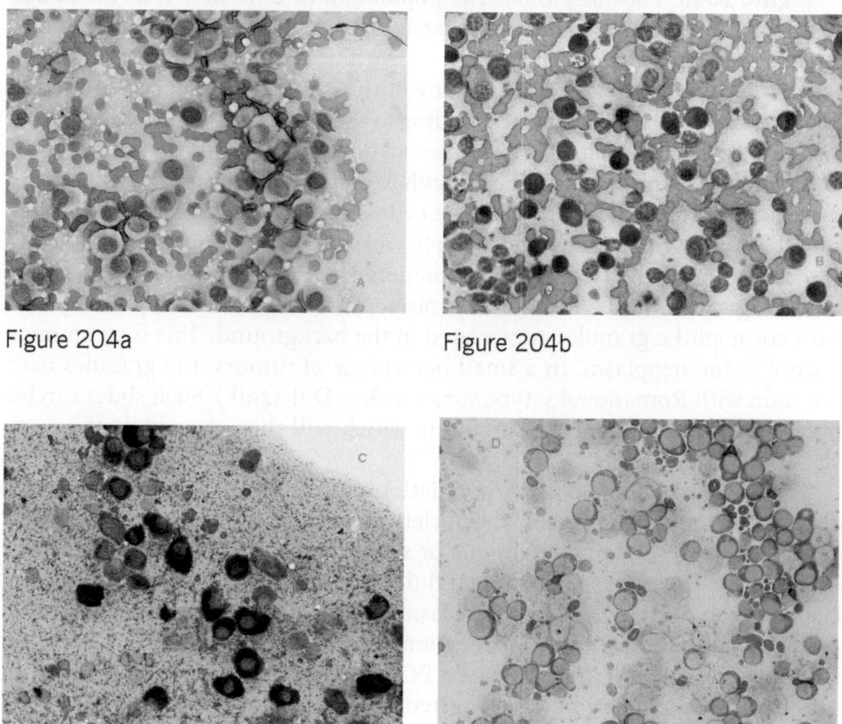

Figure 204a

Figure 204b

Figure 204c

Figure 204d

Identify the round cell tumor that each image corresponds to.

204. Figure 204a. Histiocytoma. A uniform population of large round cells with a moderate to abundant pale cytoplasm. The background fluid often stains darker, which contributes to the pale cytoplasmic appearance. The cytoplasm may also have a granular appearance, but it lacks distinct granules and vacuoles. The nuclei are round to reniform in shape with a fine chromatin pattern and contain multiple, indistinct nucleoli. The presence of small lymphocytes and other inflammatory cells will increase as tumor regression occurs.

Figure 204b. Plasmacytoma. The population of cells shown in the image has round nuclei with a uniform coarse to regular chromatin pattern. The nuclei are located toward the periphery with a moderate amount of deeply basophilic staining cytoplasm. In many of the cells, a prominent perinuclear clearing can be appreciated corresponding to the Golgi apparatus. Binucleate to multinucleated cells are another feature encountered with this neoplasm. Poorly differentiated plasma cells can be difficult to distinguish from histiocytic cells.

Figure 204c. Mast cell tumor. The cellular population present has round pale staining nuclei with distinct, deeply violet staining cytoplasmic granules. The cells also appear fragile with numerous free nuclei and granules seen in the background fluid. Additionally, numerous eosinophils may be present with eosinophilic granules appreciated in the background. This is a common feature of the neoplasm. In a small percentage of tumors, the granules may not stain with Romanowsky-type variants (i.e., Diff-Quik). Such slides can be overstained with a Giemsa-based stain, which will then accentuate the mast cell granules.

Figure 204d. Lymphoma. A population of round cells with scant pale to dark blue cytoplasm is present. The nuclei are occasionally indented, have a fine chromatin pattern, and contain one or more prominent nucleoli. Numerous cytoplasmic fragments (lymphoglandular bodies) are also observed, which is a common finding with this neoplasm. In cases where lymphoblastic cells predominate, cells may have a histiocytic appearance, which can make definitive identification difficult. In these cases, PCR techniques or histopathology with immunohistochemistry may be required to confirm the diagnosis.

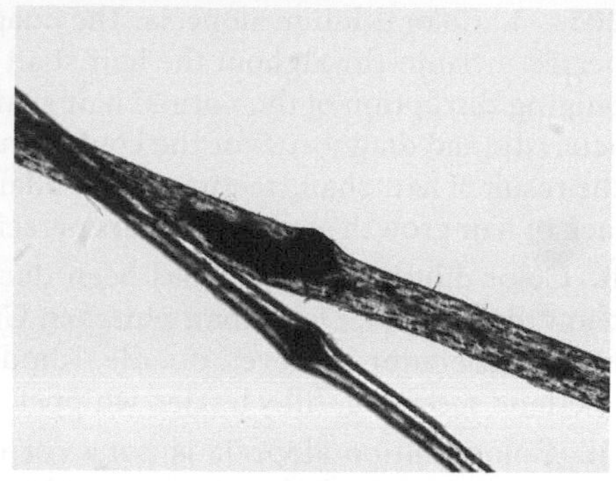

Figure 205a

205. A 2-year-old intact female Doberman pinscher presented for progressive hair thinning along her body. The owner reports that the patient is not pruritic and has not had any skin or ear infections. The patient is kept on year-round flea and heartworm preventatives. Overall, the general physical exam is fairly unremarkable except for diffuse thinning of the hair coat along the dog's dorsum and bilaterally along the thorax and flank. Taking a step back, you appreciate that the black-haired regions are affected, but the fawn hair–colored region appears normal. Given these findings, you elect to perform a trichogram, the results of which are shown in **Figure 205a**.

i. What is the patient's diagnosis?

ii. What other breeds has this condition been documented in?

iii. What recommendations should be made concerning this patient?

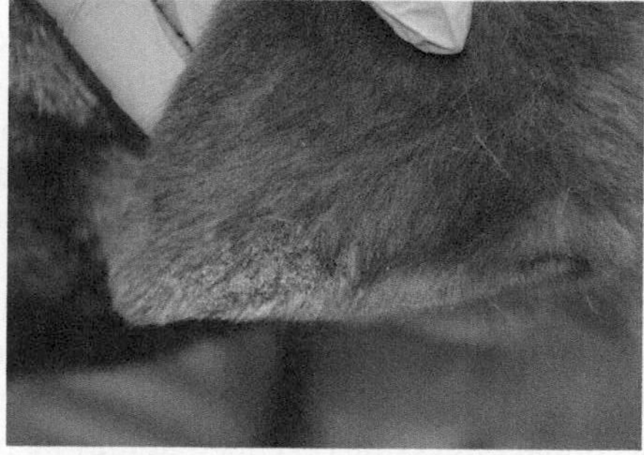

Figure 206a

206. A 2-year-old male German shepherd presented during the summer for acute head shaking and pruritus of the ears that the owner reports began 2–3 weeks prior. The patient lives on a farm and is primarily kept outdoors where he is free to roam the premises. No other symptoms or concerns are reported other than pruritus by the owners. Review of his records shows he is current on vaccinations and receives monthly preventatives that contain either milbemycin oxime for heartworm or afoxolaner for flea and tick prevention. Overall, the physical, dermatologic, and otoscopic exams are unremarkable, with the exception of the lesion shown in **Figure 206a** that is present on both ears at roughly the same spot. Lifting of the crust reveals an erythemic and slightly erosive surface.

i. What is the primary differential for this patient, what are other differentials to consider, and what diagnostics should be performed?

ii. What should treatment recommendations be for this patient?

205. i. Color dilution alopecia. The image shows a hair with irregularly dispersed melanin throughout the hair shaft and abnormal clumping leading to bulging/disruption of the normal hair shaft anatomy. These findings are characteristic and diagnostic for the condition. Alopecia in affected individuals is the result of hair shaft fracturing secondary to melanin aggregation and not a lack of hair growth as many owners perceive.

ii. Color dilution alopecia has been documented in the Chihuahua, chow chow, dachshund, Doberman pinscher, Great Dane, Irish setter, Italian greyhound, Labrador retriever, poodle, Rhodesian ridgeback, saluki, schnauzer, Shetland sheepdog, silky terrier, whippet, and Yorkshire terrier.

iii. Color dilution alopecia is not a correctable condition, so therapy tends to be symptomatic and primarily revolves around preventing secondary pyoderma and providing solar protection. Prevention of pyoderma is predominantly accomplished via routine bathing and skin nutrition. Depending on the level of alopecia, solar protection can be done through limiting solar exposure at peak UV intensity time frames, applying sunscreens, or using doggie sun suits.

206. i. The primary differential for this patient is fly-bite dermatitis or "fly-strike." The presence of a hemorrhagic crust on the distal lateral aspect of the pinnae, acute onset during the summer, a lack of necrosis or ischemia, and an overall lack of other clinical symptoms make this the most likely cause for the patient's clinical symptoms. Fly-bite dermatitis occurs in dogs who have significant outdoor exposure with lesions consisting of hemorrhagic crust and erythema that are variably pruritic and found along the tips of the ears (along the folded convex edge of dogs with pendulous ears) or face. Other potential differentials would be sarcoptic mange, trauma, or pinnal vasculitis. The use of monthly afoxolaner makes an infestation with *Sarcoptes* spp. less likely, while the symmetric presence of lesions on both ears is not consistent with trauma, and the breed is atypical for pinnal vasculitis. Diagnostics should consist of a skin scrape to look for ectoparasites and a skin impression to identify any secondary infectious agents that may be present.

ii. Treatment for fly-bite dermatitis should consist of a topical antibiotic-steroid cream/ointment applied topically one to two times a day until the lesions have resolved. Housing or lifestyle changes to avoid further exposure along with identification and elimination of fly sources should be pursued. Finally, the routine use of a flea/tick preventative that contains a repellent (i.e., permethrin) may be beneficial in preventing recurrence.

207. Recently, a series of review articles focusing on cutaneous adverse food reactions (CAFRs) have been published by Ralf Mueller and Thierry Olivry, focusing on the many aspects about this topic that veterinarians and specialists find confusing. CAFRs are a well-documented primary cause of pruritus in both dogs and cats, which require a diet elimination trial for definitive diagnosis.

i. What common food allergen sources have been identified in dogs and cats?

ii. What is the length of a diet elimination trial required to definitively diagnose a CAFR in most dogs and cats?

iii. How is a diet elimination trial performed?

207. **i.** The most frequently reported food allergens in dogs have been beef, dairy products, chicken, wheat, lamb, soy, corn, egg, pork, fish, and rice. While in cats it has been beef, fish, chicken, wheat, corn, dairy, and lamb (Mueller, Olivry, and Prelaud, 2016). When interpreting this data, it is important to remember that common food allergens in dogs and cats will reflect geographic variations in commercially produced diets and feeding habits.

ii. It is important to know that there is no consensus on the duration of a diet elimination trial required to optimally diagnose all CAFRs. However, with that said, the recent reviews have indicated that in dogs a diet elimination trial should last at least 8 weeks, at which time greater than 95% of dogs should have experienced significant improvement in their clinical symptoms if the primary cause is a CAFR. This also means that less than 5% of dogs were reported to require longer diet elimination trials for definitive diagnosis. In cats, the story is similar but slightly different. If a diet elimination trial lasts 8 weeks, only 90% of cats have been reported to achieve significant improvement in their clinical symptoms (Mueller, Olivry, and Prelaud, 2015). As a result, potentially 1/10 cats with a CAFR will be misdiagnosed if only an 8-week diet elimination trial is used, which explains why longer trials are recommended for cats. These are good general guidelines, and it is important to remember that there are always outliers, but this is a good basis for most pruritic cats and dogs.

iii. There are always slight variations to how individual specialists perform diet elimination trials, but the following is a basic outline. First a prescription novel/exotic protein, hydrolyzed diet, or a balanced home-cooked diet should be chosen based on the patient. The reason for choosing a prescription or home-cooked diet trial is that there is concern about discrepancies in labeling and ingredients in commercial pet foods (Olivry and Mueller, 2018). Once a diet is chosen, it should be fed exclusively to the patient for the defined time frame. Following feeding of the exclusion diet, the owner should be asked if their pet is better. If the patient is not better, then the current diet or another can be continued for a longer period of time to further evaluate for a CAFR or the patient can be considered not to be food allergic, and other primary causes should be considered. If the patient is better, then a provocation trial with prior foodstuffs that the patient was exposed to should be pursued and the owner informed to monitor for worsening of clinical symptoms. If no worsening is observed following provocation, then benefit seen is likely a coincidence and other primary causes for clinical presentation should again be evaluated. If clinical worsening is observed with exposure to prior foodstuffs, then the patient should again be placed on the prior/original exclusion diet and if clinical symptoms abate once again a confirmation of a CAFR can be diagnosed.

References

Aalbaek B, Bemis DA, Schjaerff M et al. 2010. Coryneform bacteria associated with canine otitis externa. *Veterinary Microbiology*, 145: 292–298.

Appelgrein A, Hosgood G, Reese SL. 2016. Computed tomography findings and surgical outcomes of dermoid sinuses: A case series. *Australian Veterinary Journal*, 94: 461–466.

Bauer JE. 2011. Timely topics in nutrition: Therapeutic use of fish oils in companion animals. *Journal of the American Veterinary Medical Association*, 238: 1441–1451.

Bauer JE. 2016. Timely topics in nutrition: The essential nature of dietary omega-3 fatty acids in dogs. *Journal of the American Veterinary Medical Association*, 249: 1267–1272.

Beale K. 2012. Feline demodicosis: A consideration in the itchy or overgrooming cat. *Journal of Feline Medicine and Surgery*, 14: 209–213.

Beco L, Guaguere E, Lorente Mendez C et al. 2013. Suggested guidelines for using systemic antimicrobials in bacterial skin infections (2): Antimicrobial choice, treatment regimens and compliance. *Veterinary Record*, 172: 156–160.

Becskei C, DeBock F, Illambas J et al. 2016. Efficacy and safety of a novel oral isoxazoline, sarolaner (Simparica™), for the treatment of sarcoptic mange in dogs. *Veterinary Parasitology*, 222: 56–61.

Becskei C, Reinemeyer C, King VL et al. 2017. Efficacy of a new spot-on formulation of selamectin plus sarolaner in the treatment of *Otodectes cynotis* in cats. *Veterinary Parasitology*, 238: S27–S30.

Bergvall K. 2004. A novel ulcerative nasal dermatitis of Bengal cats. *Veterinary Dermatology*, 15: 28.

Bitam I, Dittmar K, Parola P et al. 2010. Fleas and flea-borne diseases. *International Journal of Infectious Diseases*, 14: 667–676.

Bizikova P, Linder KE, Olivry T. 2014. Fipronil-amitraz-S-methoprene-triggered pemphigus foliaceus in 21 dogs: Clinical, histological and immunological characteristics. *Veterinary Dermatology*, 25: 103–111.

Bizikova P, Moriello KA, Linder KE et al. 2015. Dinotefuran/pyriproxyfen/permethrin pemphigus-like drug reaction in three dogs. *Veterinary Dermatology*, 26: 206–208.

Bizikova P, Olivry T. 2016. A randomized, double-blinded crossover trial testing the benefit of two hydrolysed poultry-based commercial diets for dogs with spontaneous pruritic chicken allergy. *Veterinary Dermatology*, 27: 289–e70.

Blache JL, Ryan K, Arceneaux K. 2011. Histoplasmosis. *Compendium: Continuing Education for Veterinarians*, 3: E1–E11.

Blagburn BL, Dryden MW. 2009. Biology, treatment, and control of flea and tick infestations. *Veterinary Clinics of North America: Small Animal Practice*, 39: 1173–1200.

Borio S, Colombo S, La Rosa G et al. 2015. Effectiveness of a combined (4% chlorhexidine digluconate shampoo and solution) protocol in MRS and non-MRS canine superficial pyoderma: A randomized, blinded, antibiotic-controlled study. *Veterinary Dermatology*, 26: 339–344.

Buckley L, Nuttal T. 2012. Feline eosinophilic granuloma complex(ities): Some clinical clarification. *Journal of Feline Medicine and Surgery*, 14: 471–481.

References

Buckley LM, Schmidt VM, McEwan NA et al. 2012. Positive and negative predictive values of a *Sarcoptes* specific IgG ELISA in a tested population of pruritic dogs. *Veterinary Dermatology*, 23: 36.

Budgin JB, Flaherty MJ. 2013. Alternative therapies in veterinary dermatology. *Veterinary Clinics of North America: Small Animal Practice*, 43: 189–204.

Bylaite M, Grigaitiene J, Lapinskaite GS. 2009. Photodermatoses: Classification, evaluation and management. *British Journal of Dermatology*, 161: 61–68.

Cain CL. 2013. Antimicrobial resistance in staphylococci in small animals. *Veterinary Clinics of North America: Small Animal Practice*, 43: 19–40.

Campbell KL. 1999. Sulphonamides: Updates on use in veterinary medicine. *Veterinary Dermatology*, 10: 205–215.

Cerundolo R, Mauldin EA, Goldschmidt MH et al. 2005. Adult-onset hair loss in Chesapeake Bay retrievers: A clinical and histological study. *Veterinary Dermatology*, 16: 39–46.

Classen J, Bruehschwein A, Meyer-Lindenberg A et al. 2016. Comparison of ultrasound imaging and video otoscopy with cross-sectional imaging for the diagnosis of canine otitis media. *Veterinary Journal*, 217: 68–71.

Cole LK. 2012. Primary secretory otitis media in Cavalier King Charles Spaniels. *Veterinary Clinics of North America: Small Animal Practice*, 42: 1137–1142.

Cole LK, Samii VF, Wagner SO et al. 2015. Diagnosis of primary secretory otitis media in the cavalier King Charles spaniel. *Veterinary Dermatology*, 26: 459–466.

Correia TR, Scott FB, Verocai GG et al. 2010. Larvicidal efficacy of nitenpyram on the treatment of myiasis caused by *Cochliomyia hominivorax* (Diptera: Calliphoridae) in dogs. *Veterinary Parasitology*, 173: 169–172.

Deboer DJ, Hillier A. 2001. The ACVD task force on canine atopic dermatitis (XV): Fundamental concepts in clinical diagnosis. *Veterinary Immunology and Immunopathology*, 81: 271–276.

Dryden MW, Gaafar SM. 1991. Blood consumption by the cat flea, *Ctenocephalides felis* (Siphonaptera: pulicidae). *Journal of Medical Entomology*, 28: 394–400.

Duclos DD, Hargis AM, Hanley PW. 2008. Pathogenesis of canine interdigital palmar and plantar comedones and follicular cysts, and their response to laser surgery. *Veterinary Dermatology*, 19: 134–141.

Faires MC, Gard S, Aucoin D et al. 2009. Inducible clindamycin-resistance in methicillin-resistant *Staphylococcus aureus* and methicillin-resistant *Staphylococcus pseudintermedius* isolates from dogs and cats. *Veterinary Microbiology*, 139: 419–420.

Favrot C, Steffan J, Seewaldt W et al. 2010. A prospective study on the clinical features of chronic canine atopic dermatitis and its diagnosis. *Veterinary Dermatology*, 21: 23–31.

Ferreira D, Sastre N, Ravera I et al. 2015. Identification of a third feline *Demodex* species through partial sequencing of the 16S rDNA frequency of *Demodex* species in 74 cats using a PCR assay. *Veterinary Dermatology*, 26: 239–245.

Ferreira M, Fattori K, Souza F et al. 2009. Potential role for dog fleas in the cycle of *Leishmania* spp. *Veterinary Parasitology*, 165: 150–154.

Fitzgerald JR. 2009. The *Staphylococcus intermedius* group of bacterial pathogens: Species re-classification, pathogenesis and the emergence of methicillin resistance. *Veterinary Dermatology*, 20: 490–495.

Fontaine J, Heimann M, Day MJ. 2010. Canine cutaneous epitheliotropic T-cell lymphoma: A review of 30 cases. *Veterinary Dermatology*, 21: 267–275.

Forsythe P, Paterson S. 2014. Ciclosporin 10 years on: Indications and efficacy. *Veterinary Record*, 174: 13–21.

Garosi LS, Lowrie ML, Swinbourne NF. 2012. Neurological manifestations of ear disease in dogs and cats. *Veterinary Clinics of North America: Small Animal Practice*, 42: 1143–1160.

Gaschen FP, Merchant SR. 2011. Adverse food reactions in dogs and cats. *Veterinary Clinics of North America: Small Animal Practice*, 41: 361–379.

Genovese AG, McLean MK, Khan MS et al. 2012. Adverse reactions from essential oil-containing natural flea products exempted from Environmental Protection Agency regulations in dogs and cats. *Journal of Veterinary Emergency and Critical Care*, 22: 470–475.

Glass EN, Cornetta AM, deLahunta A et al. 1998. Clinical and clinicopathologic features in 11 cats with *Cuterebra* larvae myiasis of the central nervous system. *Journal of Veterinary Internal Medicine*, 12: 365–368.

Gortel K. 2013. Recognizing pyoderma more difficult than it may seem. *Veterinary Clinics of North America: Small Animal Practice*, 43: 1–18.

Graham PA, Refsal KR, Nachreiner RF. 2007. Etiopathologic findings of canine hypothyroidism. *Veterinary Clinics of North America: Small Animal Practice*, 37: 617–631.

Greci V, Mortellaro CM. 2016. Management of otic and nasopharyngeal, and nasal polyps in cats and dogs. *Veterinary Clinics of North America: Small Animal Practice*, 46: 643–661.

Gross TL, Ihrke PJ, Walder EJ et al. 2005. Postrabies vaccination panniculitis. In: *Skin Diseases of the Dog and Cat: Clinical and Histopathologic Diagnosis*. 2nd ed. Blackwell Science Ltd., Oxford, UK, pp. 538–541.

Guillot J, Latié L, Manjula D et al. 2001. Evaluation of the dermatophyte test medium Rapid Vet-D. *Veterinary Dermatology*, 12: 123–127.

Halos L, Beugnet F, Cardoso L et al. 2014. Flea control failure? Myths and realities. *Trends in Parasitology*, 30: 228–233.

Han HS, Sharma R, Jeffery J et al. 2017. *Chrysomya bezziana* (Diptera: Calliphoridae) infestation: Case report of three dogs in Malaysia treated with spinosad/milbemycin. *Veterinary Dermatology*, 28: 239–241.

Harwick RP. 1978. Lesions caused by canine ear mites. *Archieves of Veterinary Dermatology*, 114: 130–131.

Henneveld K, Rosychuk RAW, Olea-Popelka FJ et al. 2012. *Corynebacterium* spp. in dogs and cats with otitis externa and/or media: A retrospective study. *Journal of the American Animal Hospital Association*, 48: 320–326.

Hensel P. 2010. Nutrition and skin diseases in veterinary medicine. *Clinics in Dermatology*, 28: 686–693.

Hensel P, Santoro D, Favrot C et al. 2015. Canine atopic dermatitis: Detailed guidelines for diagnosis and allergen identification. *BMC Veterinary Research*, 11: 196.

Hill CA, Platt J, MacDonald JF. 2010. Black flies: Biology and public health risk. *Purdue Extension*, E-251-W: 1–3.

Hillier A, Desch CE. 2002. Large-bodied *Demodex* mite infestation in 4 dogs. *Journal of the American Veterinary Medical Association*, 220: 623–627.

Hillier A, Lloyd DH, Weese JS et al. 2014. Guidelines for the diagnosis and antimicrobial therapy of canine superficial bacterial folliculitis (Antimicrobial Guidelines Working Group of the International Society for Companion Animal Infectious Diseases). *Veterinary Dermatology*, 25: 163–e43.

Hutt JHC, Prior IC, Shipstone MA. 2015. Treatment of canine generalized demodicosis using weekly injections of doramectin: 232 cases in the USA (2002–2012). *Veterinary Dermatology*, 26: 345–349.

References

Irwin KE, Beale KM, Fadok VA. 2012. Use of modified ciclosporin in the management of feline pemphigus foliaceus: A retrospective analysis. *Veterinary Dermatology*, 23: 403–409.

Jazic E, Coyner KS, Loeffler DG et al. 2006. An evaluation of the clinical, cytological, infectious and histopathological features of feline acne. *Veterinary Dermatology*, 17: 134–140.

Kidd LB, Salavaggione OE, Szumlanski CL et al. 2004. Thiopurine methyltransferase activity in red blood cells of dogs. *Journal of Veterinary Internal Medicine*, 18: 214–218.

Kunkle G, Halliwell R. 2002. Flea allergy and flea control. In: *BSAVA Small Animal Dermatology*, 2nd ed. A Foster, C Foil (eds). British Small Animal Veterinary Associations, Gloucester, UK, pp. 137–145.

Lenox CE. 2016. Role of dietary fatty acids in dogs and cats. *Today's Veterinary Practice Journal: ACVN Nutrition Notes*, 6(5): 83–90.

Logas D, Kunkle GA. 1994. Double-blinded crossover study with marine oil supplementation containing high dose eicosapentaenoic acid for the treatment of canine pruritic skin disease. *Veterinary Dermatology*, 5: 99–104.

Lopez RA. 1993. Of mites and man. *Journal of the American Veterinary Medical Association*, 203: 606–607.

Lower KS, Medleau LM, Hnilica K et al. 2001. Evaluation of an enzyme-linked immunosorbent assay (ELISA) for the serological diagnosis of sarcoptic mange in dogs. *Veterinary Dermatology*, 12: 315–320.

MacPhail C. 2016. Current treatment options for auricular hematomas. *Veterinary Clinics of North America: Small Animal Practice*, 46: 635–641.

Malik R, Ward MP, Seavers A et al. 2010. Permethrin spot-on intoxication of cats: Literature review and survey of veterinary practitioners in Australia. *Journal of Feline Medicine and Surgery*, 12: 5–14.

Marsella R, Sousa CA, Gonzales AJ et al. 2012. Current understanding of the pathophysiologic mechanisms of canine atopic dermatitis. *Journal of the American Veterinary Medical Association*, 241: 194–207.

Martinez M, Modric S, Sharkey M et al. 2008. The pharmacogenomics of P-glycoprotein and its role in veterinary medicine. *Journal or Veterinary Pharmacology and Therapeutics*, 31: 285–300.

Matricoti I, Maina E. 2017. The use of oral fluralaner for the treatment of feline generalized demodicosis: A case report. *Journal of Small Animal Practice*, 58: 476–479.

Mazepa ASW, Trepanier LA, Foy DS. 2011. Retrospective comparison of the efficacy of fluconazole or intraconazole for the treatment of systemic blastomycosis in dogs. *Journal of Veterinary Internal Medicine*, 25: 440–445.

Mealey KL. 2013. Adverse drug reactions in veterinary patients associated with drug transporters. *Veterinary Clinics of North America: Small Animal Practice*, 43: 1067–1078.

Mealey KL, Fidel J. 2015. P-glycoprotein mediated drug interactions in animals and humans with cancer. *Journal of Veterinary Internal Medicine*, 29: 1–6.

Meckfessel MH, Brandt S. 2014. The structure, function, ad importance of ceramides in skin and their use as therapeutic agents in skin-care products. *Journal of the American Academy of Dermatology*, 71: 177–184.

Mecklenburg L, Linek M, Tobin DJ. 2009. Canine pattern alopecia. In: *Hair Loss Disorders in Domestic Animals*. Wiley-Blackwell, Ames, IA, pp. 164–168.

Melville K, Smith KC, Dobromylskyj MJ. 2015. Feline cutaneous mast cell tumours: A UK-based study comparing signalment and histological features with long-term outcomes. *Journal of Feline Medicine and Surgery*, 17: 486–493.

Miller WH, Griffin CE, Campbell KL. 2013a. Canine scabies. In: *Muller & Kirk's Small Animal Dermatology*, 7th ed. Elsevier, St. Louis, MO, pp. 315–319.

Miller WH, Griffin CE, Campbell KL. 2013b. Thyroid physiology and disease. In: *Muller & Kirk's Small Animal Dermatology*, 7th ed. Elsevier, St. Louis, MO, pp. 502–512.

Moore PF 2014. A review of histiocytic diseases of dogs and cats. *Veterinary Pathology*, 51: 167–184.

Moriello KA. 2016. Decontamination of laundry exposed to *Microsporum canis* hairs and spores. *Journal of Feline Medicine and Surgery*, 18: 457–461.

Moriello KA, Coyner K, Paterson S et al. 2017. Diagnosis and treatment of dermatophytosis in dogs and cats. Clinical Consensus Guidelines of the World Association for Veterinary Dermatology. *Veterinary Dermatology*, 28: 26–303.

Moriello KA, DeBoer DJ. 2012. Dermatophytosis. In: *Greene's Infectious Diseases of the Dog and Cat*, 4th ed. Elsevier Saunders, St. Louis, MO, pp. 588–602.

Moriello KA, Verbrugge MJ, Kesting RA. 2010. Effects of temperature variations and light exposure on the time to growth of dermatophytes using six different fungal culture media inoculated with laboratory strains and samples obtained from infected cats. *Journal of Feline Medicine and Surgery*, 12: 988–990.

Morris DO. 2013. Ischemic dermatopathies. *Veterinary Clinics of North America: Small Animal Practice*, 43: 99–111.

Morris DO, Loeffler A, Davis MF et al. 2017. Recommendations for approaches to methicillin-resistant staphylococcal infections of small animals: Diagnosis, therapeutic considerations and preventative measures. Clinical Consensus Guidelines of the World Association for Veterinary Dermatology. *Veterinary Dermatology*, 28: 304–e69.

Mueller RS. 2004. Treatment protocols for demodicosis: An evidence-based review. *Veterinary Dermatology*, 15: 75–89.

Mueller RS, Bensignor E, Ferrer L et al. 2012a. Treatment of demodicosis in dogs: 2011 clinical practice guidelines. *Veterinary Dermatology*, 23: 86–96.

Mueller RS, Bergvall K, Bensignor E et al. 2012b. A review of topical therapy for skin infections with bacteria and yeast. *Veterinary Dermatology*, 23: 330–e62.

Mueller RS, Bettenay SV, Shipstone M. 2001. Value of the pinnal-pedal reflex in the diagnosis of canine scabies. *Veterinary Record*, 148: 621–623.

Mueller RS, Olivry T. 2017. Critically appraised topic on adverse food reactions of companion animals (4): Can we diagnose adverse food reactions in dogs and cats with *in vivo* or *in vitro* tests? *BMC Veterinary Research*, 13: 275.

Mueller RS, Olivry T, Prélaud P. 2015. Critically appraised topic on adverse food reactions of companion animals (1): duration of elimination diets. *BMC Veterinary Research*, 11: 225.

Mueller RS, Olivry T, Prélaud P. 2016. Critically appraised topic on adverse food reactions of companion animals (2): Common food allergen sources in dogs and cats. *BMC Veterinary Research*, 12: 9.

Mueller RS, Rosychuk RAW, Jonas LD. 2003. A retrospective study regarding the treatment of lupoid onychodystrophy in 30 dogs and literature review. *Journal of the American Animal Hospital Association*, 39: 139–150.

Müntener T, Schuepbach-Regula G, Frank L et al. 2012. Canine noninflammatory alopecia: A comprehensive evaluation of common and distinguishing histological characteristics. *Veterinary Dermatology*, 23: 206–221.

Negre A, Bensignor E, Guillot J. 2009. Evidence-based veterinary dermatology: A systematic review of interventions for *Malassezia* dermatitis in dogs. *Veterinary Dermatology*, 20: 1–12.

References

Njaa BL, Cole LK, Tabacca N. 2012. Practical otic anatomy and physiology of the dog and cat. *Veterinary Clinics of North America: Small Animal Practice*, 42: 1109–1126.

Nuttall T, Hill PB, Bensignor E et al. 2006. House dust and forage mite allergens and their role in human and canine atopic dermatitis. *Veterinary Dermatology*, 17: 223–235.

Nuttall T, Reece D, Roberts E. 2014. Life-long diseases need life-long treatment: Long-term safety of ciclosporin in canine atopic dermatitis. *Veterinary Record*, 174: 3–12.

Oberkirchner U, Linder KE, Dunston S et al. 2011. Metaflumizone-amitraz (Promeris)-associated pustular acantholytic dermatitis in 22 dogs: Evidence suggests contact drug-triggered pemphigus foliaceus. *Veterinary Dermatology*, 22: 436–448.

Oldenhoff WE, Frank GR, Deboer DJ. 2014. Comparison of the results of intradermal test reactivity and serum allergen-specific IgE measurement for *Malassezia* pachydermatis in atopic dogs. *Veterinary Dermatology*, 25: 507–511.

Olivry T, Mueller RS. 2018. Critically appraised topic on adverse food reactions of companion animals (5): Discrepancies between ingredients and labeling in commercial pet foods. *BMC Veterinary Research*, 14: 24.

Olivry T, Mueller RS, Prélaud P. 2015. Critically appraised topic on adverse food reactions of companion animals (1): Duration of elimination diets. *BMC Veterinary Research*, 11: 225.

Pallo-Zimmerman LM, Byrin JK, Grave TK. 2010. Fluoroquinolones: Then and now. *Compendium*, 32: E1–9.

Palm MD, O'Donoghue MN. 2007. Update on photoprotection. *Dermatologic Therapy*, 20: 360–376.

Palmeiro BS. 2013. Cyclosporine in veterinary dermatology. *Veterinary Clinics of North America: Small Animal Practice*, 43: 153–171.

Park C, Yoo JH, Kim HJ et al. 2010. Combination of cyclosporin A and prednisolone for juvenile cellulitis concurrent with hindlimb paresis in 3 English cocker spaniel puppies. *The Canadian Veterinary Journal*, 51: 1265–1268.

Pennisi MG, Hartmann K, Lloret A et al. 2013. Cryptococcosis in cats: ABCD guidelines on prevention and management. *Journal of Feline Medicine and Surgery*, 15: 611–618.

Pereira AV, Pereira SA, Gremiao IDF et al. 2012. Comparison of acetate tape impression with squeezing versus skin scraping for the diagnosis of canine demodicosis. *Australian Veterinary Journal*, 90(11): 448–450.

Peters J, Scott DW, Erb HN et al. 2003. Hereditary nasal parakeratosis in Labrador retrievers: 11 new cases and a retrospective study on the presence of accumulations of serum ("serum lakes") in the epidermis of parakeratotic dermatoses and inflamed nasal plana of dogs. *Veterinary Dermatology*, 14: 197–203.

Perters J, Scott DW, Erb HN et al. 2007. Comparative analysis of canine dermatophytosis and superficial pemphigus for the prevalence of dermatophytes and acantholytic keratinocytes: A histopathological and clinical retrospective study. *Veterinary Dermatology*, 18: 234–240.

Reinhart JM, Kukanich KS, Jackson T et al. 2012. Feline histoplasmosis: Fluconazole therapy and identification of potential sources of *Histoplasma* species exposure. *Journal of Feline Medicine and Surgery*, 14: 841–848.

Ricci R, Granato A, Vascellari M et al. 2013. Identification of undeclared sources of animal origin in canine dry foods used in dietary elimination trials. *Journal of Animal Physiology and Animal Nutrition*, 97: 32–38.

Rosales MS, Marsella R, Kunkle G et al. 2005. Comparison of the clinical efficacy of oral terbinafine and ketoconazole combined with cephalexin in the treatment of *Malssezia* dermatitis in dogs—A pilot study. *Veterinary Dermatology*, 16: 171–176.

Rosser EJ. 2006. German shepherd dog pyoderma. *Veterinary Clinics of North America: Small Animal Practice*, 36: 203–211.

Rufener L, Danelli V, Bertrand D et al. 2017. The novel isoxazoline ectoparasiticide lotilaner (Credelio): A non-competitive antagonist specific to invertebrates γ-aminobutyric acid-gated chloride channels (GABACls). *Parasites and Vectors*, 10: 530.

Rutland BE, Byl KM, Hydeskov HB et al. 2017. Systemic manifestations of *Cuterebra* infection in dogs and cats: 42 cases (2000–2014). *Journal of the American Veterinary Medical Association*, 251: 1432–1438.

Santoro D, Kubicek L, Lu B et al. 2017. Total skin electron therapy as treatment for epitheliotropic lymphoma in a dog. *Veterinary Dermatology*, 28: 246–e65.

Saridomichelakis MN, Koutinas AF, Farmaki R et al. 2007. Relative sensitivity of hair pluckings and exudate microscopy for the diagnosis of canine demodicosis. *Veterinary Dermatology*, 18: 138–141.

Sastre N, Ravera I, Villanueva S et al. 2012. Phylogenetic relationships in three species of canine *Demodex* mite based on partial sequences of mitochondrial 16S rDNA. *Veterinary Dermatology*, 23: 509–514.

Short J, Gram D. 2016. Successful treatment of *Demodex gatoi* with 10% imidacloprid/1% moxidectin. *Journal of the American Animal Hospital Association*, 52: 68–72.

Short J, Zabel S, Cook C et al. 2014. Adverse events associated with chloramphenicol use in dogs: A retrospective study (2007–2013). *Veterinary Record*, 175: 537–539.

Shumaker AK, Angus JC, Coyner KS et al. 2008. Microbiological and histopathological features of canine acral lick dermatitis. *Veterinary Dermatology*, 19: 288–298.

Simpson KM, Williams DL, Cherubini GB. 2015. Neuropharmacological lesion localization in idiopathic Horner's syndrome in golden retrievers and dogs of other breeds. *Veterinary Ophthalmology*, 18: 1–5.

Smith SH, Goldschmidt MH, McManus PM. 2002. A comparative review of melanocytic neoplasms. *Veterinary Pathology*, 39: 651–678.

Somogyi O, Meskó A, Csorba L et al. 2017. Pharmaceutical counseling about different types of tablet-splitting methods based on the results of weighing tests and mechanical development of splitting devices. *European Journal of Pharmaceutical Sciences*, 106: 262–273.

Stoll S, Dietlin C, Nett-Mettler CS. 2015. Microneedling as a successful treatment for alopecia X in two Pomeranian siblings. *Veterinary Dermatology*, 26: 387–e88.

Sula MJM. 2012. Tumors and tumorlike lesions of dog and cat ears. *Veterinary Clinics of North America: Small Animal Practice*, 42: 1161–1178.

Taenzler J, de Vos C, Roepke RKA et al. 2017. Efficacy of fluralaner against *Otodectes cynotis* infestations in dogs and cats. *Parasites and Vectors*, 10: 30.

Toma S, Comegliani L, Persico P et al. 2006. Comparison of 4 fixation and staining methods for the cytologic evaluation of ear canals with clinical evidence of ceruminous otitis externa. *Veterinary Clinical Pathology*, 35: 194–198.

Trepanier LA, Danhof R, Toll J et al. 2003. Clinical findings in 40 dogs with hypersensitivity associated with administration of potentiated sulfonamides. *Journal of Veterinary Internal Medicine*, 17: 647–652.

Van Riet-Nales DA, Doeve ME, Nicia AE et al. 2014. The accuracy, precision and sustainability of different techniques for tablet subdivision: Breaking by hand and the use of tablet splitters or a kitchen knife. *International Journal of Pharmaceutics*, 466: 44–51.

References

Vercelli A, Raviri G, Cornegliani L. 2006. The use of oral cyclosporine to treat feline dermatoses: A retrospective analysis of 23 cases. *Veterinary Dermatology*, 17: 201–206.

Vo DT, Hsu WH, Abu-Basha EA et al. 2010. Insect nicotinic acetylcholine receptor agonists as flea adulticides in small animals. *Journal of Veterinary Pharmacology and Therapeutics*, 33: 315–322.

Voie KL, Campbell KL, Lavergne SN. 2012. Drug hypersensitivity reactions targeting the skin in dogs and cats. *Journal of Veterinary Internal Medicine*, 26: 863–874.

Waisglass SE, Landsberg GM, Yager JA et al. 2006. Underlying medical conditions in cats with presumptive psychogenic alopecia. *Journal of the American Veterinary Medical Association*, 228: 1705–1709.

Wallisch K, Trepanier LA. 2015. Incidence, timing, and risk factors of azathioprine hepatotoxicosis in dogs. *Journal of Veterinary Internal Medicine*, 29: 513–518.

White SD, Brown AE, Chapman PL et al. 2005. Evaluation of aerobic bacteriologic culture of epidermal collarette specimens in dogs with superficial pyoderma. *Journal of the American Veterinary Medical Association*, 226: 904–908.

Wildermuth BE, Griffin CE, Rosenkrantz WS. 2012. Response of feline eosinophilic plaques and lip ulcers to amoxicillin trihydrate-clavulanate potassium therapy: A randomized, double-blind placebo-controlled prospective study. *Veterinary Dermatology*, 23: 110–118.

Wilson AG, KuKanich KS, Hanzlicek AS et al. 2018. Clinical signs, treatment, and prognostic factors for dogs with histoplasmosis. *Journal of the American Veterinary Medical Association*, 252: 201–209.

Yang C, Huang HP. 2016. Evidenced-based veterinary dermatology: A review of published studies of treatments for *Otodectes cynotis* (ear mite) infestation in cats. *Veterinary Dermatology*, 27: 221–234.

Zanna G, Docampo MJ, Fondevila D et al. 2009. Hereditary cutaneous mucinosis in shar pei dogs is associated with increased hyaluronan synthase-2 mRNA transcription by cultured dermal fibroblasts. *Veterinary Dermatology*, 20: 377–382.

Index

A

B

C

Index

E

F

G

Index

R

S

X

Y

Z

Printed and bound by CPI Group (UK) Ltd, Croydon, CR0 4YY
17/10/2024
01775660-0009

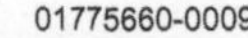